# THE NEW
# CHINESE
# MEDICINE
# HANDBOOK

An Innovative Guide to Integrating Eastern Wisdom
with Western Practice for Modern Healing

Misha Ruth Cohen, O.M.D., L.Ac.

FAIR WINDS

*This book is dedicated to all my loving friends, family, clients, teachers, mentors, students, mentees, colleagues, guides, and adversaries, living and passed on. Each one of you has helped me understand the intricate balance of Yin and Yang and to perceive wholeness and wellness as a continuous and unending journey.*

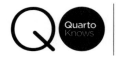

Quarto is the authority on a wide range of topics.

Quarto educates, entertains and enriches the lives of our readers—enthusiasts and lovers of hands-on living.

www.QuartoKnows.com

© 2015 Quarto Publishing Group USA Inc.
Text © 2015 Quarto Publishing Group USA Inc.

First published in the United States of America in 2015 by
Fair Winds Press, an imprint of
Quarto Publishing Group USA Inc.
100 Cummings Center
Suite 406-L
Beverly, Massachusetts 01915-6101
Telephone: (978) 282-9590
Fax: (978) 283-2742
Visit our blogs at www.QuartoKnows.com

19 18 17 16 15          1 2 3 4 5

ISBN: 978-1-59233-693-7

Digital edition published in 2015
eISBN: 978-1-62788-758-8

Library of Congress Cataloging-in-Publication Data

Cohen, Misha Ruth.
 The new Chinese medicine handbook : an innovative guide to integrating eastern wisdom with western practice for modern healing / by Misha Ruth Cohen, O.M.D., L.Ac.
    pages cm
 Includes bibliographical references and index.
 ISBN 978-1-59233-693-7 (paperback)
 1. Medicine, Chinese. 2. Qi gong. 3. Alternative medicine. 4. Self-care, Health. I. Title.
 R601.C692 2015
 610.951--dc23
                2015025993

Cover and book design by Megan Jones Design
Illustrations by William Michael Wanke

Printed and bound in the USA

*The information in this book is for educational purposes only. It is not intended to replace the advice of a physician or medical practitioner. Please see your health care provider before beginning any new health program.*

# CONTENTS

PREFACE · 4

PART ONE: A CONTEXT FOR HEALING · 10

CHAPTER 1: New Chinese Medicine · 11

CHAPTER 2: Understanding the Mind/Body/Spirit · 17

CHAPTER 3: Roots of Disharmony · 48

CHAPTER 4: Disharmony Revealed · 54

PART TWO: THE HEALING PROCESS · 75

CHAPTER 5: When You Visit a Chinese Medicine Practitioner · 76

CHAPTER 6: You Are What You Eat · 91

CHAPTER 7: Rebuilding Essential Substances and Organ Systems · 112

CHAPTER 8: Dancing with Dang Gui and Friends · 138

CHAPTER 9: Metal and Fire · 154

CHAPTER 10: Qi Gong · 175

CHAPTER 11: The Healing Touch · 190

PART THREE: WHERE THE PATHS MEET · 219

CHAPTER 12: Introduction to New Chinese Medicine's Comprehensive Programs of Healing · 220

CHAPTER 13: Strengthening Organ Qi and Protective Qi · 223

CHAPTER 14: Calming the Shen · 240

CHAPTER 15: Harmonious Cycles · 249

CHAPTER 16: Supporting the Center · 288

CHAPTER 17: Fatty Liver · 298

CHAPTER 18: Cancer Support · 315

GLOSSARY · 330

APPENDIX: How to Find Practitioners, Supplements and Herbs, and More · 332

GENERAL RESOURCES AND REFERENCES · 344

NOTES · 348

ABOUT THE AUTHOR · 356

ACKNOWLEDGMENTS · 358

INDEX · 361

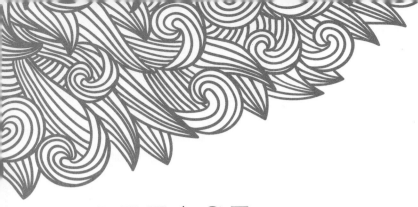

# PREFACE

## INVITATION TO A SHARED HEALING JOURNEY

If you have picked up this book, you are searching for answers to the age-old questions: How do I live life fully, how can I heal myself of sickness, and who can guide me in this complex process?

I will answer all of those questions, and more, for you in *The New Chinese Medicine Handbook: An Innovative Guide to Integrating Eastern Wisdom with Western Practice for Modern Healing*. This book is a reflection of my life journey. It is the underlying philosophy by which I live and work. I heartily invite you to join me on this journey. Let me show you how you can best use Chinese traditional medicine in the Western world.

New Chinese Medicine, the premise upon which this book was written, integrates the best of Chinese medicine and modern medicine for an innovative approach to healing. Based upon traditional Chinese philosophy, New Chinese Medicine is tempered by modern practices. New Chinese Medicine has emerged in the past forty years, integrating a wealth of extensive experience in clinical practice and research design, Eastern and Western approaches to healing, and my unique practice of Integrated Chinese Medicine.

*The New Chinese Medicine Handbook* is an essential part of your library as you walk down your healing path.

## A BIT ABOUT ME

My name is Misha Ruth Cohen, and I am a doctor of Oriental medicine and a licensed acupuncturist. In 1975, I started on the path of learning Asian medicine. I studied Shiatsu with a world-renowned master, went to acupuncture school, and practiced in the Lincoln Hospital Detox Clinic in New York's South Bronx. I moved to San Francisco in 1979, where I was fortunate to study with fabulous teachers of Chinese, Korean, Japanese, and other Asian medicine; learned Chinese herbal medicine; and attained my doctorate in Oriental medicine. In the early 1980s, I started a full-service Chinese medicine clinic for people with HIV, and I began doing research in Chinese herbal medicine.

In 1984, I cofounded Quan Yin Healing Arts Center in San Francisco, a nonprofit clinic devoted to treating low-income and indigent people as well as people who would not be treated by other clinics, such as people with AIDS.

We set up the first comprehensive program for people with AIDS, working with medical doctors and other practitioners. In the late 1980s, I performed herbal research, and I had designed herbal formulas for people with HIV. I continued to develop herbal formulas for liver disease, endometriosis, and gynecologic conditions for the first Western herb company to produce Chinese herbal pill medicines in the United States.

By the year 2000, I had designed several Chinese medicine research projects. In 2003, I joined the faculty of the University of California San Francisco (UCSF), and I eventually became the first Chinese medicine doctor to research Chinese herbal medicine as a UCSF principal investigator. From 1990 through the present time, with my colleagues, I have taught thousands of Chinese medicine and Western medicine practitioners how to create comprehensive programs, especially for HIV, hepatitis C, and cancer support. I have held leadership positions at the Society for Acupuncture Research as well as at Quan Yin Healing Arts Center. Currently, I am a member of the brainstorming team of the Hepatitis C Caring Ambassadors Program, on the board of directors of the Society for Integrative Oncology, and on the board of the Humanitarian Acupuncture Project.

For twenty-five years, I have maintained an Integrated Chinese Medicine private practice in San Francisco, auspiciously named Chicken Soup Chinese Medicine. Every day, my team provides complex consultations, integrated treatment plans, acupuncture, herbs, massage, and the full gamut of Chinese medicine and natural medicine to people who are looking for wholeness, balance, and wellness. We specialize in gynecology, cancer support, liver wellness, immune system imbalances, viral diseases, metabolic syndrome, digestive disorders, and pain management. The clinic is especially known for working with people with unusual and complex conditions and people who have unresolved illnesses or who have had unsuccessful treatment with conventional medicine.

*The New Chinese Medicine Handbook* allows me to share with you what I have learned in my years of teaching and practice—in an easy-to-read format. This book offers you an exploration of the Chinese medicine philosophy, theory, and practices as well guidance on how to use this philosophy to inform your daily life and healing practices.

Part One of *The New Chinese Medicine Handbook* walks you through the physiology and anatomy of Chinese medicine, causes of disease in Chinese medicine, and how we determine patterns of disharmony.

Part Two explains dietary principles for rebuilding and maintaining your health; includes a survey of Chinese herbs; and details the arts of acupuncture and moxibustion, Chinese exercise and meditation, Chinese Qi Gong massage, and other body therapies. Of most importance, Part Two tells you what to expect when you visit a Chinese medicine practitioner.

Part Three offers you comprehensive programs that integrate Traditional Chinese Medicine concepts and practices, natural medicine therapies, and Western medicine diagnosis and treatments. Everyone can benefit from the first comprehensive program in the book. This program addresses basic good health and how to maintain a strong immune system. Other targeted programs will help you if you suffer from stress, anxiety, or depression; need support for gynecological health or fertility; have digestive problems; need support for your liver; or if you or a loved one has been diagnosed with cancer and need support.

## BACKGROUND

When I stepped into the world of Asian medicine more than forty years ago, little did I know just how fast the public would come to embrace this medicine. I am grateful that all of us have been able to experience so much change in such a short time. This revolution has led to a great number of people experiencing the fullness of healing and wellness.

New Chinese Medicine has been an integral part of this revolution in medicine in the West. New Chinese Medicine integrates the best of Chinese traditional medicine and modern medicine, for an innovative approach to healing using traditional Chinese philosophy tempered by modern practices.

When I entered the field in the 1970s in New York City, we had no personal computers, no PowerPoint presentations, and no Chinese medicine books translated into English. To understand both Eastern and Western medicine and the then-current research, I visited medical school libraries, and I researched books that could not be taken out of the libraries for days at a time. Fortunately, in the South Bronx at Lincoln Detox and in Manhattan, I had dedicated teachers who had learned acupuncture and Shiatsu from oral traditions or highly experienced practitioners who had studied in Asia. I wrote everything my teachers taught in notebooks, which I still have! Later, in San Francisco, I had wonderful teachers who translated and taught from traditional and modern Chinese texts. I also had teachers who showed me exactly how to needle traditionally as well as how to properly create raw herbal formulas.

Today, students of Asian medicine have more than sixty accredited colleges of higher learning in the United States from which to choose. The colleges include teachers from many Asian medicine traditions and Western sciences. Students now can access smartphone apps for learning acupuncture, herbs, and bodywork.

However, it remains my opinion that oral tradition and in-person training are essential to carrying on Asian medicine traditions. Students who seek out highly experienced practitioners outside of formal schools often learn valuable techniques that otherwise might be lost, and they develop a deeper appreciation of the diversity of practice.

## INTEGRATIVE MEDICINE AND NEW CHINESE MEDICINE

Integrative medicine is a Western medicine concept. It is described by the National Center for Complementary and Integrative Medicine (NCCIM) at the National Institutes of Health (NIH) as medicine that "combines mainstream medical therapies and complementary and alternative medicine therapies for which there is some high-quality scientific evidence of safety and effectiveness."

While integrative medicine attempts to blend different practices, Western medicine remains at its foundation. In contrast, New Chinese Medicine maintains the philosophical underpinnings of Chinese traditional medicine. Chinese medicine practices have been used for centuries to improve health and establish harmony of mind/body/spirit. When new practices fit in with New Chinese Medicine philosophy and bring wholeness and wellness to a person, these practices become part of New Chinese Medicine. New Chinese Medicine thrives on integrating current knowledge and scientific discovery, and it naturally incorporates that which is new into that which is ancient and traditional. The whole cannot be separated from the parts.

In New Chinese Medicine, we do not simply cherry-pick popular techniques and import them into the Western medicine setting. For example, if I want to prescribe a scientifically proven natural nutritional supplement, I look at the current evidence, and I incorporate traditional diagnosis before prescribing the supplement. Simply speaking, when we use the philosophical framework of Chinese medicine, it allows us to create wholeness and wellness through establishing balance in the mind/body/spirit in conjunction with the external world.

Here is a case in point. When AIDS first arrived in the early 1980s, there were no viable Western treatments. Doctors sent me their patients after they had given up. I was the last resort, which was a very difficult place to be. I worked with many young people who died long before their time. At times, we were able, with Chinese medicine and other natural therapies, to help them manage their health, often extending their lives for months or even years. Some of those people are still with us today. When Western physicians were able to offer people with AIDS life-saving medications for pneumonia and other AIDS-related conditions, it was a true blessing. For people diagnosed with AIDS, those treatments extended their lives. When effective antiviral medications were developed and added to the armament, AIDS became a chronic viral disease rather than a death sentence for most people in the United States.

My experience of integrating Chinese medicine with Western practices, especially with people with AIDS, hepatitis, and cancer, gave birth to New Chinese Medicine.

## WHAT IS *NEW* IN NEW CHINESE MEDICINE?

At first glance, there is nothing new. Chinese medicine has developed continuously over thousands of years. Chinese medicine philosophy states that everything constantly changes, and nothing stays the same. Yin becomes Yang, and Yang becomes Yin. However, New Chinese Medicine takes this concept of constant change and distinguishes it by incorporating modern medicine within the ancient philosophy of Chinese medicine.

First, New Chinese Medicine is a partnership between ancient Chinese medicine wisdom and experience and the insight of Western medicine. Second, with expanded access to all kinds of research and information due to the Internet, apps, and other modern technological advances, there is much more readily available knowledge. Within this overabundance of information, there is good and bad, true and false, and at times, it is hard to tell the difference. With New Chinese Medicine, I can help you make sense of this morass of information and help you choose what actually works and what is safe. Third, you are in charge of your own healing process. New Chinese Medicine, as shown in this book, gives you tools to make your own decisions and become supported as the captain of your healing team, with practitioners as your facilitators and catalysts.

I wrote another book twenty years ago, *The Chinese Way to Healing: Many Paths to Wholeness*. What is *new* in *The New Chinese Medicine Handbook* are comprehensive programs and treatments that were not on the radar of most doctors or laypeople twenty years ago. What is *new* is that fatty liver disease has grown to enormous proportions and now affects millions of people. I was compelled by all of the people suffering with liver disease and metabolic syndrome to write a full chapter to help you address your liver health.

Twenty years ago, a limited number of people diagnosed with cancer regularly sought complementary and alternative medicine. In this book, there is a *new* chapter with a comprehensive program for people diagnosed with cancer, living with cancer, and surviving and thriving with cancer. There is also a brand *new* section in this book on natural fertility treatment. While I created fertility programs for women and men twenty years ago, this is now a major focus for Chinese medicine practitioners. This is due to the extensive research and focused practice prompted by the significant increase in infertility over the past couple of decades.

This book also includes a completely updated comprehensive program for everyone for basic good health and a strong immune system, and this book also features updated programs for people suffering with digestive disorders; from stress, anxiety, and depression; and from premenstrual syndrome (PMS) and menopausal symptoms.

## AN INVITATION TO JOIN ME ON THIS JOURNEY

I applaud you for stepping forward to take control of your own healing. Each one of our paths is unique. My personal path led me through illness, accidents, and life-transforming events to greater health and balance, to becoming a healer and a teacher of healing practices. Your path may lead you to places you cannot even imagine right now.

As you embark on your own healing journey, I thank you for allowing me to help you walk down the path of New Chinese Medicine. Together, you and I will explore ancient concepts along with modern advances in medicine. I fervently hope this will inspire you to experience a life filled with wholeness and wellness as well as provide you with harmony of mind/body/spirit.

Your path may take you anywhere. There may be many turns or roadblocks. Sometimes the path may disintegrate before your eyes. Yet, when you go inside and pay close attention, you can visualize your internal path. That allows you to continue on the external one just a little bit farther, one step at a time.

—Misha Ruth Cohen, San Francisco, October 2015

# PART ONE

## A CONTEXT
## FOR HEALING

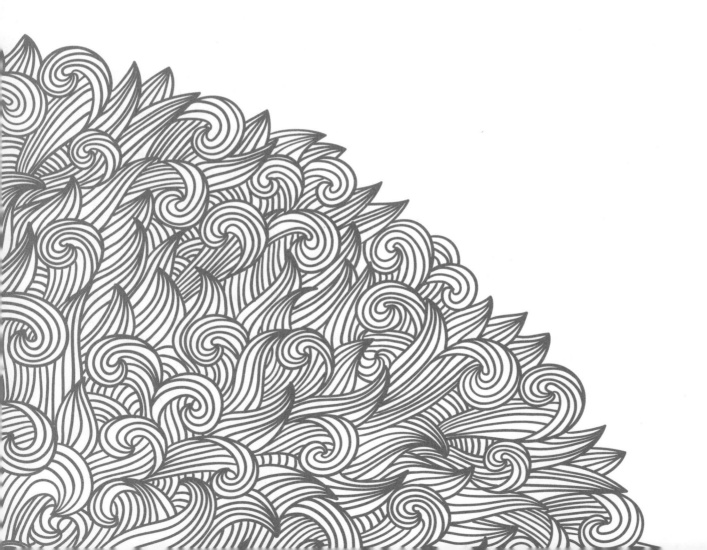

# 1

# NEW CHINESE MEDICINE
## Creating Your Own Path to Wholeness

Marcia wouldn't take no for an answer. She refused to believe, "No, we can't figure out what's causing your nausea and pain. No, we can't do much for your depression besides give you drugs."

Marcia initially came to the Chicken Soup Chinese Medicine clinic to enlist our help with her gynecological problems. For six months, she worked with me, using acupuncture and herbs, to ease her monthly pain and nausea.

"From the beginning, I could feel the improvement, but it still sort of snuck up on me, just how much of a difference it was making," Marcia said. After several months of weekly treatments, she no longer had to miss a day of work every month. She rarely had any discomfort, and pain was a thing of the past.

Marcia was pleased that she'd sought out a solution and that it had worked. She'd been bouncing from doctor to doctor for years, and they never found a reason for her symptoms. But Chinese medicine looked at Marcia's mind/body/spirit, not one isolated part of her body, and it offered her treatments based on an understanding of her whole being.

However, despite Marcia's improved gynecological health, she was spiraling into depression. Her much-loved brother was diagnosed with HIV/AIDS, and she felt helpless and angry that she couldn't do more for him. Marcia had trouble sleeping, lacked energy, and lost interest in doing activities that she used to enjoy.

"I couldn't think of how to do anything helpful. It all seemed useless," she said, looking back on her sinking mood. "I guess I was always troubled a bit by depression, because my body had been out of balance for so long, but my brother's illness pushed me over the edge."

Although Marcia was scared, she didn't give up. She created her own path to wholeness by putting together a team of health care providers and making sure they worked together within the context of Chinese medicine's understanding of the unity of the mind/body/spirit.

"At first, I went to a psychiatrist for my depression," Marcia said. "Then it occurred to me. I knew that acupuncture and herbal medicines were effective; they cured my recurring gynecological troubles. I thought maybe Chinese medicine combined with psychiatry could help my depression."

Marcia said that she wanted me to talk with her other doctor so we could coordinate our treatments. She was in charge of her healing process; she guided us toward each other. The results were tremendous.

The psychiatrist and I compared diagnoses and treatment. I had determined Marcia suffered primarily from Liver Qi Stagnation, which was causing her gynecological problems, as well as disturbances of the Shen or spirit, which were producing depression. The doctor said Marcia was in a clinical depression, and she had decided she didn't want to take antidepressants. The doctor concurred with her and said it would help Marcia's growth if she could battle her psychological problems without drugs. That led the doctor to ask if I could provide treatments that would ease the physiological aspects of depression. I drew up a revised herb and acupuncture program and shifted the focus of Marcia's treatment from primarily the body to primarily the spirit.

Marcia then expanded her healing team to include several other practitioners. She used both Feldenkrais and Rolfing body therapies to quiet her anxiety and tension, and she began seeing a nutritionist to reshape her diet so it provided more energy.

In a matter of weeks, Marcia's whole demeanor changed. She began to believe that she might see some real improvement in her life. Her depression lifted.

"Things are better now," she said. "When I'm feeling bad, I don't think it's the end of the world. When I feel good, it doesn't worry me."

Marcia has been directing her combined therapies for eight months now. Her initial regime of acupuncture and herbs, along with her weekly visits to the psychiatrist and the other therapies, resolved the depression.

"I feel terrific," Marcia said. "It worked."

For maintenance, Marcia receives acupuncture once every two weeks, takes herbs, and sees her psychiatrist once a month.

Marcia's determination to regain harmony in mind/body/spirit inspired her to create a comprehensive healing program. It's to Marcia—and to everyone who won't take no for an answer—that this book is dedicated.

*The New Chinese Medicine Handbook* is your guidebook to pursuing health in mind/body/spirit. In this book, I demonstrate how you—like Marcia—can take control of your healing process and maintain or restore harmony in all aspects of your life, using Chinese medicine as the great vessel that transports you toward wholeness while bringing in many other healing arts as adjunct therapies.

This eclectic approach to healing, grounded in the philosophy and practice of Chinese medicine, and embracing the wisdom and benefits of many other forms of healing, is what I call the New Chinese Medicine.

New Chinese Medicine evolved over the first two decades at my clinic, Chicken Soup Chinese Medicine, and at Quan Yin Healing Arts Center, of which I was cofounder and then director of research and education. The underpinning of New Chinese Medicine is Chinese traditional medicine. Chinese medicine has evolved over several thousand years without interruption to its modern forms.

What is now named Traditional Chinese Medicine (TCM) in China and in Western schools of TCM is a post-revolution compilation of the ancient Chinese medical theories of acupuncture, herbal therapy, dietary therapy, and Qi Gong exercise/meditation. In addition to TCM, my practice harks back to the roots of Chinese medicine and places a great emphasis on treatment of disharmony in the mind, emotions, and spirit. Chinese

## THE POWER OF CHINESE MEDICINE

If you expand your concept of healing to include the Chinese way of thinking about the human condition, you may experience a subtle but powerful change in how you take care of yourself.

- Chinese medicine theory will give you a new way of describing illness. You don't catch a cold; you develop a disharmony.

- Chinese medicine will allow you to imagine a new way of overcoming illness. You don't kill a bug with a drug; you use acupuncture and herbs to dispel disharmony.

- Chinese medicine offers a unique approach to treating physical problems and emotional upheaval. When you have a broken arm, you don't treat only the body. And when you have a broken heart, you don't treat only the spirit.

The mind/body/spirit is treated as a whole.

medicine is the root of this healing approach because it provides us with a powerful way to view human beings in all facets of our physical and spiritual being.

At my clinic, we recommend other healing approaches in addition to Chinese medicine treatments. We encourage clients to use whatever other healing therapies are necessary to create balance, wholeness, and wellness. These therapies may come from Ayurvedic medicine, Tibetan medicine, naturopathic medicine, standard Western medicine, homeopathy, chiropractic, psychotherapy, bodywork practices such as Shiatsu and deep tissue massage, Bach Flower therapy, aromatherapy, and body realignment therapies, such as Alexander Technique, Pilates, and Feldenkrais. The list goes on and on. Chinese medicine theory and practice—in conjunction with Western medicine and various modalities—is the essence of New Chinese Medicine.

## APPLYING NEW CHINESE MEDICINE

You don't need to see a Chinese medicine practitioner or come to our clinic to reap the benefits of New Chinese Medicine. You can use many self-care techniques to help you get started along your path to wholeness *today*. These techniques and therapies include Chinese dietary guidelines; various forms of meditation and exercise from Chinese Qi Gong to aerobics; Western nutritional supplementation; self- and partnered massages from Japan, China, and the West; and soaks, saunas, and compresses.

Self-care practices can make a dramatic and immediate difference in the quality of your life even before you have explored the Chinese medicine concepts on which New Chinese Medicine is based. Self-care therapies are *not* second best. I believe that they should be 80 percent of all care. They're the most important part of any journey toward wholeness. You can't arrive there unless you bring yourself along.

## THE BENEFITS OF NEW CHINESE MEDICINE

New Chinese Medicine offers the opportunity to maximize your pursuit of wholeness.

- You will have an opportunity to explore the basics of Chinese medicine philosophy and practices.

- You will learn about many self-care techniques that give you control over the harmony of your mind/body/spirit.

- You will become familiar with the comprehensive programs for maintaining general good health; managing digestive problems; supporting the liver; handling stress, anxiety, and depression; managing women's gynecological health; and helping people with cancer to survivorship. Each comprehensive program in this book sets out a specific plan for using Chinese medicine, standard Western medicine, and various other Eastern and Western healing therapies to restore balance and harmony in the mind/body/spirit.

## TAKING CHARGE OF YOUR PURSUIT OF WHOLENESS

Why did I develop this New Chinese Medicine that encompasses so many traditions and healing arts? I developed it because many of my clients demanded control over their own healing process and access to the widest array of health-seeking therapies. Their vision of healing gave birth to New Chinese Medicine, and their determination proved a person can move toward wholeness—even in the face of devastating illness.

Twenty-four years ago, Jennifer came to see me because her Western doctor had diagnosed her with endometriosis. She had emergency surgery, which made her symptoms worse, and she could not tolerate the proffered drug therapy because of her sensitivity to similar medication. Jennifer was extremely skeptical about Chinese medicine, but she was desperate to find some relief from the severe pain of her condition. I prescribed her a regimen of herbs, acupuncture, and nutritional supplements. Slowly, she began to become sensitive to how her mind/body/spirit were affected by the disease and could contribute to the cure. She began to meditate and practice visualization while we continued her healing regimen.

After one year, Jennifer returned to her original Western doctor for an examination. He did another laparoscopy to check on the disease. There was no sign of endometriosis! Jennifer had combined Western and Chinese medicine, and she had both cured the physical disorder and propelled herself along a path to mind/body/spirit healing.

New Chinese Medicine can also be a powerful healing tool when a cure, in a Western sense, is impossible. In fact, the people whom I have seen become the most balanced and whole are not necessarily those who have become perfectly physically well. The most balanced are people who have gained maturity through growth and continual attention to the inner self. They may not have chosen to become ill, but they did exercise a choice about how they became well. Instead of allowing other people to make decisions for them, they took control of their lives and healing processes.

Let me give you an example.

Nick, a client with AIDS, came to me in 1987. He had been diagnosed with AIDS-related lymphoma, and his medical doctor told him that he had two treatment choices: chemotherapy or no chemotherapy. When Nick asked what the results of treatment might be, he was told that with chemotherapy he could live six months but would feel horrible, and without chemotherapy he could live three to six months without feeling especially sick. Nick decided not to pursue any Western therapies for AIDS or cancer. He began a self-designed regimen of vitamin C and the use of crystals for healing.

When Nick arrived in my office six months after beginning his self-treatment, he challenged me to say what I could offer him. I said I could not necessarily extend his life, but I could offer him a healing process. My role would be to provide all of the tools of Chinese medicine and, sometimes, to recommend that he seek Western therapies. We started a program of acupuncture and herbal remedies, and he agreed to use Western treatments for the various syndromes and diseases associated with AIDS if it became necessary. I told Nick he would have to be part of the process. He agreed (not liking the Western part), and insisted that he must be in charge of his treatment.

Sometimes, Nick listened to exactly what I told him, and other times he ignored me completely. At all times, Nick listened to his inner self, continuing to meditate and sit in front of his altar with its crystals and other objects that he thought were healing for him.

Nick had one of the strongest spirits and the most irascible personalities I have ever experienced. He lived for another five and a half years. This was a man who took full responsibility for his own healing, and he died a healed man.

These are but some of the paths to wholeness. As you search for your own path, it is my hope that *The New Chinese Medicine Handbook* will help you in your healing journey. Use this book as a resource. Take what you need and leave the rest. You may return to this book again and again, or you may sit with it and explore the deeper meanings in Chinese medicine. Your spirit will guide you. Healing will follow.

# 2

# UNDERSTANDING THE MIND/BODY/SPIRIT
## The Physiology and Anatomy of Chinese Medicine

Chinese medicine is a system of preserving health and curing disease that treats the mind/body/spirit as a whole. Its goal is to maintain or restore harmony and balance in all parts of the human being and also between the whole human being and the surrounding environment.

Each of Chinese medicine's healing arts—from dietary therapy and exercise/meditation to acupuncture and herbs—is designed to be integrated into daily life. Together, they offer the opportunity to live in harmony and to maintain wholeness. In fact, for all of Chinese medicine's power to heal the body, its focus is on preventive care. In ancient China, doctors were paid only when their patients were healthy. When patients became ill, obviously the doctors hadn't done their job.

## THE ROLE OF THE TAO

Chinese medicine's focus on maintaining wholeness and harmony of the mind/body/spirit emerges from the philosophy of the Tao, which is sometimes translated as "the infinite origin" or the "unnameable."

The guiding principles of the Tao are:

- Everything in the universe is part of the whole.

- Everything has its opposite.

- Everything is evolving into its opposite.

- The extremes of one condition are equal to its opposite.

- All antagonisms are complementary.

- There is no beginning and no end, yet whatever has a beginning has an end.

- Everything changes; nothing is static or absolute.

This dynamic balance between opposing forces, known as Yin/Yang, is the ongoing process of creation and destruction. It is the natural order of the universe and of each person's inner being.

To Westerners, Yin/Yang is most easily understood as a symbol for equilibrium, but in Chinese philosophy and medicine, it is not symbolic. It is as concrete as flesh and blood. It exists as an entity, a force, a quality, and a characteristic. It lives within the body, in the life force (Qi), in each Organ System.

## YIN AND YANG ORGAN SYSTEMS

When the dynamic balance of Yin/Yang is disturbed, disharmony afflicts the mind/body/spirit, and disease can take root.

| YIN ORGAN SYSTEMS | YANG ORGAN SYSTEMS |
| --- | --- |
| Liver System | Gallbladder System |
| Heart System | Small Intestine System |
| Spleen System | Stomach System |
| Lung System | Large Intestine System |
| Kidney System | Urinary Bladder System |
| Pericardium System | Triple Burner System |

## YIN AND YANG DISEASE

| YIN DISEASE | YANG DISEASE |
| --- | --- |
| This generally relates to interior chronic conditions and is associated with: | This generally relates to exterior disease located in the skin, muscles, or bone and is associated with: |
| 1. Pain in the body or trunk | 1. Acute chills, fever, and body aches |
| 2. Changes in tongue shape, size, and color | 2. Aversion to cold or wind |
| 3. No aversion to cold or wind | 3. Changes in tongue coat/fur |
| 4. A deep pulse | 4. A floating pulse |
| 5. Changes in urine or bowels | 5. No internal organ changes |

Each symptom of Yin/Yang disharmony tells the trained practitioner about what's going on in the inner workings of a person's body. Once a disharmony is identified, the Chinese medicine practitioner addresses the entire web of interconnected responses in mind/body/spirit that are triggered by the presence of disharmony. Healing is achieved by rebalancing Yin and Yang and restoring harmony in the whole person.

# APPLYING THE TAO TO PHYSIOLOGY AND ANATOMY

Chinese medicine conceives of wellness and disease differently than Western medicine does, and it also describes the internal workings of the body in ways you may not be used to. In place of individual organs, blood vessels, and nerves, Chinese medicine identifies the body's Essential Substances, Organ Systems, and Channels. These terms describe the internal working of the body in ways that are significantly distinct from Western ideas.

## BASICS OF CHINESE MEDICINE ANATOMY AND PHYSIOLOGY

Essential Substances are those fluids, essences, and energies that nurture the Organ Systems and keep the mind/body/spirit in balance. They are identified as:

- *Qi*, the life force

- *Shen*, the spirit

- *Jing*, the essence that nurtures growth and development

- *Xue*, which is often translated as blood, but which contains more qualities than blood and transports Shen and Qi

- *Jin-Ye*, which is all of the fluids that are not included in Xue

Organ Systems, unlike the Western concept of organs, define the central organ plus its interaction with the Essential Substances and Channels. For example, the Heart System is responsible for the circulation of what in the West is called blood, and it also acts as the ruler of Xue and is in charge of storing Shen.

Channels, or meridians, are the conduits in the vast aqueduct system that transports the Essential Substances to the Organ Systems.

# ESSENTIAL SUBSTANCES

The Essential Substances, which have an impact on and are impacted by both the Organ Systems and the Channels, are called Qi, Shen, Jing, Xue, and Jin-Ye.

## Qi

Qi (*chee*) is the basic life force that pulses through everything in the universe. Organic and inorganic matter are composed of and defined by Qi. Within each person, Qi warms the body, retains the body's fluids and organs, fuels the transformation of food into other substances such as Xue, protects the body from disease, and empowers movement, including physical movement, the movement of the circulatory system, thinking, and growth.

We use the Chinese word for this substance because there is no precise English translation for the word or the concepts it contains. If you want to think of Qi as the energy that creates and animates material and spiritual being, the life force, or the breath of life, you will come close to understanding Qi. As you delve more deeply into Chinese medicine, you will begin to identify how Qi lives within you and fuels your very existence. You'll find Qi is most accurately defined by its function and its impact.

Where does Qi come from and where does it go? We are all born with Qi. We can preserve, create, or deplete it by the air we breathe, the food we eat, and the way in which we live within our mind/body/spirit. There are many forms of Qi, which all work together.

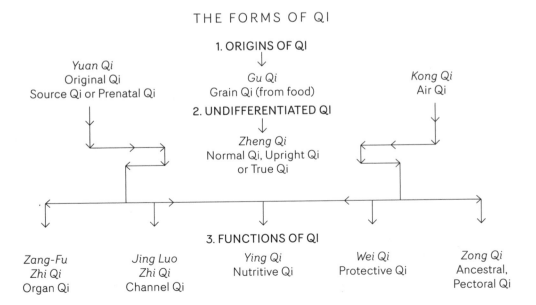

THE FORMS OF QI

1. ORIGINS OF QI

Yuan Qi
Original Qi
Source Qi or Prenatal Qi

Gu Qi
Grain Qi (from food)

Kong Qi
Air Qi

2. UNDIFFERENTIATED QI

Zheng Qi
Normal Qi, Upright Qi
or True Qi

3. FUNCTIONS OF QI

Zang-Fu
Zhi Qi
Organ Qi

Jing Luo
Zhi Qi
Channel Qi

Ying Qi
Nutritive Qi

Wei Qi
Protective Qi

Zong Qi
Ancestral,
Pectoral Qi

**Original Qi or Yuan Qi** is transmitted by parents to their children at conception and is stored in the Kidney System. It is partially responsible for the person's inherited constitution. We possess a fixed amount of Original Qi, which can be used up.

**Grain Qi or Gu Qi** is taken in with food, and it is released from the digestion of food in the stomach.

**Air Qi or Kong Qi** is extracted by the lungs from the air we breathe.

**Normal Qi or Zheng Qi** is produced when Yuan Qi, Gu Qi, and Kong Qi intermingle within the body. This is what is generally meant by the term Qi. It has five major functions:

1. Creates all body movement.

2. Protects the body by resisting the entrance of External Pernicious Influences.

3. Transforms food into Xue, Qi itself, plus tears, sweat, and urine.

4. Governs the retention of body substances and organs, keeping everything in and in its place.

5. Warms the body.

**Organ Qi or Zang-Fu Zhi Qi** defines, influences, and promotes each Organ System's proper functioning.

**Channel Qi or Jing Luo Zhi Qi** moves through the Channels (meridians), bringing Qi to the Organ Systems and linking the Organ Systems and the Xue, and helping them to function harmoniously. Acupuncture adjusts Channel Qi.

**Nutritive Qi or Ying Qi** moves the blood through the vessels and transforms pure food elements into blood. It also moves with the Xue and helps it nourish body tissue.

**Protective Qi or Wei Qi** resists and combats External Pernicious Influences. It is the most Yang manifestation of Qi in the body. It moves within the chest and abdominal cavities and travels between the skin and the muscles. It regulates the sweat glands and pores, moistens and protects skin and hair, and warms the organs. When Protective Qi is Deficient, we are susceptible to the deleterious effects of environmental factors, such as Cold or Wind, which are called External Pernicious Influences.

**Ancestral Qi, Pectoral Qi, or Zong Qi** gathers in the chest, where it forms the Sea of Qi. Ancestral Qi travels up to the throat and down to the abdomen. It is responsible for breathing, speaking, and regulating heartbeat and respiration. Meditation can strengthen Ancestral Qi, and it is particularly beneficial for maintaining or restoring harmony.

## Shen

Shen (*shen*) or spirit is as palpable to a Chinese medicine doctor as the heart or the left hand. Shen is consciousness, thoughts, emotions, and senses, which make us uniquely human. Its harmonious flow is essential to good health. Originally transmitted into a fetus from both parents, Shen must be continuously nourished after birth.

## Jing

Jing (*jing*) is often translated as *essence*, the fluid that nurtures growth and development. We are born with Prenatal or Congenital Jing, inherited from our parents. Jing defines our basic constitution, along with Original Qi. Acquired Jing is transformed from food by the Stomach and Spleen, and it constantly replenishes the Prenatal Jing, which is consumed as we age.

Prenatal Jing gives rise to Qi, but during our lifetime, as Jing changes, it is dependent on Qi. Qi is Yang; Jing is Yin. Qi and Jing are joined in the process of aliveness. While Qi is the energy associated with any movement, Jing is the substance associated with the slow movement of organic change. Jing is the inner essence of growth and decline.

Prenatal Jing is our genetic capability, but whether we reach our genetic capability depends on how much Qi we are able to nurture. Think of a child whose parents are 6 feet (1.8 m) tall. If that child is malnourished, he or she will never reach the height conveyed by genetic potential. But if there is an ample supply of food, the child can grow fully. In the same way, if there is enough Qi, the possibilities of Jing can become realized.

Prenatal Jing evolves through the stages of life. According to the ancient Chinese medicine text, the *Nei Jing*, in women, its changes accompany seven stages of life:

> *The Kidney energy of a woman becomes in abundance at the age of seven, her baby teeth begin to be replaced by permanent ones and her hair begins to grow longer. At the age of fourteen, a woman will begin to have menstruation, her conception meridian begins to flow, the energy in her connective meridian begins to grow in abundance, and she begins to have menstruation, which is the reason why she is capable of becoming pregnant. At the age of twenty-one, the Kidney energy of a woman becomes equal to an average adult, and for that reason, her last tooth begins to grow with all other teeth completed. At the age of twenty-eight, tendons and bones have become hard, the hair grows to the longest, and the body is in the top condition. At the age of thirty-five, the bright Yang meridians begin to weaken with the result that her complexion starts to look withered and her hair begins to turn grey. At the age of forty-two, the three Yang meridians are weak above [in the face], the face is dark, and the hair begins to turn white. At the age of forty-nine, the energy of*

*the conception meridian becomes Deficient, the energy of the connective meridian becomes weakened and scanty, the sex energy becomes exhausted, and menstruation stops with the result that her body becomes old and she cannot become pregnant any longer.* [1]

The *Nei Jing* also states that men's development corresponds to eight stages of Jing:

*As to man, his Kidney energy becomes in abundance, his hair begins to grow longer, and his teeth begin to change at the age of eight. At the age of sixteen, his Kidney energy has become even more abundant, his sex energy begins to arrive, and he is full of semen that he can ejaculate. When he has sexual intercourse with a woman, he can have children. At the age of twenty-four, the Kidney energy of a man becomes equal to an average adult with strong tendons and bones, his last tooth begins to grow with all other teeth completed. At the age of thirty-two, all tendons, bones, and muscles are already fully grown. At the age of forty, the Kidney energy begins to weaken, hair begins to fall off, and the teeth begin to wither. At the age of forty-eight, a weakening and exhaustion of Yang energy begins to take place in the upper region with the result that his complexion begins to look withered and his hair begins to turn grey. At the age of fifty-six, the Liver energy begins to weaken, the tendons become inactive, the sex energy begins to run out, and the semen becomes scanty. The Kidney becomes weakened with the result that all parts of the body begin to grow old. At the age of sixty-four, hair and teeth are gone.* [2]

## Xue

The Chinese word Xue (*sch-whey*) is a much more precise description of this bodily substance than blood, which is the common English translation. Xue is not confined to the blood vessels, nor does it contain only plasma and red and white blood cells. Xue carries the Shen. Xue also moves along the Channels in the body where Qi flows.

Xue is produced by food that is collected and mulched in the Stomach, refined by the Spleen into a purified Essence (Acquired Jing), and then transported upward to the Lung, where Nutritive Qi begins to turn Jing into Xue. At the Lung, Jing combines with air and produces Xue. Qi propels Xue through the body.

## THE PRODUCTION OF XUE

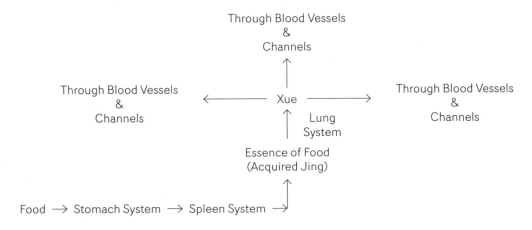

Xue is intertwined with many body functions:

- The Heart System rules Xue. Xue depends on the Heart System for its harmonious, smooth circulation.

- The Liver System stores Xue.

- The Spleen System governs Xue. The retentive properties of Spleen Qi keep Xue within its designated pathways.

- Qi creates and moves Xue and holds it in place. The Chinese saying is, "Qi is the commander of Xue."

- Xue in turn nourishes the Organ Systems that produce and regulate the Qi. It is also said that Xue is the mother of Qi.

## Jin-Ye

Jin-Ye (*jin-yee*), the Chinese word for all fluids other than Xue, includes sweat, urine, mucus, saliva, and other secretions such as bile and gastric acid. Jin-Ye is produced by digestion of food. Organ Qi regulates it. Certain forms of what is called Refined Jin-Ye help produce Xue.

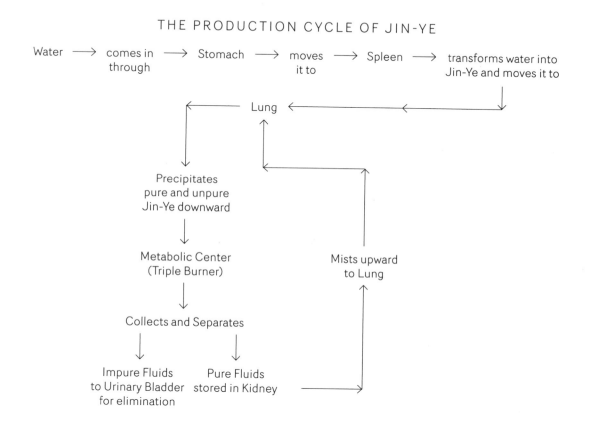

THE PRODUCTION CYCLE OF JIN-YE

These Five Essential Substances are the primordial soup from which life emerges and in which harmony and disharmony coexist. In Chinese medicine, reading the condition of these substances is an important part of diagnosis and treatment.

# THE ORGAN SYSTEMS

Chinese medicine talks about Organ Systems—not the individual, anatomical organs that are identified by Western medicine. Although the Organ Systems are responsible for organ functions that are familiar to Western medicine, they also embrace the organ's impact on the whole body. Each Organ System governs specific body tissues, emotional states, and activities, and each Organ System is associated with and influenced by the Essential Substances and Channels.

- Every Organ System is governed by Organ Qi and influences the balance of Qi. This energy creates the Organ Systems' impact on the mind/body/spirit.

- The Essential Substances—Qi, Shen, Jing, Xue, and Jin-Ye—infuse each Organ System with energy and shape its characteristics.

- Some Organ Systems are Yin, and other Organ Systems are Yang. Together, they are called the Zang-Fu Organs, and they form a harmonious balance that sustains life.

## ZANG (YIN) AND FU (YANG) ORGAN SYSTEMS

| ZANG (YIN) | FU (YANG) |
|------------|-----------|
| Heart | Small Intestine |
| Spleen | Stomach |
| Lung | Large Intestine |
| Kidney | Urinary Bladder |
| Liver | Gallbladder |
| Pericardium | Triple Burner |

In general, Zang Organs are associated with pure substances—Qi, Xue, Jing, Shen, and Jin-Ye. Fu Organ Systems govern the digestion of food and the elimination of waste. But the division between Zang (Yin) and Fu (Yang) organs is not black and white. In the East, there is no great compulsion to say, "This is X, and it is always X. This is Y, and it shall never be X." Each organ, whether Zang (Yin) or Fu (Yang), has nourishing Yin and active Yang qualities within it. The dual unit of Yin/Yang exists within all life. For example, the Heart System stores Shen—that's a Yin function—but it also rules Xue—that's a Yang function. The Liver System stores Xue—that's a Yin function—and it regulates and moves the Qi—that's a Yang function. This characteristic association with either Yin or Yang and with both Yin and Yang is true of each Organ System—and of Yin and Yang itself, which is the unity of opposites.[3]

## The Zang (Yin) Organs

The Zang (Yin) Organs are the Kidney System, Spleen System, Liver System, Lung System, and Heart System. Let's talk about each in turn.

**Kidney System:** The Kidney System manages fluid metabolism, which the West associates with the kidneys and the adrenal glands. In addition, however, the Kidney System is responsible for storing surplus Qi. The Kidney System also rules birth, maturation, reproduction, growth, and regeneration.

The bones, inner ear, teeth, and lower back are also associated with the Kidney System, as is regulation of the growth of bone, marrow, and the brain.

The Kidney System stores Jing, and it provides it to other Organ Systems and body tissue. Also, the Kidney System is the root of eight important Channels that connect the Organ Systems to one another.

The Kidney opens up to the external world through the ear. Kidney harmony is revealed through acuity of hearing.

**Spleen System:** The Spleen System creates and controls Xue, as it is involved with the blood in Western medicine. It is also responsible for extracting Gu (Grain) Qi and fluids from food, transforming these substances into Ying (Nutritive) Qi and Xue, and storing Qi that is acquired by the body after birth.

The Spleen System also maintains the proper movement of ingested fluids and food throughout the body. The Spleen System transmits the Gu (Grain) Qi upward and the pure fluids to the Lung and Heart Systems. Balanced fluid movement lubricates the tissues and joints. This prevents excess dryness, and it keeps fluids from pooling or stagnating and creating Dampness. The Spleen likes dryness, and it is negatively affected by Dampness. The Spleen System also is associated with muscle mass and tone and with keeping the internal organs in place.

When the Spleen is balanced, the transformation and transportation of fluids is harmonious, Qi and Xue permeate the whole body, and the digestive tract functions well. The Spleen System's connection to the external world is through the mouth, and the Spleen's vigor is mirrored in the color of the lips.

**Liver System:** The Liver System stores the Xue, and it is responsible for the proper movement of Qi and Xue throughout the body. The Liver System regulates the body by making sure Qi moves smoothly through the Channels and Organ Systems. It regulates the secretion of bile to aid digestion, balances emotions, protects against frustration and sudden anger, and stores Xue. You can think of the Liver System as a holding tank where the Xue retreats when you are at rest. The Liver System also nourishes the eyes, tendons, and nails. The Liver System opens up to the world through the eyes, and the health of the Liver System is reflected in the sharpness of eyesight.

**Lung System:** The Lung System rules Qi by inhaling the Kong (Air) Qi from outside of the body, which, along with Gu (Grain) and Yuan (Original) Qi, forms Zheng (Normal) Qi. As in Western medicine, the Lung System administers respiration, but it also regulates water passage to the Kidney System, which stores pure fluids. The Lung System also disperses water vapor throughout the body, especially to the skin, where it is associated with perspiration. In addition, the Lung System is in charge of Zong (Ancestral) Qi, which gathers in the chest, providing the Heart System with Qi. It also rules the exterior of the body through its relationship with Wei (Protective) Qi, providing resistance to External Pernicious Influences. (See "The Six Pernicious Influences" on page 48.) The nose is the gateway of the Lung System, and the health of the Lung System is reflected in the skin.

## UNDERSTANDING THE POWERS OF THE ORGAN SYSTEMS

We can learn about the power of the Organ Systems through the following two examples.

**Organ removal:** If an organ is removed (a woman may have a hysterectomy, for example), the body does not lose the entire Organ System or its contribution to the harmony of the mind/body/spirit. The energetics of the Organ System and its associated Channel remain. Although the removal of an organ creates an imbalance, it can be addressed with acupuncture, herbs, dietary adjustments, and exercise/meditation.

**Intangible organ systems:** In Chinese medicine, there's an Organ System—the Triple Burner—that you couldn't find if you were to cut open the body and search for it. This is possible because Organ Systems, similar to much in Chinese medicine, are defined by function, not location. The term *Organ System* in Chinese medicine describes a nexus of functions that are concrete and have identifiable traits. That's all the information that's needed to be able to chart the development of disharmony in an Organ System and to remedy it.

**Heart System:** The Heart System is associated with the heart, the movement of the Xue through the vessels, and the storing of Shen. It is the ruler of the Xue and the blood vessels. When the Heart's Xue and Qi are in harmony, the Shen is at peace, and a person has an easy time dealing with what the world dishes out. The emotional states of joy, lack of joy, and charisma are associated with the Heart.

The Heart opens into the tongue, and abundant Heart Xue is revealed by moist and supple facial skin.

**Pericardium:** The Pericardium is considered by some to be a distinct Organ System because it disperses Excess Qi from the Heart and directs it to a point in the center of the palm where it can exit the body naturally. The Pericardium is the covering or protector of the heart muscle, and it provides the outermost defense of the Heart against external causes of disharmony. Although the Pericardium has no physiological function separate from the Heart, it has its own acupuncture Channel. Not all systems of Chinese medicine consider the Pericardium to be a separate Organ System.

## The Fu (Yang) Organs

The Fu Organs' main purposes are to receive food, absorb usable nutrition, and excrete waste. Fu Organs are considered less internal than the Zang Organs because they are associated with impure substances: food, urine, and feces. The Fu Organs and Channels can play a major role in acupuncture. The Fu Organs are the Gallbladder System, Stomach System, Small Intestine System, Large Intestine System, Urinary Bladder System, and the Triple Burner System.

**Gallbladder System:** Working with the Liver System, the Gallbladder System stores and secretes bile into the Large Intestine and Small Intestine Systems to help digestion. Any disharmony of the Liver System impacts the Gallbladder System, and vice versa.

**Stomach System:** The Stomach System receives and decomposes food so the Spleen System can transform the fluids and food essence into Qi and Xue. The Stomach System is also responsible for moving Qi downward and sending waste to the Intestines. The Spleen moves Qi upward, and harmony between the Stomach and Spleen is vital.

**Small Intestine System:** Working with the Stomach System, the Small Intestine System helps produce Qi and Xue. The Small Intestine separates and refines the pure from the impure in fluids and food and in the mind.

**Large Intestine System:** Moving the impure waste down through the body, the Large Intestine System extracts water and produces feces.

**Urinary Bladder System:** The Urinary Bladder System excretes urine, which is produced by the Kidney and Lung Systems and from intestinal wastewater.

**Triple Burner System:** This Organ System, which is divided into three parts—the Upper Burner, Middle Burner, and Lower Burner—does not exist in Western medicine. In Chinese texts, it is called *San Jiao*, and it is said to have a "name without shape." The best way to understand the Triple Burner is to examine its function, which is to mediate the body's water metabolism. Don't worry about where it lives, but seek to understand what it does.

- The Upper Burner is identified in the ancient Chinese text *Ling Shu* as an all-pervasive, light fog that distributes the Qi of water and food throughout the body. This part of the Triple Burner is associated with the head and chest and the Heart and Lung Organ Systems.

- The Middle Burner, identified as a froth of bubbles, is associated with the Spleen, Stomach, and, according to some texts, the Liver. It's involved with digestion, absorption of Essential Substances, evaporating fluids, and imbuing Xue with Nutritive Qi. The froth of bubbles refers to the state of decomposing, digested foods.

- The Lower Burner, which is called a drainage ditch, designates an area below the navel and includes the Kidney, Large and Small Intestines, Urinary Bladder, and Liver—due to the location of the acupuncture Channel. It governs the elimination of impurities. The Lower Burner helps regulate the Large Intestine System, and it helps the Kidney System process waste.[4]

## The Extraordinary or Ancestral Fu Organs

The Marrow, Bones, Brain, Uterus, Blood Vessels, and Gallbladder are called the Extraordinary Organs. The ancient Chinese medical text *Nei Jing* states that they resemble the Fu (Yang) organs in form and the Zang (Yin) organs in function.

**Marrow and Bones:** The Marrow, which includes the spinal cord, bone, and brain, are wedded to the Kidney System, and their existence depends on Jing, which gives rise to Brain and Marrow. The Marrow nourishes the bones.

**The Brain:** This is the Sea of Marrow, and it is nourished by the Marrow. Consciousness is also associated with the Brain. The five senses, plus memory and thinking, are associated with other Organ Systems, but they are influenced by the Brain. Although the Heart stores the Shen, the Brain is also associated with it.

**The Uterus:** The Uterus, called *Bao Gong* (palace of the child), usually functions as a storage organ. However, in relation to menstruation and labor, its function is to discharge. While the Uterus is the anatomical source of menstruation and the location of gestation, its functioning is governed by other Organ Systems.

Both the Conception (Ren) and Penetrating (Chong) Channels (see page 40) arise from the Uterus. Menstruation depends on these Channels' harmonious functioning, on the strength of the Kidney Jing, and on the Xue functions of the Spleen and Liver Systems. Kidney Qi dominates the Uterus's reproductive function because reproduction is related to the Kidney. When the functions of the Heart, Liver, Spleen, and Kidney Systems are balanced, menstruation is normal. When the Heart and Kidney functions are strong, conception is easy.

Men are said to possess the energetic area of the Uterus. It contributes to their harmony, and it affects the flow of Essential Substances through the Conception and Penetrating Channels.

**The Blood Vessels:** These transport most of the Xue through the body. Although the distinction between Xue circulating in the Blood Vessels and in the Channels is not delineated, it's generally accepted that Blood Vessels carry more Xue than Qi, and Channels carry more Qi than Xue.

Understanding how the Blood Vessels function cannot be separated from understanding the relationship between the Xue and the Zang Organ Systems. Heart rules the Xue, keeping the heartbeat regular and balanced; the Liver stores and regulates the Xue, keeping an even flow of Xue throughout the body; and the Spleen governs the Xue, keeping it within the Blood Vessels and Channels. Disharmony of the Blood Vessels may be corrected by treating one of these Organ Systems.

**The Gallbladder:** This Organ System is considered both a Fu Organ and an Extraordinary Organ because it contributes to the breakdown of impure food—a Yang function—but unlike any other Yang Organ, it contains a pure fluid, bile.

## THE CHANNELS

The Channels, which are sometimes called meridians or vessels, are a great aqueduct system that transports the Essential Substances—Qi, Jing, Xue, Jin-Ye, and Shen—to each Organ System and to every part of the body. By tuning into the way Qi moves through the body's Channels, Chinese medicine practitioners can "read" the harmony or disharmony of the body's Essential Substances and Organ Systems. Practitioners can also manipulate the flow of Qi and other Essential Substances through the Channels to keep the flow irrigating the body evenly.

Acupuncture controls the flow of the Essential Substances by needling acupuncture points that are positioned along the network of Channels like a series of gates. At these points, the flow of Essential Substances, particularly Qi, comes close to the surface of the skin, and the needling stimulates or retards their passage through the Channels.

According to Traditional Chinese Medicine (TCM), the functions of the Channels are to:

- Transport Xue and Qi and regulate Yin and Yang
- Resist pathogens and reflect symptoms and signs of disease and disharmony
- Transmit curative sensations that occur during acupuncture, such as the spreading of warmth and relaxation through the body, the sense of Qi moving, and a feeling of concentrated heaviness
- Regulate Excess and Deficiency conditions

The major Channels are divided into the Twelve Primary Channels, the Eight Extraordinary Channels, and the Fifteen Collaterals. There are also the less-often-discussed, although important medically, Twelve Divergent Channels, Twelve Muscle Regions, and Twelve Cutaneous Regions. Let's talk about each in turn.

## The Twelve Primary Channels

Each Primary Channel is linked to an Organ System, transports Qi and other Essential Substances, and helps maintain harmony in mind/body/spirit. The *Ling Shu*, part of the *Nei Jing*, explains, "Internally, the twelve regular meridians connect with the Zang-Fu organs and externally with the joints, limbs, and other superficial tissues of the body."

The Twelve Primary Channels are Lung, Large Intestine, Stomach, Spleen, Heart, Small Intestine, Urinary Bladder, Kidney, Pericardium, Triple Burner, Gallbladder, and Liver.

Each Channel is defined by whether it starts or ends at the hand or foot, whether the Channel is Yin (runs along the center of the body) or Yang (runs along the sides of the body), and whether it is related to a Zang Organ System (the Lung, Kidney, Spleen, Heart, Liver, or Pericardium) or a Fu Organ System (Large Intestine, Stomach, Small Intestine, Urinary Bladder, Triple Burner, or Gallbladder).

Each Yin Channel and Zang Organ is paired with a Yang Channel and a Fu Organ. The Lung is paired with the Large Intestine, the Spleen with the Stomach, the Kidney with the Urinary Bladder, the Pericardium with the Triple Burner, and the Liver with the Gallbladder. This association means that if one of the paired Organs becomes unbalanced, the other one may be thrown into disharmony as well.

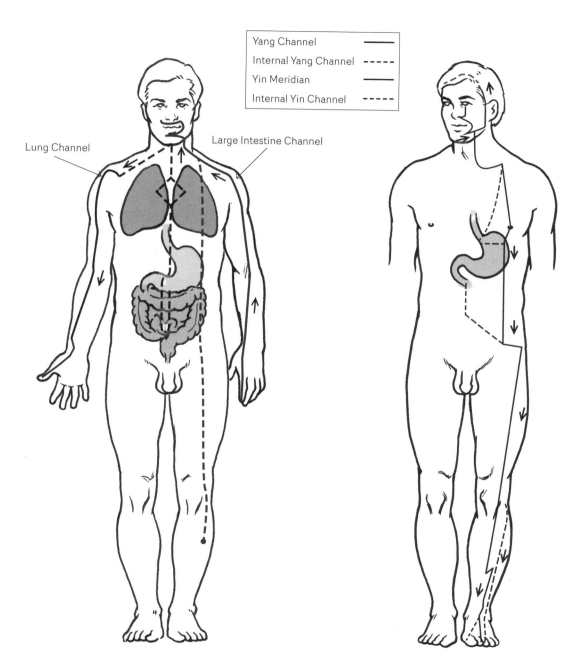

*The Lung Channel of Hand—Taiyin,*
*The Large Intestine Channel of Hand—Yangming*

*The Stomach Channel of Foot—Yangming*

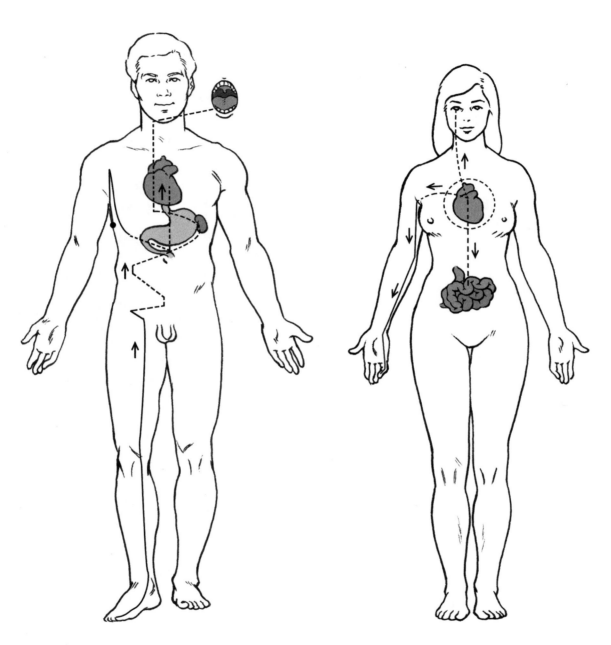

*The Spleen Channel of Foot—Taiyin*          *The Heart Channel of Hand—Shaoyin*

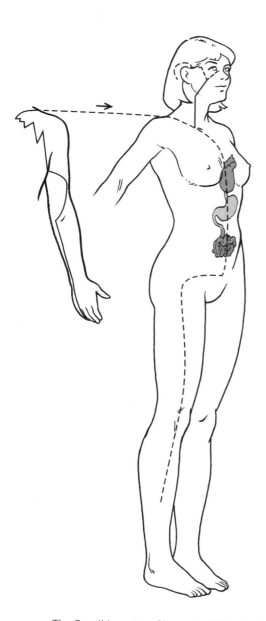

*The Small Intestine Channel of Hand—Taiyang*

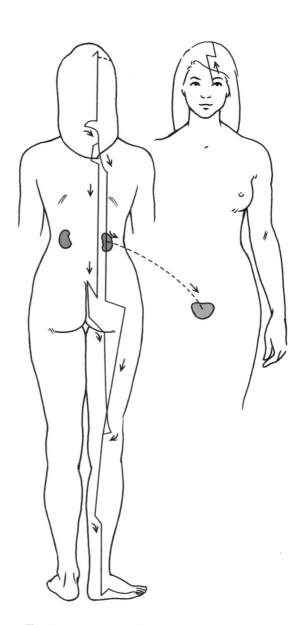

*The Urinary Bladder Channel of Foot—Taiyang*

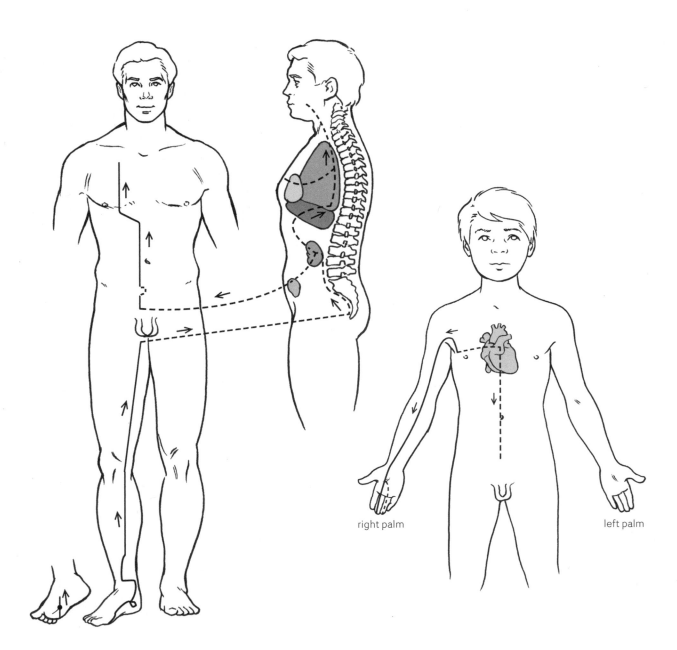

*The Kidney Channel of Foot—Shaoyin*

right palm  left palm

*The Pericardium Channel of Hand—Jueyin*

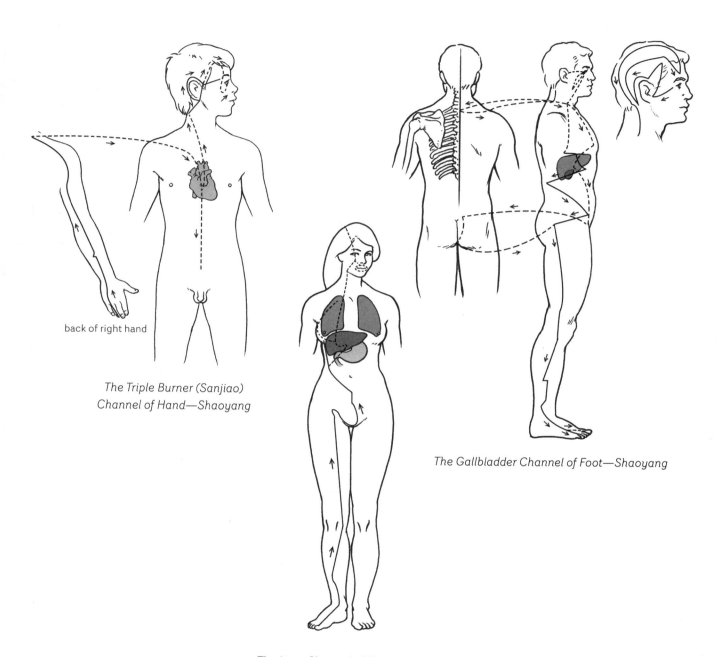

back of right hand

*The Triple Burner (Sanjiao)*
*Channel of Hand—Shaoyang*

*The Liver Channel of Foot—Jueyin*

*The Gallbladder Channel of Foot—Shaoyang*

## THE CYCLICAL FLOW OF QI IN THE TWELVE REGULAR CHANNELS

⟶  The channels and the direction of their flow
⟵  Organ System Pairs

ZANG ORGANS, YIN CHANNELS      FU ORGANS, YANG CHANNELS

⟶ 1. Lung ——————————⟶ 2. Large Intestine
    (3–5)     ⟷     ↓ (5–7)

4. Spleen ⟵—————————— 3. Stomach
↓ (7–9)     ⟷     (9–11)

5. Heart ——————————⟶ 6. Small Intestine
(11–13)     ⟷     ↓ (13–15)

8. Kidney ⟵—————————— 7. Urinary Bladder
↓ (15–17)     ⟷     (17–19)

9. Pericardium ——————————⟶ 10. Triple Burner
(19–21)     ⟷     ↓ (21–23)

12. Liver ⟵—————————— 11. Gallbladder
↓ (23–1)     ⟷     (1–3)

*Note: The time of day when each Channel is most open and active is noted under each organ. The time is given in twenty-four-hour time.*

## The Eight Extraordinary Channels

In addition to the Twelve Primary Channels, there are Eight Extraordinary Channels. According to another ancient medical text, the *Nan Jing*, "The twelve organ-related Qi Channels constitute rivers, and the eight extraordinary vessels (channels) constitute reservoirs." Unlike the Twelve Primary Channels, the Eight Extraordinary Channels aren't associated with any of the twelve Organ Systems. But they are extremely important because they augment the communication between the Twelve Primary Channels, act as a storage system for Qi, and exert a strong effect on personality. These reservoirs collect Excess Qi, releasing it into the various Twelve Primary Channels if they become Qi Deficient because of mental or physical stress or trauma. They also have their own special functions. Some French acupuncturists call them "miraculous meridians" because they are used for therapeutic effects when other techniques prove to be ineffective.

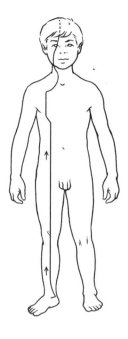

The Yinqiao Channel

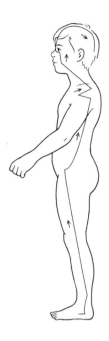

The Yangqiao Channel

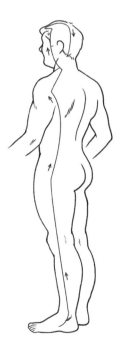

The Yangwei Channel

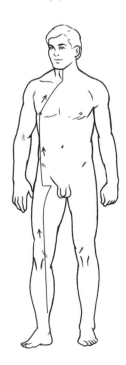

The Yinwei Channel

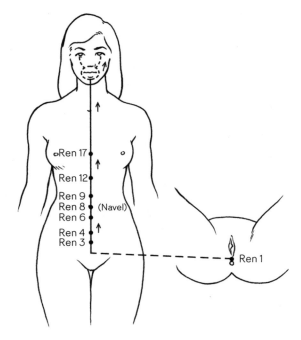

*The Ren Channel*

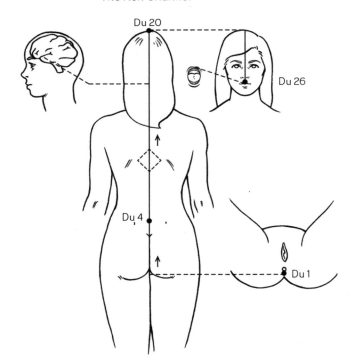

*The Du Channel*

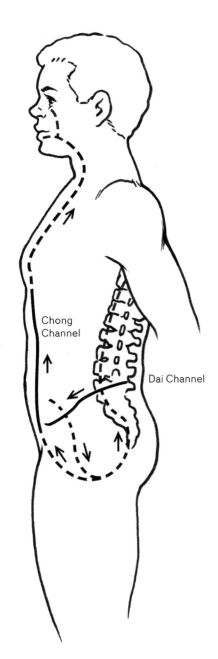

*The Chong and Dai Channels*

Four of the Extraordinary Channels are located in the trunk of the body. They are solitary, unpaired Channels with special functions. They are the Chong Mai, the Ren Mai, the Du Mai, and the Dai Mai.

**The Chong Mai** (*chong-my*), or Penetrating Channel, is known as the Sea of Qi and Xue. It regulates the Qi and Xue of the Twelve Primary Channels, and it distributes Jing throughout the body. It brings the Kidney Qi upward to the abdomen and chest. The Chong Mai is the root of the other Extraordinary Channels.

**The Ren Mai** (*ren-my*), or Conception Channel, regulates the six Yin Channels and Yin throughout the body. It's in charge of the Jin-Ye and Jing, and it regulates the supply of body fluids to the fetus. Along with the Chong Mai, this Channel originates in the Uterus, supporting and supplying the Uterus and regulating the seven-year life cycle in women and the eight-year life cycle in men. (In men, the energetic area of the Uterus exists even without the presence of the physical organ.)

**The Du Mai** (*doo-my*), or Governing Channel, also rises from the Uterus, and it links the Spinal Cord and the Brain and all of the Yang Channels. (The Uterus area of the body exists in both men and women.) The Du Mai is the master of all of the Yang energy. Along with the Ren Mai, it regulates the balance of Yin/Yang, which in turn regulates the balance of Qi and Xue.

**The Dai Mai** (*die-my*), or Belt Channel, encircles the middle of the body like a belt. It links together all of the other Channels. It controls the Chong, Ren, and Du Mai, and it strengthens their links to the Uterus.

The last four Extraordinary Channels are located in the trunk and legs and are paired.

**The Yangqiao Mai** (*yang-chow-my*), or Yang Heel Channel, connects with the Governing Vessel. The Qi supplying this Channel is generated through leg exercises, and it rises upward to nourish the Yang Channels.

**The Yinqiao Mai** (*yin-chow-my*), or Yin Heel Channel, connects with the Kidney Channel. Qi enters the Channel through the transformation of Kidney Jing into Qi.

**The Yangwei Mai** (*yang-way-my*), or Yang Linking Channel, regulates Qi in the Yang Channels, including the Du Mai. Yangwei connects and networks the Exterior Yang of the whole body.

**The Yinwei Mai** (*yin-way-my*), or Yin Linking Channel, connects with the Kidney, Liver, and Spleen Yin Channels, the Ren Mai, and the Interior Yin of the whole body.

**The Fifteen Collaterals**

These are branches of the Twelve Primary Channels. They run from side to side along the exterior of the body, and they have the same acupuncture points as the Twelve Primary Channels. They also take their names from the Twelve Primary Channels, plus the Du Mai, the Ren Mai, and the Great Collateral of the Spleen.

The Fifteen Collaterals are responsible for controlling, joining, storing, and regulating the Qi and Xue of each of the Twelve Primary Channels.

# ANOTHER VIEW OF HOW THE MIND/BODY/SPIRIT WORKS

You may have heard of the Five Phases (*Wu Xing*)—or as they are sometimes called, the Five Elements. This is the philosophical basis for the systems used by Worsley School acupuncturists, many Classical Chinese Medicine practitioners, and many Japanese and Korean practitioners both to describe the physiology of the mind/body/spirit and to guide diagnosis and treatment.

Strictly speaking, Traditional Chinese Medicine (TCM) does not use the Five Phases for treatment. However, many TCM practitioners also incorporate the Five Phases into their diagnosis and treatment because many aspects of the Phases provide powerful diagnostic tools. I often use Five Phases–based treatment plans for problems that are primarily emotional or that I intuitively sense would benefit from the approach.

The Five Phases—Wood, Fire, Metal, Water, and Earth—describe the dynamic system of matter's transformation through growth, decline, decay, rebirth, and balance. This continual cycle of growth and dormancy exists in both the external world and the world within human beings.

A person may be characterized as being predominantly Wood, Earth, Fire, Water, or Metal, or a combination of Phases. A disharmony may manifest the influence of one or more Phases as well.

Around the outside of the illustration on the next page is the Shen Cycle, or cycle of creation. Wood burns Fire, which, when turned to ashes, forms the Earth, from which Metal is derived, which in turn if heated becomes liquid, like Water. Water then creates Wood, and the Shen Cycle is whole.

The Destruction, or Ko cycle, connects the Phases (see the arrows in the center of the diagram). This cycle controls and balances the Phases. Wood controls Earth, Earth controls Water, Water controls Fire, Fire controls Metal, and Metal controls Wood.

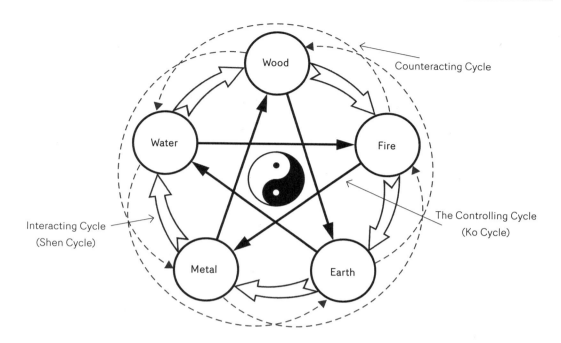

The tension between creation and destruction and the interrelationships of the Five Phases maintain the natural flow and harmony. Disharmony in one Phase impacts the associated Phases.

Each Phase is associated with and describes a stage of transition, direction, color climate, human sound, emotion, taste, Yin Organ, Yang Organ, sense organ, tissue, smell, and grain. These associations aid diagnosis, providing detailed clues about the nature of disharmonies.

Emotions are of particular importance in the Five Phases system, and many practitioners spend a great deal of time in their initial interview with a client asking about the Seven Emotions: Joy, Anger, Grief, Sadness, Fear, Fright, and Pensiveness/Worry. Every disharmony or illness in a Phase is associated with an emotion. That emotion is a strong indication of where in the body to look for illness and which Channels to treat with acupuncture. The Five Phases practitioner will also evaluate facial colors, smell, touch, and pulses, although these are sometimes different in character from TCM.[5] Each Phase is associated with acupuncture Channels, and disharmony in a Phase or Phases indicates which Channel(s) to treat to help restore harmony.

To help you understand how the Five Phases translates into practical medical care, you may want to familiarize yourself with the following basic principles of the Five Phases: Wood, Fire, Metal, Water, and Earth.

## The Wood Phase

Wood is associated with functions in the growing stage of life. Like a strong, rooted tree that grows upward and outward, a Wood person is firmly anchored with clear, strong Qi. If the Qi is not clear, you feel off-balance, uprooted. Sufficient Qi does not nourish your limbs. You may have spinal problems.

The Liver System, associated with Wood, governs the flow of Qi. People who are Liver dominant are critical thinkers and problem solvers, well focused, and take charge of business. The psychic sense of Liver is that it carries things into the future. When Liver is over-dominant, a person may become compulsive, rigid, irritable, and judgmental. The Gallbladder is also associated with Wood. It is also related to the decision-making ability.

The emotion of anger is associated with Wood, and it can be Excess or Deficient. The climate connected with the Liver is Wind. That has an impact on health because, as the ancient texts explain, if Wind enters the body and depletes the breath, then a person's Essence (Jing) is lost, and evil influences will injure the Liver.

## The Fire Phase

This Phase is associated with life in all of its passion and vitality. In the cycle of birth, growth, and decay, Fire is warm and nourishing, keeping life moving forward. When there is a lack of Fire, you cannot give or receive warmth in your life. Your life spark is dimmed. This may result in hot, painful joints, as if Fire were stuck. Fevers may flare up, and circulation may become poor, making parts of the body cold, while others are hot. Varicose veins and digestive problems are possible results.

The Organ Systems that are aligned with Fire are the Small Intestine, Heart, Triple Burner, and Circulation Sex, which corresponds to the Pericardium in TCM.

The Small Intestine, paired with the Heart, separates the pure from the impure, physiologically, emotionally, and spiritually. Excess or Deficient Fire affects Xue, and the blood vessels are associated with Fire as well. Furthermore, because the Heart is home to the Spirit Path or Gate, where Shen resides, people who have Fire as the dominant Phase are usually charismatic, open-minded, and empathetic. They seek similarities between people instead of differences. But if Heart becomes too dominant, a person may be come easily confused, uncertain, and oversensitive. They may become afraid of not knowing where or who they are. In cases of extreme disharmony, the person becomes disturbed, even psychotic. When Fire is unbalanced, the Shen is wounded, and joy, the emotion associated with Fire, is lost or destroyed.

Circulation Sex is paired with the Triple Burner, and it has a powerful effect on the psyche. According to the Five Phases, Circulation Sex is associated with the vascular system and the circulation of fluids. The Organ has no specific location. The Triple Burner is associated in Five Phases with temperature maintenance and regulation. It impacts family relationships and social ties, plus sympathy and antipathy.

## The Metal Phase

This Phase represents functions that are declining. Metal is involved in the communication networks in the body that allow the intake of air and fuel and assimilate them into energy. A Deficiency of Metal causes a breakdown in the mind/body/spirit.

The Lung System is associated with Metal, and an imbalance in Metal is associated with asthma, bronchitis, or emphysema. The Lung System also fuels emotions—consider how overwhelming beauty is said to be "breathtaking." A Metal imbalance can produce grief and deep sadness. A person who is Lung dominant is said to be ethereal, creative, intuitive, and even psychic. When Lung becomes overly dominant, the emotions may veer out of control, and the person may have difficulty dealing with change and may swing between being a passive victim and a tyrannical dictator.

The Large Intestine is associated with Metal. Its function is to remove waste from the body. Any imbalance of Metal may make it difficult for the body to rid itself of toxic substances and emotions.

## The Water Phase

The Water Phase takes the shape of whatever contains it, and it can be hot, cold, liquid, solid, clear, or murky. In the body, water enlivens every cell and the blood, tears, urine, sweat, and other liquids.

The Kidney System is associated with Water. It is the storehouse of what is called the Vital Essence (Jing), and it acts as the gateway to the Stomach. A person who is Kidney dominant is often a visionary, imagining future possibilities and seeing her or his own destiny clearly. If knocked down, this person gets right back up and fights again. However, if the Kidney becomes too dominant, the person may slide into suspiciousness, fear of getting close to others, and a sense of separation or falling apart. When the Kidneys are in disharmony, the Shen is volatile. You may feel like you are drowning in your fears. Physically, Kidney-dominant people may experience lethargy and edema and urinary and back problems. It is also associated with hypertension.

## The Earth Phase

This Phase denotes balance. Healthy Earth provides a feeling of contentedness and purpose. When it is unbalanced, disruption of the basic cycles of sleep, menstruation, appetite, breathing, and fertility may occur.

Earth's role as the center is revealed in its association with the Spleen System, which is the source of life for all of the other Organ Systems. It is also aligned with the Stomach, which influences formation of ideas and opinions. People who are Earth dominant are characterized as reliable, sedate, nurturing, and supportive. They have excellent memory for details, and they like to be the center of things. When Earth becomes overly dominant, they can become obsessive, they may drown in their own mental contents, and they may lose the ability to associate ideas logically. Physically, they may experience trouble with digestion and absorption of food.

### IDENTIFYING YOUR FIVE PHASES CHARACTERISTICS

Understanding your Five Phases characteristics can help you balance your mind/body/spirit and guide your healing process. To identify your primary Phase, answer the following two questions.

1. Would you characterize yourself as:
   A. Ethereal and creative
   B. Open-minded and empathetic
   C. Able to imagine your destiny clearly
   D. Reliable and nurturing
   E. A take-charge kind of person

2. Which emotion do you feel is the strongest in you?
   A. Sadness
   B. Joy
   C. Fear
   D. Worry/pensiveness
   E. Anger

A answers have constitution characteristics associated with Metal, while B associates with Fire, C with Water, D with Earth, and E with Wood.

## FIVE PHASES ASSOCIATIONS

|  | WOOD | FIRE | EARTH | METAL | WATER |
|---|---|---|---|---|---|
| Transitions | Birth | Growth | Transformation | Harvest | Storing |
| Direction | East | South | Center | West | North |
| Color | Green | Red | Yellow | White | Black |
| Climate | Wind | Heat | Damp | Dry | Cold |
| Human Sound | Shout | Laugh | Sing | Weep | Groan |
| Emotion | Anger | Joy | Worry/ Pensiveness | Grief/ Sadness | Fright/Fear |
| Taste | Sour | Bitter | Sweet | Pungent | Salty |
| Yin Organ | Liver | Heart/ Pericardium | Spleen | Lung | Kidney |
| Yang Organ | Gallbladder | Small Intestine, Triple Burner | Stomach | Large Intestine | Urinary Bladder · |
| Sense Organ | Eye | Mouth | Tongue | Nose | Ear |
| Tissue | Tendons | Blood | Muscles | Skin/Hair | Bones |
| Smell | Goatish | Burning | Fragrant | Putrid | Rotten |
| Grains | Wheat | Corn | Millet | Rice | Beans |
| Season | Spring | Summer | Late Summer/ Change of Seasons | Fall | Winter |

# ROOTS OF DISHARMONY
## Causes of Disease in Chinese Medicine

Ancient Chinese medicine does not talk about viruses or bacteria as triggers of disease or disorders. Instead, it talks about influences, which cause disharmony in Yin/Yang, the Essential Substances, the Organ Systems, the Channels, and the Five Phases.

Several categories of influences produce disharmony: the Six Pernicious Influences, Epidemic Factors, the Seven Emotions, and other factors, such as poor nutrition.

### THE SIX PERNICIOUS INFLUENCES

The Six Pernicious Influences—Cold, Heat, Dampness, Dryness, Summer Heat, and Wind—are external climatic forces that can invade the body and create disharmony in the mind/body/spirit. For example, if you are exposed to excess Heat, Cold, or Wind for a long time, or if you are exposed to such Influences when your body is already weak, you may develop an illness. This illness, triggered by External Pernicious Influences, can migrate inward and become more serious. For example, a slight cold may become pneumonia. This happens when the External Pernicious Influences overpower the body's natural protection against disease.

#### Cold

When hypothermia hits a skier or a mountain climber, muscle control fades, motion becomes slow and awkward, fatigue sets in, and the body shuts down. That's the same effect that the Cold Pernicious Influence has. It saps the body's energy, and it makes movements cumbersome. The tongue becomes pale; the pulse is slow. A person may develop a fear of cold and feel like sleeping in a curled-up position. Cold is Yin, and when it invades the body, it chills all or part of it. If there's pain, it's eased by warmth.

When External Cold attacks the body, acute illness may develop, along with chills, fever, and body aches. When the External Cold moves inward and becomes an Interior Cold disharmony, it is associated with a chronic condition that produces a pale face, lethargy and grogginess, a craving for heat, and sleeping for longer than usual periods of time.

## Heat

Heat disorders feel like you've been playing tennis for two hours in the blazing sun. You're weary, and at the same time, you feel strangely cranked up. You can't stop talking about the game, but your words stick in your mouth. You won't feel like yourself again until you cool down and quench your thirst.

Heat disorders cause overactive Yang functions or insufficient Yin functions. They are generally associated with bodily heat, a red face, hyperactivity and talkativeness, fever, thirst for cold liquids, and a rapid pulse. Symptoms include carbuncles and boils, dry mouth, and thirst. Confused speech and delirium arise when Heat attacks the Shen.

## Dampness

Think about what happens to your backyard when it rains for two days. It becomes soggy, and water collects in stagnant pools. That is how Dampness affects the body. Damp pain is heavy and expansive, blocks the flow of Qi, and causes a stuffy chest and abdomen.

When External Dampness invades, it enters the Channels and causes stiff joints and heavy limbs. When Dampness invades the Spleen, it can cause an upset stomach, nausea, lack of appetite, a swollen abdomen, and diarrhea.

Interior Dampness—caused by either the penetration of External Dampness to the Interior or by a breakdown in the Spleen's transformation of fluids—may transform into Phlegm, which in Chinese medicine is more than simply a bodily secretion. It can cause obstructions and produce tumors and coughing. If Phlegm invades the Shen, it can lead to erratic behavior and insanity. Once Dampness has taken root, it is hard to displace. Severe Dampness is known as Phlegm.

## Dryness

Dryness is a frequent partner with Heat. Think about the cracked bottom of a dried-up riverbed. But where Heat creates redness and warmth, Dryness creates evaporation and dehydration. External Dryness invading the body may create respiratory problems, such as asthmatic breathing and a dry cough, acute pain, and fever.

## Summer Heat

Summer Heat feels like the humid, oppressive weather that creates the dog days of August. It attacks the body after exposure to extreme heat and causes a sudden high fever and total lethargy. It is an External Influence and often arises with Dampness.

## Wind

Wind animates the body, stirring it from repose into motion just as wind moves the leaves of a tree. When Wind enters the body, it is usually joined to another influence, such as Cold or Dampness.

If the body is infiltrated by Wind, the first symptoms usually appear on the skin, in the lungs, or on the face. Tics, twitches, fear of drafts, headaches, and a stuffed-up nose are symptoms.

When External Wind invades the body more deeply or when Wind arises due to internal problems, it is identified as Internal Wind. This can be associated with seizures, ringing in the ears, and dizziness.

## Stages of Heat- and Cold-Induced Patterns of Disharmony

When Heat or Cold invade the body, they create stages of disharmony. The symptoms associated with these stages help in the process of diagnosis and treatment. (Remember, Chinese medicine is not linear. These stages can appear in any order, or not at all.)

When there is a Cold invasion, it may pass through the following six stages:

- **Taiyang** (*tie-yang*) is characterized by cold, fever, headache, a stiff neck, and what is called a floating pulse.

- **Yangming** (*yang-ming*) is characterized by fever, no fear of cold/aversion to heat, irritability, thirst, possible digestive symptom such as fullness and constipation, and a full pulse. This is a stage of Interior Heat disharmony because Cold induces Heat in both the first and the second stages.

- **Shaoyang** (*shau-yang*) is characterized by malaria-like alteration of cold and fever, no appetite, a bitter taste in the mouth, tenderness along the sides, the urge to vomit, and a wiry pulse.

- **Taiyin** (*tie-yin*) is characterized by vomiting, loss of appetite, pain, and diarrhea, but no thirst. This is associated with a Deficient Spleen System.

- **Shaoyin** (*shau-yin*) is characterized by profound sleepiness, cold, and a weak pulse. Fever disappears. This is associated with Deficient Yang of the Kidney System. Rarely, it is associated with Yin Deficient Heat conditions.

- **Jueyin** (*zh-way-yin*) is characterized by upper body Heat and lower body Cold.

When a Heat-induced disharmony moves into the body, it may pass in some order through one or more of the following four stages:

- **The Wei** (*way*) **stage:** The body's natural defenses are attacked, and the result may be fever, slight fear of cold, coughing, headache, a reddish tongue, and a quick floating pulse.

- **The Qi** (*chee*) **stage:** The Pernicious Influence penetrates the protective defenses of the body. The main symptom is usually high fever without chills, but symptoms vary, depending on which Organ System is affected. For example, Lung Heat produces high fever and coughing, while Stomach Heat produces high fever, abdominal pain, and constipation.

- **The Ying** (*ying*) **stage:** Deeper penetration by Pernicious Heat increases the disharmony in mind/body/spirit. The symptoms of this stage include a bright red tongue, an easily disturbed spirit, restlessness or even mania, a rapid pulse, dark yellow urine, less thirstiness than in the Qi stage, and possible skin eruptions.

- **The Xue** (*sch-whey*) **stage:** In the fourth and deepest stage, the Pernicious Influence of Heat enters the Xue (Blood), exacerbating the Ying-stage symptoms. Severe rashes, skin eruptions, high fever, and even coma may result. Blood in the urine or vomit may appear. Heat can injure the Yin, producing symptoms such as low fever, hot palms, dry teeth, a thin pulse, and stiffness and unresponsiveness.

# EPIDEMIC FACTORS

In addition to the Six Pernicious Influences, infectious Epidemic Factors are associated with various pestilences in Chinese medicine. The Epidemic Factors trigger symptoms that are similar to the External Pernicious Influences, but they are severely toxic. They cause the sudden onset of diseases, such as cholera and plague. These Epidemic Factors enter the body through the orifices, and each pestilence is associated with its own Epidemic Factor.

Some diseases—particularly viral diseases, such as HIV—that do not always have an apparent sudden onset are also triggered by Epidemic Factors. In Chinese medicine, Epidemic Factors are known as *Li Qi*.

# THE SEVEN EMOTIONS

While the Six Pernicious Influences are generally external triggers of disharmony, the Seven Emotions—Joy, Anger, Fear, Fright, Sadness, Grief, and Pensiveness/Worry—are internal causes of disease.

The Seven Emotions are as real a source of disharmony in the mind/body/spirit as the External Pernicious Influences are. In Chinese medicine, a disease is never dismissed as being "all in your head." Chinese medicine does not divide diseases or disorders into neat little packages: This one is physical, that one is emotional, this one is psychological, and that one is spiritual. Rather, Chinese medicine views the human being as a whole. There is no separation between the body and the emotions, between the body and the spirit, and between the body and the forces that shape the quality of daily life.

Despite this recognition of the importance of the Seven Emotions in diagnosing disharmony, TCM, as practiced in post-revolutionary China, does not place as large an emphasis on the Seven Emotions as it does on the Pernicious Influences. On the other hand, the Five Phases System pays special attention to emotions. It offers the TCM practitioner useful insights when diagnosing emotion-based disharmonies.

## Disharmonies of the Seven Emotions

An Excess or a Deficiency of any emotion is indicative of disharmony in the mind and spirit, and it alerts the Chinese medicine practitioner to disharmonies in Organ Systems as well. The Heart and Liver are the most susceptible to emotions. The Heart stores the Shen, and unharmonious emotions can disturb the Shen and cause sleeplessness, muddled thinking, inappropriate crying or laughing, and, in extreme cases, fits, madness, and hysteria. Excess or Deficient Joy especially impacts the Heart.

The Liver, which is responsible for the movement of Qi, Xue, and all of the emotions, is associated with anger. If the Liver Qi is stuck or in disharmony, the emotions become suppressed. If the emotions become suppressed, they suppress the function of the Liver. Sadness and grief, which are associated but distinct states, take their toll on the Lung System. If a person worries or overthinks, the Spleen System will become unbalanced.

Fear and fright, which are also related but distinct emotions, interfere with the smooth functioning of the Kidney System.

# OTHER SOURCES OF DISHARMONY

Several other factors can produce disharmony. Some examples include poor nutrition, unharmonious sex, and excess physical activity.

## Poor Nutrition

A balanced diet is an essential component of good health. In Chinese medicine, a balanced diet is used as a powerful therapeutic tool. The Chinese system recognizes that diet exerts a strong influence over the mind/body/spirit. Digestive problems, depletion of energy, depression, and many specific disharmonies can be triggered by eating too much or too little, by eating too frequently or not often enough, by eating food that is too cold, by eating too many raw foods, and by eating food that is impure or unsanitary. This happens, in part, because the Stomach and Spleen Systems, which receive and transform food, are the most sensitive to diet. When they become imbalanced, many associated components of the mind/body/spirit are affected.

Eating a diet that helps counter the disharmonies can restore harmony. For example, if you are suffering from Interior Cold Deficiency, your practitioner may suggest you eat foods that are warming and sweet to help rebuild your Qi. (See chapters 6 and 7, pages 91 and 112.)

## Unharmonious Sex

Excessive sex can cause Deficiency disorders, especially in men. For women, similar problems arise from multiple pregnancies.

## Excess Physical Activity

Obsessive exercise, overworking, and high-stress situations all deplete the mind/body/spirit. They make the body vulnerable to disharmony and disease.

# 4

# DISHARMONY REVEALED
## The Eight Fundamental Patterns of Disharmony and the Pathology of Essential Substances, Organ Systems, and Channels

Chinese medicine texts do not discuss diseases or disorders as we know them in the West. You don't catch an illness; you develop a disharmony.

In the beginning, that may make it difficult to understand how your Chinese medicine practitioner describes what ails you. For example, when you go for help because you have migraines, the practitioner may offer to treat you for disharmonies such as Stagnant Liver Qi, Liver Heat, Dampness, Deficient Qi and Xue, or Excess Yang. The Chinese diagnosis depends on the signs and symptoms that accompany your headache. The headache is viewed as a symptom and not the underlying disorder that requires treatment.

This chapter is designed to help you clarify the differences between Chinese and Western concepts of illness and disharmony. Therefore, I outline the Eight Fundamental Patterns of Disharmony, and I explain how Chinese medicine describes disturbances in Organ Systems, Channels, and Essential Substances.

## WESTERN DISEASES AND ASSOCIATED CHINESE MEDICINE DISHARMONIES

In Chinese medicine, the diagnosis of a disharmony is highly individualized: Two people with the same Western ailment may not have the same disharmony. A disharmony—unlike a disease—is not defined only by its physical manifestations but also by how it influences the harmony of the Essential Substances, Organ Systems, and the mind/body/spirit as a whole.

## DISEASES AND ASSOCIATED DISHARMONIES

This table offers examples of Western diseases and syndromes and associated Traditional Chinese Medicine patterns of disharmony.

| Western Diagnosis | Possible Chinese Medicine Patterns |
|---|---|
| Common cold | Wind-Heat, Wind-Cold, Taiyang Stage Cold Disease, or Qi Stage Hot Disease |
| Depression | Shen Disturbance, Stagnant Liver Qi, or Deficient Heart Xue |
| Essential hypertension | Hyperactive Liver Yang, Deficient Kidney Yin, Deficient Qi and Xue, or Deficient Yin/Excess Yang |
| Food poisoning | Summer Heat or Food Stagnation in Stomach |
| Hepatitis | Liver/Gallbladder Damp-Heat, Spleen Damp-Heat, Spleen Damp-Cold, Stagnant Liver Qi, Deficient Spleen Qi, Deficient Xue, or Stagnant Xue |
| Menopausal syndrome | Deficient Kidney and Liver Yin, Deficient Kidney Yang, Deficient Liver Xue, or Deficient Kidney Yin and Yang |
| Irritable bowel syndrome | Deficient Spleen Qi, Dry Large Intestine, Deficient Spleen Yang, Heat in Large Intestine, Spleen Dampness, Stagnant Liver Qi, or Large Intestine Damp-Heat |
| Sinusitis | Wind-Damp, Wind-Damp-Heat, Wind-Damp-Cold, Lung Phlegm-Heat, or Spleen Dampness |

# THE EIGHT FUNDAMENTAL PATTERNS

The Eight Fundamental Patterns, which are paired as Interior, Exterior; Heat, Cold; Excess, Deficiency; and Yin, Yang, describe the way in which the External Pernicious Influences and the Seven Emotions create disharmony in the mind/body/spirit. They also reveal the dynamic association of complementary yet opposed forces (Yin/Yang) within the body that have been thrown off balance by the presence of an influence or other disharmony.

**Interior and Exterior** patterns tell the practitioner where the disease resides.

Interior patterns of disharmony are indicated if the disharmony is chronic, produces changes in urine and stool, if there is discomfort or pain in the torso, and if there is no aversion to Cold or Wind.

Exterior patterns of disharmony often come on suddenly and are acute. Common signs include chills, fever, a dislike of cold, and an achy feeling overall.

**Heat and Cold** describe the activity of the body and the nature of the disease. Deficient Yang or an External Pernicious Cold Influence cause Cold Patterns. With Cold, everything slows down, and a person becomes withdrawn and sleeps in a curled-up position. Pain is relieved by warmth, bodily secretions are thin and clear, and there is a desire for warm liquids. Heat Patterns are caused by invasion of an External Pernicious Heat Influence, the depletion of Yin substances, as well as Excess Yang. With Heat, the body's processes speed up, and a person may talk excessively, have a red face and a hot body, and prefer cold beverages. Secretions become thick, putrid, and dark.

**Excess and Deficiency** express the impact of the disharmony on the body's resistance to disease (Normal Qi). With Deficiency, there is underactivity in the Organ System(s), weakness and tentative movement, a pale or ashen face, sweating, incontinence, shallow breathing, and pain that is relieved by pressure. Excess is associated with overactivity of bodily functions; heavy, forceful movements; a loud, full voice; heavy breathing; and pain increased by pressure.

## BODY SIGNS

You can enhance your ability to harmonize your mind/body/spirit by learning to "read" your body and to then associate what you observe with Chinese medicine's way of describing balance and imbalance.

Take a minute to think over your medical history. Have you ever had an illness that you could identify as Excess? As Deficient? Can you recall having an illness that made you have an aversion to the cold? How about one in which cold did not bother you?

**Yin and Yang** encompass the other six Fundamental Patterns. Yin encompasses Interior, Cold, and Deficient. Yang encompasses Exterior, Heat, and Excess.

To determine Yin/Yang disharmony, the doctor searches for clues about whether your disharmony is Interior or Exterior, for clues about patterns of Heat and Cold, and for clues about patterns of Deficiency and Excess. These can be translated into clinical symptoms. Patterns of Heat and Excess, for example, show themselves in fast, forceful movements and pain that is intensified by pressure and soothed by cold. If these qualities are observed during your consultation, the doctor will then diagnose you with a Heat Excess Yang condition. (See chapter 5, page 76, for details.)

After we examine the effect of the Eight Pernicious Influences and the Seven Emotions and the patterns of disharmony, the next step is for us to explore the pathologies of the Essential Substances, Organ Systems, and Channels. This will demonstrate how these lead to disharmony, the many ways that disharmonies can manifest themselves, and what disharmonies do to the balance of the mind/body/spirit.

# THE PATHOLOGY OF THE ESSENTIAL SUBSTANCES

Now we need to explore the pathology of the Essential Substances: Qi, Shen, Xue, Jing, and Jin-Ye. We'll talk about disharmonies of each in turn.

## Qi Disharmonies

When Qi moves harmoniously throughout the body, there is wholeness and good health. When Qi is disrupted, disharmony and illness can arise. Unbalanced Qi may become Excess, Rebellious, Deficient, or Sinking or Collapsed.

**Excess Qi** almost always collects and pools and becomes Stagnant. Excess Qi and Stagnant Qi are associated with blockages in the Channels and Organ Systems. These blockages interfere with the circulation of Qi and cause it to pool up, deprive some areas of the body, and flood other areas. The blockages may occur due to suppressed emotions, External Pernicious Influences, poor diet, or traumatic injury. Symptoms of Excess and Stagnant Qi are pain that worsens with pressure and is not easy to pinpoint, a feeling of fullness, and belching may relieve the pain. You may ache all over and have trouble sitting still. Often the pain waxes and wanes, and it is related to your emotional state.

When Stagnant Qi becomes more severe, it may actually reverse direction and become **Rebellious Qi**. This disharmony causes vomiting, belching, hiccups, coughing, asthma, liver disturbances, and fainting.

**Deficient Qi** occurs when bad diet, lack of exercise, respiration problems, and/or disharmony of the spirit and mind use up Qi and don't replenish it. It can trigger spontaneous sweating, fatigue, weakness, lack of a desire to move, a weak voice, a pale but bright face, disharmony of a particular Organ System, and symptoms that become worse when you exert yourself. Deficient Qi is relatively Yin.

If the condition worsens, Deficient Qi may become **Sinking or Collapsed Qi**, which develops if Deficient Qi is left unchecked for a period of time. Sinking or Collapsed Qi is associated with organ prolapses (when it sags or falls down, such as a prolapsed uterus or bladder), dizziness, lack of stamina, and a bright, pale face.

## Shen Disharmonies

Shen disharmonies are usually triggered by emotional disharmonies (an imbalance of the Seven Emotions). They are often accompanied by Stagnant Qi (often found in depression) and disharmony of the Heart and Liver Systems. With Deficient Heart Xue leading to Disturbed Shen, there may also be an underlying Deficient Spleen condition.

**Disturbed Shen** causes forgetfulness, disorientation, memory lapses, insomnia, and lackluster eyes. Extreme disharmony is associated with madness.

**Lack of Shen** is associated with a flat affect and inability to communicate. The classic phrase "The lights are on, but no one's home," describes this state.

To a Chinese medicine doctor, it makes no sense to heal the corporal body without healing the Shen. The physical and spiritual are inseparable parts of the human being. Disharmony in your Shen is often the first hint of developing disharmonies and disease. Feeling out of sorts, fatigued, blue, grumpy, and dispirited may indicate that an illness is developing. If the practitioner and the client intercede early, when your Shen is only mildly unbalanced, the development of full-blown disorders and disease may be forestalled for you.

## Xue Disharmonies

**Deficient Xue** is associated with malnutrition, loss of blood, Deficient Spleen, depletion of Qi, and emotional stress. It can trigger insomnia, dry skin, dizziness, hair loss, palpitations, menstrual irregularities, and blurry vision. When there is Deficient Xue, your body doesn't receive sufficient nourishment, often in one or more Organ Systems. When the whole body is Deficient in Xue, your skin has a pallor and is dry.

**Excess or Stagnant Xue** (also called Xue Stasis) is either caused by direct damage to the body's tissues (such as falling while skateboarding) or is a result of Stagnant Qi, Deficient Xue, and Cold Obstructing Xue. Symptoms include sharp, stabbing, fixed pain, tumors, or swollen organs. Pregnancy is a unique time in which an increase in Xue and Jin-Ye is part of a normal healthy body and is not necessarily associated with an Excess disharmony.

## Jing Disharmonies

We are born with Jing, and we can either deplete or replenish it throughout our lives. It always tends toward Deficiency. **Deficient Jing** symptoms include congenital disabilities, improper maturation, premature aging, sexual problems, and infertility. Disharmony of Jing is associated with Deficient Kidney.

## Jin-Ye Disharmonies

Jin-Ye may be either Deficient or Excess. **Deficient Jin-Ye** is associated with dry lips, hair, eyes, and skin. **Excess Jin-Ye** is related to accumulation of fluids and produces edema and swelling.

# THE EFFECTS OF DISHARMONY ON THE ORGAN SYSTEMS

When External and Internal Pernicious Influences create disharmony, they upset the balance within and between each Organ System and the various Channels. Each Organ System has its own patterns of disharmony and associated symptoms.

## Disharmonies in the Zang (Yin) Organ Systems

Each of the Zang (Yin) Organ Systems—the Kidney System, Spleen System, Liver System, Lung System, Heart System, and Pericardium System—can experience disharmony.

### KIDNEY SYSTEM

When the Kidney System becomes imbalanced, it may have one of four patterns of disharmony: Deficient Yang, Deficient Qi, Deficient Yin, or Deficient Jing. Such disruptions are often associated with the emotional state of Fear and with the exercise of (or lack of ability to exercise) the will.

**Deficient Kidney System Yang** is associated with impotence, hearing loss, and incontinence. It is often associated with cold limbs, lack of Shen, swollen limbs, profuse clear urine, sore lower back, and loose teeth.

**Deficient Kidney System Qi** may trigger frequent urination, incontinence, bedwetting, asthmatic breathing, and low back pain.

**Deficient Kidney System Yin** is associated with hot palms and soles, dry mouth, thirst, constipation, red cheeks, afternoon fevers, night sweats, insomnia, ringing in the ears, premature ejaculation, forgetfulness, and low back pain.

**Deficient Kidney System Jing** may lead to infertility, premature aging, retarded growth, lack or retardation of initial menstrual periods, and stiff joints.

## ANYA'S STORY

Anya, a thirty-three-year-old woman who was unable to become pregnant, came to the clinic after having been given the hormones progestin and Clomid by her gynecologist, which made her ill. She hadn't had her period for six years since going off birth control pills. As a teenager, she had painful periods associated with vomiting. Anya said she was cold most of the time.

I diagnosed her with Deficient Kidney Qi, and I treated her with Korean constitutional acupuncture, moxibustion, and herbs.

After several treatments, Anya reported she felt warmer. After two months, her pulse changed from slow, which is associated with Cold, to wiry, which is associated with Stagnant Qi. She became angry and depressed for a while, as her body went through a series of adjustments. We then had to change the treatment to regulate the Qi. At the same time, Anya started ovulating, and she began to have regular menstrual periods.

Twelve months after beginning treatment, Anya became pregnant, and she then gave birth to a healthy baby boy. Three years later, she came in again for some acupuncture support, and she had another healthy baby, this time a girl.

## SPLEEN SYSTEM

Spleen System disharmony in general manifests in loose stools, abdominal fullness and distention, nausea, and poor appetite. Anxiety and the inability to concentrate are also associated with Spleen System imbalance. Congenital weakness, malnutrition, chronic diseases, and excessive mental activity are caused by Interior Spleen disharmonies.

**Deficient Spleen System Qi** symptoms are loose stools, poor appetite, abdominal distention and pain, pale complexion, fatigue and lethargy, weight gain due to fluid retention, edema, shortness of breath, and a pale bright face.

**Sinking Spleen System Qi** is a subset of Deficient Spleen Qi. Muscular weakness and prolapsed organs—particularly of the uterus, bladder, and rectum—characterize this disharmony.

**Spleen System Not Able to Govern the Xue**, another subset of Deficient Spleen Qi, is associated with Xue circulating outside its proper pathways. The symptoms are chronic bleeding such as bloody stools, nosebleeds, varicose veins, hemorrhoids, excessive menstrual bleeding, non-menstrual uterine bleeding, easy bruising, and purpura—purple spotting indicative of bleeding beneath the skin.

## ESTHER'S STORY

One of the most persistent cases of Deficient Spleen Qi leading to Spleen Not Being Able to Govern the Xue was found in Esther, a young woman in her thirties. She had gone to her Western doctor for spotting between periods, easy bruising, varicose veins, excessively heavy periods, fatigue, and abdominal distention. He was unable to solve her problems.

I recommended that Esther switch to a diet with no raw foods and use moxibustion on certain acupuncture points to help reduce bleeding and eradicate the pain of the varicose veins. After six weeks, the spotting stopped, and her energy returned.

**Deficient Spleen System Qi Leading to Dampness** is a Deficiency condition leading to Excess.

**Deficient Spleen System Yang** develops from chronic Deficient Spleen Qi and Cold. The symptoms are the same as for Deficient Spleen Qi, plus clear copious urine, cold extremities and body, edema, weak digestion, and the desire for hot beverages.

**Deficient Spleen System Yin** appears in end-stage, life-threatening illness, such as AIDS and diabetes without the benefit of insulin. The symptoms include severe dryness, especially of the skin and lips, unquenchable thirst, loss of lean muscle mass, and severe wasting. Fever appears every afternoon and often in the evenings.

Externally caused **Excess Spleen System** patterns are often a result of an underlying Deficient Spleen System condition. They include Damp-Cold and Damp-Heat in the Spleen System.

- Damp-Cold occurs when Spleen Yang becomes trapped by exposure to excessive Dampness. This can happen if you are being drenched by rain, wade through cold water, or are exposed to damp and cold temperatures for a prolonged time. The associated symptoms are lack of appetite, watery stools, fatigue, no thirst, and a lusterless, yellow face.

- Damp-Heat occurs when External Dampness and Heat invade the body or when Deficient Spleen System Qi leads to Excess Damp and combines with Heat. It results in the slowing of bodily functions, and it causes an accumulation of fluids. The symptoms are lack of appetite, a feeling of fullness in the stomach, fatigue, and scanty, dark urine. Sometimes it is associated with thirst without the desire to drink, itchy skin, and fever. It may also be associated with acute viral hepatitis.

## LIVER SYSTEM

Repression of emotions is the most frequent cause of Liver System problems, which can manifest themselves in various patterns.

**Stagnant Liver System Qi** is the most common and usually the first Liver System disorder to appear when the system becomes imbalanced. It is an Excess condition, and it is relatively Yang. The main causes of Stagnant Liver Qi are emotional suppression and trauma. This leads to depression, uncomfortable feelings, and discomfort and pain between the ribs and in the chest, breast, and diaphragm. There may also be abdominal distention, restlessness, premenstrual congestion or distention, and a quick temper.

**Stagnant Liver System Xue** is characterized by fixed, sharp, stabbing pains and palpable masses. It often develops from Stagnant Liver Qi as well as Deficient Xue. In women, it is associated with missed menstrual periods, menstrual clotting and cramps, or severe trauma. In men, this pattern's appearance is almost always the result of severe trauma or severe illness.

**Liver System Yang (or Fire) Rising** develops when Stagnant Liver System Qi becomes more congested and severe. It is associated with an accumulation of heat. Symptoms include headaches, eye pain, red eyes, sharp chest pain, scanty yellow urine, vertigo, nosebleeds, fits of anger, and dry stools. If left unchecked, this pattern can develop into a more serious condition—**Interior Liver System Wind**—that is associated with strokes, high fever with convulsions, paralysis, and loss of consciousness.

**Deficient Liver System Xue** is characterized by general dryness without any Heat symptoms. The symptoms are dryness of the eyes and nails, blurry vision, dizziness, muscle spasms, reduced menstrual periods, twitching, and a pale, lusterless face.

**Deficient Liver System Yin** includes all of the symptoms of Deficient Liver System Xue, plus red cheeks and eyes, restlessness, hot flashes, headaches, dizziness, numb limbs, night sweats, dry mouth and throat, ringing in the ears, and a quick temper.

## BEATRICE'S STORY

Beatrice, a thirty-eight-year-old woman, in her first month of pregnancy, came for treatment of severe nausea that lasted all day and was uncontrolled by food intake. The symptoms were clear signs of Stagnant Liver Qi. In addition, Beatrice was an enthusiastic jogger. She used it to control stress, but she was unable to continue running. This only increased her disharmony.

Beatrice was put on a program of diet therapy and acupuncture. We asked her to eliminate chicken and turkey for the duration of the pregnancy because they congest Liver Qi and cause Qi Stagnation. She also received one acupuncture treatment and a short course of herbal therapy. Within two days, the nausea stopped. A month later, when she tried to eat chicken, her nausea returned briefly.

**Damp-Heat of Liver System** can occur when the diet is of poor quality and food is heavily spiced and fatty. It can also result from invasion of an Epidemic Factor, which is now known as viral hepatitis. The symptoms are discomfort in the top of the shoulders and rib cage, a bitter taste in the mouth, poor appetite, jaundice, fever and chills, and scanty, dark urine. Damp-Heat of the Liver System is associated with hepatitis and inflammation of the gallbladder.

**Cold Obstructing the Liver Channel** tends to be a male disharmony. Symptoms include a swollen scrotum and distention in the groin that is relieved by warmth.

**Deficient Liver System Qi** is rare. It creates Deficient Qi in the whole body, leading to a breakdown in joint function, general lethargy, shallow breathing, a lack of forcefulness in voice, and spontaneous sweating.

## LUNG SYSTEM

General symptoms of Lung System disharmonies include dry skin or skin eruptions, shortness of breath on exertion, cough, asthma, allergies, nose and throat disorders, low resistance to External Pernicious Influences, and reduced energy. Grief and the inability to let go at the proper time are also associated with the Lung System. There are also symptoms associated with specific types of Lung System disharmonies.

Exterior Excess Lung System patterns include the following.

**Wind Cold** is associated with chills, head and body aches, a lack of sweating, and frothy, thin, clear or white phlegm.

**Wind Heat** is associated with fever, slight chills, sore throat, some sweating, a coarse cough, and thick, yellow, sticky phlegm.

**Wind Dryness** is associated with a fever with chills, headache, dry throat and nose, and scant, dry phlegm.

Patterns of the Interior Excess Lung System include the following.

**Dampness** is generally triggered by a pre-existing lack of Spleen and Kidney function. It is associated with a full, high-pitched cough, chest inflammation, difficulty breathing when lying down, wheezing, copious phlegm, no thirst, and a swollen face.

**Heat** is generally triggered by overactive Liver and Heart Systems or the penetration of an External Pernicious Influence. When the Liver Invading the Lung causes it, the symptoms are dryness, pain in the chest or ribs, chest distention, and choking cough with thick green phlegm. When the Heart System causes it, the symptoms are insomnia, restlessness, cough, agitation, and confusion. When caused by an External Pernicious Influence, the symptoms are fever, sweating, cough, shortness of breath, and a rapid, superficial pulse.

Deficient Lung System patterns include the following.

**Deficient Lung System Qi** appears when the External Excess Pernicious Influence remains in the Lung and injures the Qi or when there are other Interior disharmonies that affect the Lung. The symptoms include a whispering voice, reluctance to speak, weak respiration, susceptibility to colds, weak cough, spontaneous sweating, shortness of breath that is worse with exertion, lack of warmth, and thin white phlegm.

## JON'S STORY

Jon, a forty-year-old man who had suffered with asthma since he was a child, came to the clinic after a bout of mononucleosis, which had lowered his resistance to pollens and molds. He was fatigued, and his asthma had become so severe that he had to give up regular exercise and was constantly using two kinds of inhalers. Jon was coughing up white phlegm, and he was short of breath and quite lethargic.

I diagnosed Jon with Deficient Lung Qi with Dampness due to Deficient Spleen. His prescribed treatment included acupuncture and moxibustion to the Lung System points on his upper back along with other Organ System tonification points. For acute asthma attacks, I prescribed herbal pills for him to use as needed. For the underlying Deficiency, he was given a constitutional herbal formula.

"After a few months, I noticed that the herbs had reduced the phlegm," Jon said. "I was able to wean myself off of the inhalers. During the last allergy season, which was a pretty intense one, I felt great."

**Deficient Lung System Yin** is associated with Deficient Jin-Ye of the Lung. The causes are Internal Dryness, chronic Deficient Kidney Yin, and the External Pernicious Influence of Heat remaining in the Lung and causing Dryness. Symptoms are fatigue; weakness; dry cough with no phlegm; restlessness; insomnia; afternoon fevers; night sweats; dry mouth and throat; weak voice; red cheeks; varicose veins; a feverish sensation in the palms, soles, and chest (Five Centers Heat); and sometimes scanty phlegm, streaked with blood.

## BODY SIGNS

Have you ever experienced Deficient Spleen System Qi—fatigue, lethargy, abdominal distention, fluid retention, and a pale complexion? Or Excess Lung System Wind/Cold—chills, head and body aches, clear or white phlegm, and lack of sweating? In Western medicine, these symptoms may be associated with irritable bowel syndrome and influenza, respectively.

## HEART SYSTEM

Deficiency patterns of the Heart System include the following.

**Deficient Heart System Xue** is often associated with Deficient Spleen Qi, because the Spleen is responsible for making the Xue. The symptoms include a pale lusterless face, dizziness, anxiety, confusion, excessive crying or laughing, and difficulty falling asleep.

**Deficient Heart System Yin** includes the symptoms of Deficient Heart Xue plus Heat symptoms, such as palpitations, agitation, insomnia, waking up at night, warm palms and soles, emotional lability, increased dreams, poor memory, night sweats, and physical and emotional hypersensitivity. It is often associated with Deficient Kidney Yin.

**Deficient Heart System Qi** is associated with the physiological problems of circulation, such as irregular pulse, arrhythmia, shortness of breath, fatigue, edema, and heart failure. Symptoms become worse with exercise.

**Deficient Heart System Yang** includes the symptoms of Deficient Heart Qi plus Cold symptoms, such as pain and distention in the chest, cold limbs and/or coldness throughout the whole body, purplish lips, and a slower, weaker heartbeat. It often appears with Deficient Kidney Yang and Deficient Lung Qi.

A subset of Deficient Heart System Yang is **Collapse of Yang**, in which Yin and Yang can separate, and the person is near death. Symptoms include profuse sweating, extremely cold limbs, purple lips, and confusion.

## HAROLD'S STORY

Harold, a sixty-eight-year-old man with congestive heart failure and arrhythmia, came into the clinic because his cardiologist had not been able to do anything to stabilize his irregular heartbeat or shortness of breath. He also had severe fatigue and swelling in the ankles. Harold was diagnosed as having Deficient Heart Qi, and we started him on a once-a-week program of acupuncture, moxibustion, and leg and foot massage to stabilize his heartbeat and reduce swelling. In addition, he was on crutches because he needed a hip replacement, which made his treatment more difficult. The constant pain and physical strain aggravated his Deficient Qi.

After six months of therapy, the swelling had gone away, and Harold's Western doctor reported that there had been no further deterioration of his congestive heart problem.

Patterns diagnosed as Excess include the following.

**Excess Heart System Fire** is caused by extreme emotional excitement, sunstroke, or excess consumption of hot, pungent foods, drinks, or herbs. Symptoms include insomnia, restlessness, red face, inflammation or soreness of the tongue and mouth, thirst, and scanty, burning urine with blood.

**Excess Phlegm Obstructing Heart System or Misting of the Orifices** may arise from Spleen Dampness or simply from a general internal lack of proper fluid circulation. The symptoms include Shen disharmony, aberrations of consciousness, coma or semi-coma (in Chinese medicine it's called "dumb like a wooden chicken"), excessive weeping or laughing, depression or dullness, mania, incoherent speech, muttering to oneself, drooling, and predisposition to stroke.

There are two types of Phlegm: Cold and Hot. **Excess Cold Phlegm** symptoms are a withdrawn, inward manner, muttering, staring at walls, and sudden blackouts. **Excess Hot Phlegm** symptoms include hyperactivity, agitation, aggression, incessant talking, and violent lashing-out behavior.

**Heart System Stagnant Qi** is associated with a stuffy chest and difficulty breathing. If it is the result of Stagnant Phlegm, there are the same symptoms plus excess phlegm expectoration, abdominal fullness, nausea, and vomiting.

**Heart System Stagnant Xue** is associated with angina and pectoral pain, and it results from Deficient Heart Qi or Deficient Heart Yang. Symptoms include palpitations, shortness of breath, irregular pulse, fixed stabbing pain, and a purple face.

## PERICARDIUM SYSTEM

Only one major pattern is associated with the Pericardium System, and it is not an independent pattern: **Excess Phlegm Obstructing Heart System or Misting of the Orifices** (see page 66).

## Disharmonies in the Fu (Yang) Organ Systems

Each of the Fu (Yang) Organ Systems—the Stomach System, Triple Burner System, Gallbladder System, Small Intestine System, Large Intestine System, and Urinary Bladder System—also can experience disharmony.

### STOMACH SYSTEM

The patterns of disharmony that may afflict the Stomach include the following.

**Food Retention in Stomach System** is due to irregular eating habits, overeating, or eating hard-to-digest foods. Retention blocks passage of Qi in the abdomen, triggering distention, fullness, and pain in the abdomen; foul belching; regurgitation; anorexia; vomiting; and difficult bowel movements.

**Retention of Fluid in Stomach System Due to Cold** is associated with a constitutional Deficiency of Stomach and Spleen Qi, complicated by the invasion of the External Pernicious Influence of Cold. Eating too much cold or raw food can trigger this pattern. Symptoms include fullness and pain in the stomach relieved by warmth, reflux of clear fluid, or vomiting after eating. This pattern is associated with prolonged disease.

**Hyperactivity of Fire in Stomach System** (also called **Stomach Heat**) may arise from eating too many hot, fatty foods and from depression. The symptoms include burning and pain in the stomach, thirst for cold beverages, bleeding gums, and scant, yellow urine. It's often associated with stomach ulcers, excessive appetite, constipation, and mouth ulcers.

**Deficient Stomach System Yin** occurs when hyperactivity of Fire in the Stomach consumes the Stomach Yin or when Stomach Jin-Ye dries up because of persistent Heat due to a prolonged disease with fever. Symptoms include burning stomach pain, hunger without appetite, dry heaves, hiccups, dry mouth and throat, constipation, and an empty, uncomfortable feeling in the stomach.

### TRIPLE BURNER SYSTEM

One theory of disharmonies in the Triple Burner identifies the External Pernicious Influence of Damp Heat as the cause of disease.

**Damp Heat in the Upper Burner** can happen when Damp invades the body and stays in the muscles and upper body, damaging Spleen Qi. Symptoms include extreme dislike of cold, mild or no fever, feeling like there is a soft band around the head, heavy arms and legs, a feeling that an elephant is standing on your chest, lack of thirst, distended abdomen, noisy bowels, loose stools, and lack of facial expression.

**Damp Heat in the Middle Burner** can arise from the External Pernicious Influences of Summer Heat and Damp. It can also occur when Damp Heat from the Upper Burner sinks into the Middle Burner. Poor nutrition is also a trigger. Symptoms are similar to those for invasion of Damp and Heat in the Stomach and Spleen: heavy arms, legs, and trunk; full, distended chest and stomach; nausea; vomiting; anorexia; loose but difficult stools; dark urine; feeling thirsty with little desire to drink; and a fever that can't be felt at the first touch of the skin but that becomes evident after the skin is felt for a rather long time. In severe cases, the Shen is disturbed, and mental abilities are affected.

**Damp Heat in the Lower Burner** affects the Intestine Systems and Urinary Bladder System. It is associated with difficulties with urination and elimination. Symptoms include constipation, thirstiness with little inclination to drink, and a hard, distended lower abdomen.

## THE GALLBLADDER SYSTEM

Disharmony with the Gallbladder System manifests similar to disharmony with the Liver System, specifically Liver Damp-Heat. The symptoms associated with that pattern include discomfort in the chest, a bitter taste in the mouth, poor appetite, fever and chills, jaundice, and scanty, dark urine. General Gallbladder dysfunction can cause you to become angry and impulsive, along with an inability to make up your mind and exhibiting general weakness of character.

## SMALL INTESTINE SYSTEM

**Pain Due to Disturbance of Small Intestine System Qi** may result from poor nutrition, carrying overly heavy loads, and wearing clothing that's inappropriate for the weather, making you vulnerable to External Pernicious Influences. Symptoms include acute lower abdominal pain, abdominal distention, noisy bowels, and a heavy, downward-pushing sensation in the testes accompanied by lower back pain.

**Heart Fire Moving to the Small Intestine System** includes the symptoms of Heart Fire (see "Excess Heart System Fire" on page 66), plus irritability, cold sores, sore throat, frequent painful urination, and a full feeling in your lower abdomen.

## LARGE INTESTINE SYSTEM

**Large Intestine System Damp-Heat** is sometimes called **Damp-Heat Dysentery**. This pattern often occurs in hot climates in the summer and autumn when the External Pernicious Influences of Summer Heat, Dampness, and Toxic Heat invade the Stomach and Intestines. It also arises when a person eats too much raw, cold food, or unsanitary food or eats at irregular times. Symptoms include abdominal pain, a feeling of urgency along with difficult bowel movements, watery diarrhea, bloody stools with mucus, burning anus, and dark-colored urine. Sometimes it is accompanied by fever and thirst.

**Consumption of Jin-Ye of Large Intestine System** is often seen in the elderly, after childbirth, and in the later stages of disease with fever. Symptoms include constipation, dry stools, and dry mouth and throat.

**Intestinal Abscess** is known in Western medicine as appendicitis. The symptoms include acute pain in the lower right quadrant, aversion to touch, and possibly a fever.

## URINARY BLADDER SYSTEM

**Damp Heat in the Urinary Bladder System** is the main pattern of disharmony associated with the Urinary Bladder System. This pattern can arise from the invasion of External Pernicious Damp and Heat or from a diet of excessively hot, greasy, and sweet foods. Symptoms include painful, frequent, urgent urination; cloudy, dark urine; back pain; blood in the urine; feeling of fullness in the lower abdomen; burning pain in the urethra; and difficult urination.

## Disharmonies of the Extraordinary Organs

Each of the Extraordinary Organs—the Marrow and Brain and Uterus—also can experience disharmony.

**Marrow and Brain:** When the Marrow is Deficient, the Brain becomes unbalanced. Symptoms include ringing in the ears, vertigo, shakiness, poor eyesight, and difficulty thinking. Weak bones and retarded bone growth can also occur.

**Uterus:** If there is Deficient Heart Xue, the Heart Qi does not descend to the Uterus, and the menstrual periods may become irregular or stop altogether. Failure of Kidney Jing to descend to the Uterus can result in infertility, irregular periods, or complete cessation of menstruation. Disturbances of the Extraordinary Channels, such as the Chong Mai and Ren Mai (which arise in the Uterus), can also cause Uterus disharmonies.

Because of the interdependence of the Uterus on other Organ Systems and Channels, treatment for all menstrual and reproductive problems is through the Liver, Kidney, Spleen, or Heart Organ System and related Primary and Extraordinary Channels.

# THE EFFECT OF DISHARMONY ON THE CHANNELS

Channels are affected by disharmonies that are distinct from those afflicting Organ Systems and the Essential Substances. Some practitioners who solely practice acupuncture will primarily diagnose and devise treatments through the diagnosis of Channel disharmonies.

When a pathogen causes disharmony in a Channel, the acupuncture points become tender to the touch. The tender spots are useful in diagnosis because they clue the practitioner to the location and nature of the imbalance along the Channel and in the associated Organ System(s).

The following are the pathologies identified by the TCM school of thought that correspond to the Twelve Primary Channels, Eight Extraordinary Channels, and Fifteen Collaterals. (Not all schools of acupuncture accept these indications for diagnosis and treatment, however.) Let's talk about each in turn.

## Pathologies of the Twelve Primary Channels

Each of the Twelve Primary Channels is associated with distinct disharmonies. These disharmonies, which arise when the flow of Qi is disrupted, create symptoms in the part of the body through which the Channel flows. Each Channel has exterior and interior pathways. The exterior pathways are relatively near the surface of the skin, and they contain the acupuncture points. The interior pathways are relatively deep, and they cannot be needled directly.

**Lung Channel of Hand—Taiyin:** Symptoms associated with disharmonies of the Lung Channel include cough, asthmatic breathing, coughing up blood, congested and sore throat, the feeling that a baby elephant is standing on your chest, pain in the neck, pain in the upper chest, and pain running along the lower section of the inside of the arm.

**The Large Intestine Channel of Hand—Yangming:** Symptoms associated with disharmonies of the Large Intestine Channel include nosebleeds, runny nose, toothaches, congested and sore throat, neck pain, pain in the front of the shoulder and the front edge of the arm, noisy bowels, abdominal pain, diarrhea, and dysentery.

**The Stomach Channel of Foot—Yangming:** Symptoms associated with disharmonies of the Stomach Channel include noisy bowels, distended abdomen, edema, vomiting and stomach pain, hunger, bloody nose, a droopy mouth, congested and sore throat, chest and abdominal pain, pain along the outside of the leg, fever, and mania.

SONIA'S STORY

After a decade of performing surgery, Sonia developed chronic pain in her right wrist. An orthopedist diagnosed it as repetitive use syndrome, and Sonia was told her options were to have surgery or to suffer progressive nerve damage.

"I'm a Western doctor, through and through," Sonia said. "But I figured I had nothing to lose by trying acupuncture. I never thought it would really work, but I was desperate."

Sonia came to the clinic from out of town, saying she could only stick around for one treatment. She was diagnosed with an injury to the Large Intestine Channel due to trauma. I suggested that she get a wrist splint and make changes in her surgical schedule. I gave her an herbal trauma salve to apply to her wrist daily. Sonia then had a thirty-minute acupuncture treatment with electro-stimulation and moxibustion on her wrist.

A week later, Sonia called the clinic to report that she was 80 to 90 percent better—after only one treatment. Six weeks later, she received another treatment, and after that she reported a 95 percent improvement. Sonia vowed that every time she came to San Francisco, she'd get a tune-up treatment. She also learned how to use self-care to avoid re-injury.

**The Spleen Channel of Foot—Taiyin:** Symptoms associated with disharmonies of the Spleen Channel include belching, vomiting, stomach pain, distended abdomen, loose stools, jaundice, overall feeling of lethargy and heaviness, inflexibility and pain where the tongue attaches to the mouth, and swelling and cold along the inside of the knee and thigh.

**The Heart Channel of Hand—Shaoyin:** Symptoms associated with disharmonies of the Heart Channel include heart pain, palpitations, chest and rib pain, insomnia, night sweats, dry throat and thirst, hot palms, and pain along the inside of the upper arm.

**Small Intestine Channel of Hand—Taiyang:** Symptoms associated with disharmonies of the Small Intestine Channel include deafness, yellowing of the whites of the eyes, sore throat, swollen cheeks and throat, pain along the back edge of the shoulder and arm, and lower abdomen distention and pain.

**Urinary Bladder Channel of Foot—Taiyang:** Symptoms associated with disharmonies of the Urinary Bladder Channel include bed-wetting or trouble urinating, depression and mania, blocked and stuffy nose, teary eyes (particularly in the wind), runny nose, eye pain, bloody nose, headache, and pain along the Urinary Bladder Channel from the nape of the neck to the middle of the backs of the legs.

**The Kidney Channel of Foot—Shaoyin:** Symptoms associated with disharmonies of the Kidney Channel include bed-wetting, too-frequent urination, nocturnal emission, impotence, asthmatic breathing, coughing up blood, dry tongue, congested and sore throat, edema, lower back pain, irregular periods, pain along the back edges of the insides of the thighs, weak legs, and hot soles of the feet.

**Pericardium Channel of Hand—Jueyin:** Symptoms associated with disharmonies of the Pericardium Channel include heart pain, palpitations, tight chest and trouble breathing, emotional restlessness, depression and mania, flush face, swelling in the armpits, arm spasms, and hot palms.

**The Triple Burner (Sanjiao) of Hand—Shaoyang:** Symptoms associated with disharmonies of the Triple Burner Channel include distended abdomen, bed-wetting, painful urination, deafness, ringing in the ears, pain at the outer edge of the eyes, swollen cheeks, congested and sore throat, pain behind the ears, shoulder pain, and pain in the backs of the arms and elbows.

**The Gallbladder Channel of Foot—Shaoyang:** Symptoms associated with disharmonies of the Gallbladder Channel include headache, pain at the outer edges of the eyes, jaw pain, blurry vision, a bitter taste in the mouth, swelling and pain in the upper chest and armpits, pain along the outside of the chest and rib area, and pain in the outsides of the thighs and lower legs.

**The Liver Channel of Foot—Jueyin:** Symptoms associated with disharmonies of the Jueyin Channel include low back pain, fullness in the chest, pain in the lower epigastric area, hernia, pain on the top of the head, dry throat, hiccups, bed-wetting, painful urination, and mental disharmony.

## Pathologies of the Eight Extraordinary Channels

These Channels are closely related to the Liver System, Kidney System, Uterus, and Brain and Marrow, and they serve to connect the Twelve Primary Channels and regulate their Qi and Xue. The pathological manifestations listed here are based on the physiological functions and the area of each Channel's influence. You can work with them during self-massage and acupressure. These Channels have a big role in disharmonies of women's reproductive cycles.

**Du Mai (Governing Channel):** Symptoms associated with disharmonies of the Du Mai include stiff, painful spine, severe muscle spasm causing arching of the back, headache, and epilepsy.

**Ren Mai (Conception Channel):** Symptoms associated with disharmonies of the Ren Mai include vaginal discharge, irregular periods, infertility in women and men, hernia, nocturnal emission, bed-wetting, urinary retention, stomach pain, lower abdominal pain, and genital pain.

**Chong Mai (Penetrating Channel):** Symptoms associated with disharmonies of the Chong Mai include spasm and pain in the abdomen, irregular periods, asthmatic breathing, infertility in women and men, and in my observations, emotional and physical problems arising from various forms of abuse.

**Dai Mai (Belt Channel):** Symptoms associated with disharmonies of the Dai Mai include weak lower back, vaginal discharge, uterine prolapse, trouble moving the hips and legs, weakness and muscular atrophy of lower limbs, and an unaccountable feeling like one is sitting in water.

**Yangqiao Mai (Yang Heel Channel):** Symptoms associated with disharmonies of the Yangqiao Mai include insomnia, redness and pain at the inside corners of the eyes, pain in the back and lower back, turning out of the foot, spasm of the lower limbs, and epilepsy.

**Yinqiao Mai (Yin Heel Channel):** Symptoms associated with disharmonies of the Yinqiao Mai include epilepsy, lethargy, leg spasms, turning in of the foot, lower abdomen and lower back pain, and hip pain that causes referred pain in the pubic region.

**Yangwei Mai (Yang Linking Channel):** Symptoms associated with disharmonies of the Yangwei Mai include External symptoms, such as chills and fever.

**Yinwei Mai (Yin Linking Channel):** Symptoms associated with disharmonies of the Yinwei Mai include Internal symptoms, such as chest and heart pain and stomachaches.

## Pathologies of the Fifteen Collaterals

The Fifteen Collaterals branch off of the Primary Channels with which they are associated. They strengthen the relationships between the paired Channels, and they move Qi and Xue to organs and tissue in the body. When disharmony occurs, the Collaterals compound the symptoms of the Primary Channel with which they are associated.

**Collateral of the Lung Channel of Hand—Taiyin:** Symptoms associated with disharmonies of this Channel include hot palms and wrists, shortness of breath, bed-wetting, and frequent urination.

**Collateral of the Large Intestine Channel of Hand—Yangming:** Symptoms associated with disharmonies of this Channel include toothache, deafness, cold teeth, and a stifling feeling in the chest and diaphragm.

**Collateral of the Stomach Channel of Foot—Yangming:** Symptoms associated with disharmonies of this Channel include depression and mania, atrophy of muscles and weakness in the lower legs, congested and sore throat, and sudden attacks of hoarseness.

**Collateral of the Spleen Channel of Foot—Taiyin:** Symptoms associated with disharmonies of this Channel include spasm of the abdomen, vomiting, and diarrhea.

**Collateral of the Heart Channel of Hand—Shaoyin:** Symptoms associated with disharmonies of this Channel include chest and diaphragm fullness and aphasia.

**Collateral of the Small Intestine Channel of Hand—Taiyang:** Symptoms associated with disharmonies of this Channel include weak joints, muscular atrophy, impaired movement in the elbows, and skin warts.

**Collateral of the Urinary Bladder Channel of Foot—Taiyang:** Symptoms associated with disharmonies of this Channel include stuffed-up sinuses, runny nose, headache, back pain, and bloody nose.

**Collateral of the Kidney Channel of Foot—Shaoyin:** Symptoms associated with disharmonies of this Channel include low back pain, urinary retention, mental restlessness, and a stifling sensation in the chest.

**Collateral of the Pericardium Channel of Hand—Jueyin:** Symptoms associated with disharmonies of this Channel include (physical) heart pain and mental restlessness.

**Collateral of the Triple Burner (Sanjiao) of Hand—Shaoyang:** Symptoms associated with this Channel include flaccidity or spasm on the insides of the elbows.

**Collateral of the Gallbladder Channel of Foot—Shaoyang:** Symptoms associated with this Channel include cold feet, paralysis of the legs, and the inability to stand upright.

**Collateral of the Liver Channel of Foot—Jueyin:** Symptoms associated with this Channel include constant erection, itching in the pubic area, swollen testes, and hernia.

**Collateral of the Ren Mai:** Symptoms associated with this Channel include abdominal pain that exerts an outward pressure and itching of the abdominal skin.

**Collateral of the Du Mai:** Symptoms associated with this Channel include stiff spine, heavy sensation in the head, and head tremor.

**The Great Collateral of the Spleen:** Symptoms associated with this Channel include overall achiness, muscle pain, and weakness in the arms and leg joints.

# PART TWO
# THE HEALING PROCESS

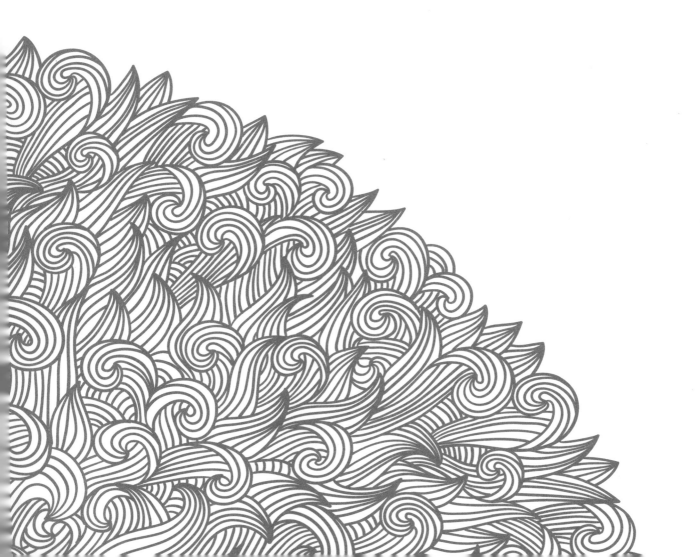

# 5

# WHEN YOU VISIT A CHINESE MEDICINE PRACTITIONER
## Evaluation and Diagnosis

When you go to see a Chinese medicine practitioner—whether it's to treat an illness, resolve acute pain, or begin a program of preventive care—your doctor will follow a system of evaluation and diagnosis that depends on observation and questioning.

In accordance with the philosophy of the Tao, diagnosis is a process of perceiving signs and symptoms and relating them to one another to reveal how they form patterns of harmony or disharmony. Each symptom or sign has meaning only in relationship to other symptoms and signs and to the whole of your mind/body/spirit.

## THE FOUR EXAMINATIONS

To begin to develop an accurate picture of your whole being, the Chinese medicine practitioner will examine you. She or he will use traditional Chinese methods called the Four Examinations: Inquiring, Looking, Listening/Smelling, and Touching. (Listening and Smelling are two seemingly different acts that are grouped together. In Chinese, they are the same character.)

This process of examination reveals which of the Eight Fundamental Patterns of disharmony are at work and what type of disharmony of the Essential Substances, Organ Systems, and Channels you may have.

The Four Examinations are often done formally. However, often the practitioner also uses intuition and casual observation to create a vivid profile of a patient. Every gesture, word, and attribute provides clues to your health and well-being.

Let's look at each step in the diagnostic process in more detail, breaking down the Four Examinations into their components, so you'll know what to expect for your visit.

## Examination One: Inquiring

Although the Four Examinations can be done in any order, and in fact some things are done simultaneously, often the practitioner begins with inquiring. There's one step within the Inquiring Examination.

### STEP ONE: ASKING QUESTIONS

The Chinese medicine doctor will take a great deal of time to ask you about yourself. Your answers allow the practitioner to benefit from the knowledge that you have, because no one can know your body as well as you do. Questioning also allows the practitioner to observe your emotions, voice, and self-presentation.

His or her basic questions will likely focus on the following:

- Your reaction to heat and cold
- Your patterns of perspiration
- If and when you experience headaches or dizziness
- What type of pain you have, if any
- Your bowel and bladder function
- Your thirst, appetite, and tastes
- Your sleep patterns
- Your sexual functioning, sexual activity, and reproductive history
- Your general medical history
- Your general physical activity
- Your emotions

## Examination Two: Looking

Generally, the practitioner will focus on the Looking Examination next. There are three steps in this examination: evaluation of the tongue, body language, and facial color.

### STEP TWO: EVALUATION OF THE TONGUE

The tongue is the mirror of the body. Harmony and disharmony are reflected in your tongue's color, moisture, size, coating, and the location of abnormalities.

Healthy Organ Systems and a lack of External Pernicious Influences produce a healthy tongue, which is pinkish red, neither too dry nor too wet, fits perfectly within your mouth, moves freely, and has a thin white coating.

Imbalances in the Organ Systems and/or invasion by External Pernicious Influences produce an unhealthy tongue. External Pernicious Influences primarily produce changes in the tongue coating. Interior problems, such as Organ System or Essential Substance disharmonies, produce changes in the tongue body.

When examining your tongue, the Chinese medicine doctor looks at the color of the tongue body, its size and shape, locations of abnormalities, moistness or dryness, presence or absence of tongue fur, and the color and thickness of the coating or fur. These signs reveal overall state of health, and they also correlate to specific Organ System functions and disharmonies, especially in the digestive system. To evaluate the tongue accurately, we do the examination in natural light whenever possible.

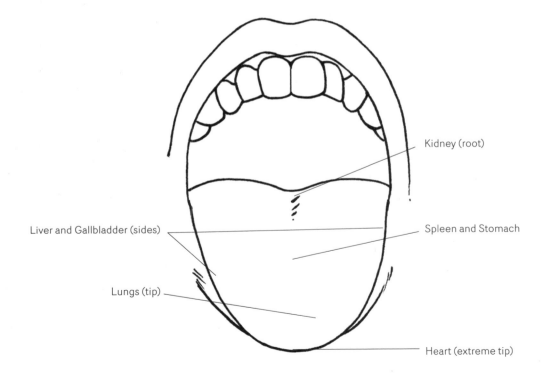

**Tongue body:** The tongue body is a fleshy mass, and it has color, texture, and shape independent from the apparent qualities of the tongue coating.

- A pale tongue body indicates Deficient Xue, Qi, Yang, or Excess Cold.

- An overly red tongue body indicates Excess Heat.

- A purple tongue indicates that Qi and/or Xue are not moving harmoniously, and they are stagnant.

- A pale purple tongue means the stagnation is related to Cold.

- A reddish purple tongue color is related to stagnation of Heat.

- When the tongue is black or gray, it indicates extreme stagnation.

- If the tongue is black and dry, it indicates extreme Heat Stagnation; if black and wet, it indicates extreme Cold Stagnation.

- A bright red tongue indicates Deficient Yin or Excess Heat.

- Dark red indicates Excess Heat.

- Cracks in a red tongue indicate Deficient Yin or Heat Injuring the Jin-Ye.

- If the tongue is pale and cracked, Deficient Qi or Xue is present.

- Thorny eruptions of the "buds" on the tongue alert the doctor to Heat or Stagnant Xue.

**Tongue fur:** The tongue's coating is best described as moss or fur. It arises when the Spleen causes tiny amounts of impure substances to drift upward to the tongue. When the Spleen and Stomach are in balance, there is a uniform density of fur, with a slightly thicker area in the center of the tongue.

- Thick fur indicates Excess.

- Thin fur is related to Deficiency during illness, but it is normal if you are well.

- Fur that is wet indicates Excess Jin-Ye and/or a Deficient Yang.

- Dry fur is a sign of Excess Yang or Deficient Jin-Ye.

- A greasy fur is a sign of Phlegm or Dampness in the body.

- If the fur looks peeled off or missing, it reveals Deficient Spleen, Deficient Yin, or Deficient Jin-Ye.

- White, moist fur indicates Cold.

- Yellow fur means Heat. However, white fur resembling cottage cheese points to Stomach Heat.
- Gray/black fur with a red tongue body is associated with extreme Heat. Gray/black fur with a pale tongue body is a sign of extreme Cold.

**Tongue size and shape:** A healthy tongue rests comfortably in the mouth, and it is neither too small nor too large.

- If a tongue is enlarged and flabby, it indicates Deficient Qi.
- If in addition to being enlarged and flabby, the tongue has scalloped (or tooth marked) edges, it indicates Dampness due to Deficient Qi or Stagnant Jin-Ye.
- If the tongue is enlarged and hard, it is a sign of Excess.
- If it swells so that it fills the mouth and is deep red, that means Excess Heat in Heart and Spleen.
- A small, thin tongue can indicate Deficient Yin or Xue.

**Tongue movement:** A healthy tongue sits in the center of the mouth, and is neither too hard nor too soft.

- A trembling, pale tongue indicates Deficient Qi.
- A flaccid tongue that is pale often reveals extreme Deficient Qi or Xue.
- A flaccid tongue that is deep red reveals severe Deficient Yin.
- A trembling, red tongue indicates Interior Wind.
- If the tongue sits off center in the mouth, early or full-blown Wind stroke may be present.
- A rigid tongue accompanies an External Pernicious Influence and fever, and it may indicate the invasion of the Pericardium by Heat and Phlegm Obstructing the Heart Qi.

**Location of tongue abnormalities:** The location of disturbances on the tongue is a vivid indication of where disharmonies in the mind/body/spirit are located. Certain Organ Systems are associated with the Upper, the Middle, and the Lower Burner, which are in turn associated with the front, middle, and back sections of the tongue.

For example, if there are red spots on the front third of the tongue, which is associated with the Upper Burner, this indicates that there is Heat in the Lung. If the tip of the tongue is red, that indicates Heart Fire. Menstrual cramps, associated with Stagnant

Xue, are often accompanied by purple spots on the edges of the tongue in the Liver/Gallbladder area.

Not all tongue irregularities are indications of disharmony, however. Food and drugs may change the coating or color of the body of the tongue. For example, coffee yellows the coating, and Pepto-Bismol turns the tongue black.

Furthermore, some people have minor, unchanging cracks on their tongue, which are considered normal. Other people are born with what is called a geographic tongue, which is covered with severe cracks and covered with hills and valleys. Some practitioners consider this to be normal, while others see it as a sign of congenital disharmony.

The way a tongue appears is not an absolute indicator of the location of the disharmony. But when features of the tongue are taken as part of an overall pattern that includes a complete evaluation, it offers strong clues to the location of disharmony.

## STEP THREE: EVALUATION OF BODY LANGUAGE—STYLES OF MOVEMENT, POSTURE, AND SELF-PRESENTATION

Seeking clues to possible External Pernicious Influences, the practitioner looks for signs of Heat or Cold Influences, Excess or Deficiency, and Yin or Yang disharmonies. If a person has a heavy-footed walk and a loud voice and sits in a sloppy, spread-out posture, it may indicate Excess. If a person acts frail and weak, sits with shoulders slumped, and is shy and receding, it may indicate a Deficiency. On the other hand, fast, jerky, impulsive movement and an outgoing personality indicate Heat. If combined with a full red face, high energy, and a loud voice, then both Heat and Excess may be at work. Cold, as you might suspect, is associated with slow but not sloppy movements and a pale face. When coupled with a low voice, shortness of breath, and passivity, Cold and Deficiency may be at work.

## STEP NUMBER FOUR: EVALUATION OF FACIAL COLOR

When you are feeling off balance or have a specific disharmony, facial colors offer clues to the nature and the severity of your imbalance.

There are several different methods of facial diagnosis, including Korean, Japanese, Worsley school, and macrobiotic. The following evaluation of facial colors is derived from a combination of Traditional Chinese Medicine (TCM) and the Five Phases[6] principles. I have found this system provides accurate analysis.

> **TIP**
>
> To obtain a clear idea of what the various facial colors look like, always use natural light when you examine your face in a mirror.

**Understanding the significance of facial colors:** When examining facial color, keep the following principles in mind:

- If the facial color is bright and fresh, the disease is called "floating," and it is on a superficial level.
- If the color is moist, neither wet nor dry, the disease is not severe, and it will be easy to treat.
- If the color is shallow and scattered over a large area, the number of days of the disease will be short.
- If the color is dark and cloudy, the disease is sinking into the inner organs.
- If the color is dark, cloudy, and dry, the disease is severe, and it will be difficult to cure.
- If the color is deep and accumulated in one spot, the disease is a long-term one.

**Reading between the lines:** Five colors appear on the face: red, green, yellow, white, and black. Depending on a person's constitution, a healthy face may have one color that is more predominant than others, but several may be visible. To determine which colors are present in your face, always examine it in natural light. Look for the overall color tone, study your skin to see which tones appear from under the surface, and look at any visible veins. For contrast, hold the back of your hand up alongside your face.

- Red is the color associated with the Heart Organ System and Xue. If the face is a fresh red, the Xue is Hot. If the face is dark red, the Xue is Stagnant. If it is light red, the Xue is Deficient.
- Green is the color associated with the Liver System and circulation of the Xue. If veins on the face appear greenish purple, the Xue is Hot. If the veins appear greenish black, the Xue is Stagnant. If the condition is severe, the veins on the face appear black.
- Yellow is the color associated with the Spleen System. If the face appears light yellow, the Spleen system is Damp and Cold. If the face appears deep yellow, Heat

has accumulated. If it is dark yellow, Heat is the result of Stagnant Xue. Withered yellow indicates Deficient Heat.

· White is the color associated with the Lung System, which regulates Qi, the breathing in of oxygen, and the exhalation of carbon dioxide. If a person is not able to exhale completely—as in emphysema—her or his face will take on a grayish white color. If the person inhales inadequately, the face will appear pale and lusterless.

· Black is the color associated with the Kidney System. If the face is cold and black, the Kidney System is not properly filtering Xue. If the face color is black but bright and moist, the condition can be treated. If the face is not shining, the condition is not good. If the black is withered, the Kidney System Yin is dry. If the face is cloudy and dark, the Kidney System Yang is dying.

When there are combinations of colors, this further refines the evaluation of your diagnosis. For example, if the color of your face is red and white, both the Heart and the Lung Channels are involved.

## BODY SIGNS

Take a couple of minutes to evaluate your facial color and tongue body and fur. For both facial colors and tongue, it helps to do an evaluation with a friend so you can compare the differences in your skin tone and tongue qualities.

On your face, do you see black, white, green, yellow, and/or red? Is the color bright, moist, floating, shallow, cloudy, dark, or dry?

Is your tongue trembling and pale, flaccid or red? Is it enlarged and flabby or scalloped? Or is it enlarged and hard or thin and small?

## Examination Three: Listening/Smelling

The third examination, the pair of listening and smelling, is composed of two steps: evaluation of voice and smell.

### STEP FIVE: EVALUATION OF VOICE

Listening to the sound of your speech, breathing, and cough can help us identify a disharmony that results from one or more External Pernicious Influences and patterns of disharmony. For example, if your voice is too loud and strident, it indicates Excess, as does the sudden onset of a violent cough. A weak, low voice that doesn't project and a weak cough indicate Deficiency. Losing your voice or hoarseness can indicate either Deficiency or Excess. Wheezing arises from Dampness.

## STEP SIX: EVALUATION OF SMELL

According to Chinese medicine theory, two main odors clue a doctor to the origin of disharmony: A strong stench from secretions or excretions indicates Excess and Heat. A weaker odor indicates Deficiency and Cold.

Five Phases practitioners (see page 42) generally rely on smell more than TCM practitioners do. Each smell is associated with a Phase, and it can indicate disharmony with the associated Organ or among Organs that are related through the Five Phases cycle. The following smells are used in Five Phases diagnosis:

- Goatish, which smells like goat milk, associated with Wood
- Burning or scorched, associated with Fire
- Fragrant or sweet, associated with Earth
- Rank or rotten, associated with Metal
- Putrid, associated with Water

## Examination Four: Touching

This last step of the examination is usually made up of two steps: evaluation of pulses and evaluation of sensitivity to touch.

## STEP SEVEN: EVALUATION OF PULSES

Twenty-eight pulse qualities are essential to Chinese medicine's process of evaluation and diagnosis. Learning to read pulses requires years of study and practice and is not something that can be done at home on yourself. However, your Chinese medicine practitioner will talk to you about your pulse diagnosis, and you will want to have a passing familiarity with the terminology that's used.

The most common pulse descriptions are floating, slippery, choppy, wiry, tight, slow, rapid, thin, big, empty, and full. (For a more detailed explanation of pulse diagnosis, see *The Web that Has No Weaver*, by Ted Kaptchuk or Chinese texts listed in the appendix on page 332.)

Most of the time, pulses are evaluated at the radial artery on your wrist, although some systems of pulse diagnosis use other locations, such as the carotid pulse on the neck and the tibial pulse on the ankle.

Disharmonies of the pulses indicate the condition of Qi, Xue, and Jin-Ye; Organ System imbalance(s); the location of the imbalance(s); the nature (Hot or Cold) of the disease; and many other qualities.

For example, a wiry pulse may indicate that the Liver System has Stagnant Qi. However, pulses do not have absolute meanings. They contribute to diagnosis only when they are viewed in context with other diagnostic techniques.

STEP EIGHT: EVALUATION OF SENSITIVITY TO TOUCH

When we palpate acupuncture points and Channels, we can trigger, increase, or reduce pain as well as indicate disharmony in the associated Channels and Organ Systems.

- If you have a pain you can't pinpoint, it indicates Stagnant Qi. Pain that moves around also indicates stagnant Qi.

- If the pain is fixed, it may indicate Stagnant Xue.

- Pain that feels better with pressure is due to Deficiency.

- Pain the feel worse with pressure is due to Excess.

- Pain that feels better with warmth is associated with Cold.

Palpation on the body does not have to be confined to the Twelve Channels, Fifteen Collaterals, or Eight Extraordinary Channels and their associated acupuncture points. Ear acupuncture points are also powerful tools for diagnosis, and they provide refined clues to the sources of disharmony. They are also useful for self-massage (see page 202). Reflexology, while not a traditional Chinese method of diagnosis and treatment, is also a useful tool at this stage of diagnosis (see page 210).

## SELECTING A PRACTITIONER

Now that you have an understanding of the basics of Chinese medicine and what to expect at a visit with a practitioner, you may be ready to make an appointment to see a Chinese medicine practitioner. The following guidelines may help you find a qualified practitioner.

When you are selecting an acupuncturist, an herbalist, or a Chinese medicine doctor, the two most important factors to consider are the training of the practitioner and your goals.

## Practitioner Training

To gain the full benefit of Chinese medicine therapy, the practitioner who administers the treatment(s) should have reputable training and a keen sense of the philosophical underpinning of Chinese medicine.

The best way to determine if a practitioner meets those standards is to ask questions about her or his training, length of practice, scope of practice, specializations, attitudes about wellness and disharmony, and understanding of Chinese medicine philosophy.

**Meeting basic standards:** The Taoist belief system is not some fancy window dressing that can be cast aside. Traditionally, it is part and parcel of Chinese medicine. Some practitioners are trained outside this context. However, it is my opinion that no particular Chinese medicine therapy, such as acupuncture or herbal remedies, can deliver its full healing potential if it is separated from the philosophical context of the Tao.

In addition, you want to find a practitioner who is schooled in the Chinese medicine therapies that you want to use. Some practitioners are licensed or certified acupuncturists but do not offer herbal therapy. Other practitioners are Chinese herbalists but provide no acupuncture. Still others are licensed acupuncturists also have training as herbalists. And still other practitioners have attained advanced degrees, such as a Doctor of Acupuncture and Oriental Medicine (D.A.O.M.), Oriental Medicine Doctor (O.M.D.), Doctor of Acupuncture and Chinese Medicine (D.A.C.M.), and Doctor of Oriental Medicine (D.O.M.), who provide advanced evaluations, integrative medicine as well as acupuncture and herbal therapy, and access to the whole breadth of Chinese medicine.

In 2013, the national Accreditation Commission for Acupuncture and Oriental Medicine (ACAOM) approved the first professional doctorate degree as the entry level for becoming a Chinese medicine practitioner. Before then, a master's degree was the only entry-level degree for becoming a licensed practitioner. Now schools will be able to apply for the doctorate degree as entry-level. Therefore, new doctoral degrees offered by nationally accredited Chinese medicine colleges will meet the new ACAOM criteria for a first professional doctorate and offer new doctorate degrees.[2]

Choose a practitioner who holds the required licenses, registrations, or certifications. According to the National Certification Commission for Acupuncture and Oriental Medicine (NCCAOM), as of October 2014, forty-four states plus the District of Columbia have acupuncture practice acts. These are laws that govern how people are allowed to practice acupuncture in those states. For example, the act might require licensure, registration, or certification before a person can perform acupuncture. Currently, forty-three states require passage of NCCAOM national examinations or NCCAOM certification for initial licensure. NCCAOM offers acupuncture, herbal, and Oriental medicine certifications on a national level. Currently, California requires passage of its own state examinations for licensure, and it does not accept the NCCAOM. You may contact the NCCAOM for a listing of certified practitioners in your area.[3] (See "NCCAOM" in the appendix on page 332.)

If you live in a state without a practice act, and it is legal for an acupuncturist to practice without a license, it is particularly important that your practitioner(s) have NCCAOM certification.

In most states, herbal medicine is not part of acupuncture licensure. Your Chinese herbalist (who may also be your acupuncturist) should have either a certificate of training or a long-standing reputation and years of documented experience. Many professional Chinese medicine schools train people in herbal medicine, but there is generally no independent licensing for Chinese herbalists. Only a few states require acupuncturists to pass an herbal exam to practice Chinese medicine or acupuncture.

## Your Goals

When choosing a practitioner, take some time to consider your goals. You want to decide if you are looking for a primary care practitioner, someone to work with your Western or other primary care doctor, or simply someone who can provide short-term treatment for a specific complaint.

If you are looking for a primary care doctor, I recommend you find someone who is knowledgeable about all aspects of Chinese medicine and Western medical procedures. Look for someone who will know when to refer you for Western evaluations and testing and who is willing to work with a Western doctor, if doing so provides you with the best therapy.

To sum up what to look for in a primary care Chinese medicine practitioner, consider the following:

- Someone who does not make promises to cure disorders and diseases for which there is no cure. (This applies to all practitioners, Eastern or Western, no matter what you use them for.)

- A practitioner who understands that there may be many different modalities that work for an individual and does not insist that his or her way is the only right or good way to go.

- Someone who has a bedside manner that pleases you. (What pleases some people most is ability, and they don't care about personality at all. That's fine. For others, a more personal relationship is important. You should make that individual decision.)

- Someone who is able to explain what she or he is doing from both a Chinese and a Western viewpoint—or is at least willing to find out about the alternative perspective when necessary.

- A practitioner who is not unconditionally opposed to any drug therapy in conjunction with acupuncture or herbal treatment, and who understands the interactions of drugs and herbs.

- Someone who will work with your medical doctors and other practitioners.

**In cases of serious illnesses,** you want to select a practitioner who understands Western medical terminology and concepts of the immune system, gynecology, viruses, and cancer, as well as Chinese concepts—if you are going for treatment of these problems.

**If you have HIV, hepatitis B, or other chronic viral infections,** be sure that the practitioner's attitude is that you can live with this chronic, manageable viral infection and that acupuncture and herbs may help you, along with Western medicine, to be more successful in that process.

## RECEIVING TREATMENT

When you select a practitioner and go for treatment, you shouldn't surrender control over your health. In the best practice of Chinese medicine, there is recognition that each individual possesses the tools he or she needs to preserve or reclaim good health. The good (or excellent) practitioner simply acts as the guide or catalyst—helping you to coax your body's own defenses to prevent or mend disharmony.

The practitioner may suggest one or more of the following five basic healing techniques: dietary therapy; acupuncture and moxibustion; acupressure, massage, and body therapy; Chinese herbal medicine; or Qi Gong exercise/meditation. A brief description of each follows here, and each therapy is discussed in detail in the following chapters.

## Dietary Therapy

Chinese dietary therapy uses foods to strengthen digestion, increase energy, and balance the body's Qi. Dietary therapy is often used prior to or in conjunction with other therapies to increase the effectiveness of these treatments.

## Acupuncture and Moxibustion

Classic acupuncture is the art of inserting fine, sterile, metal filiform needles into certain points along the Twelve Channels and Fifteen Collaterals (tributaries of the Channels) to control the flow of the Qi. These days, practitioners also use electrostimulation of the needles, lasers, and even ultrasound to stimulate the points.

Acupuncture is well known for its effectiveness for pain relief. But even more powerful is its ability to alter the flow of the Qi so that the body can heal itself when attacked by pathogens that trigger disharmony.

Moxibustion, the burning of the herb moxa (Chinese mugwort) over Twelve Channel points and certain areas of the body, is used to warm, tonify, and stimulate. It also induces the smooth flow of the Essential Substances, prevents diseases, and preserves health. Doing moxa regularly on specific acupuncture points is said to promote strength and longevity. In fact, an old Chinese saying is, "Never take a long journey with a person who does not have a moxa scar on [the acupuncture point called] Stomach 36." (It's important to note that moxibustion as it is generally used today does not cause scars. A particular type of moxa, called scarring moxa, was used by the ancient Chinese for longevity and stamina. Scarring moxa is not covered by our malpractice insurance today, but it is still used by some practitioners.)

## Acupressure, Massage, and Body Therapy

Acupressure and massage are often used in conjunction with acupuncture. Also, acupressure, massage, and other body therapies are an important part of daily self-care routines, whether self-administered or professionally provided.

Another related body therapy is Gua Sha, is a traditional Chinese medical treatment in which the skin is scraped to produce light bruising.

## Chinese Herbal Medicine

Chinese herbal medicine includes more than herbs. Although the overwhelming majority of medicinal substances come from plants, some are derived from minerals (such as oyster shell), and others come from animals (such as snake and deer antler). Whatever their origin, they are used to balance the mind/body/spirit as well as to reverse disease processes. Most Chinese herbs should only be taken under the supervision of a trained herbalist.

## Qi Gong Exercise/Meditation

Qi Gong, the Chinese art of exercise/meditation, uses dynamic movements and still postures in combination with mental and spiritual concentration to influence the flow of Qi. It is a powerful preventive therapy, and it can help remedy disharmony in the Organ Systems and the Twelve Channels.

# 6

# YOU ARE WHAT YOU EAT
## The Four Principles of Chinese Medicine Dietary Practices

Wholeness = **Dietary Guidelines** + Herbs + Acupuncture + Bodywork + Qi Gong

Diet, herbs, acupuncture, bodywork, and exercise/meditation are the therapeutic tools of Chinese medicine. They are used to build, maintain, and restore wholeness in mind/body/spirit.

Diet is extremely important because every day what you eat either nourishes or dilutes your Essential Substances. Here's why.

**Grain (Gu) Qi enters your body through food.** Combined with Respiratory (Kong) Qi, which enters the body through breathing, and Prenatal (Yuan) Qi, which is inherited from parents, it forms Normal (Zheng) Qi, which is the wellspring and companion of all movement in the body. Normal Qi assists the release of stored Nutritive (Ying) Qi from food. This process underlies the far-reaching power of diet therapy.

**What you eat shapes your Shen.** Shen, the spirit, is the driving force that makes us uniquely human. It enters the body from the parents before birth. After birth, Shen is dependent on Qi and on what you eat to retain its vitality.

**Your diet has an impact on your Jing.** Jing is the basis of life. Qi emerges from Jing, but Qi also transforms food into Postnatal Jing so that life can be nurtured and continue to blossom. Because a balanced diet builds healthy Qi, Jing is affected by what you eat.

**A balanced diet maintains the unique relationship between Qi and Xue.** This allows Qi to influence Xue and Xue to nurture Qi.

There are four dietary principles.

### Dietary Principle One: You Are What You Eat—and What You Don't Eat

Food has tremendous powers in Chinese medicine—powers that extend far beyond the Western concept of food as fuel, providing calories, carbohydrates, protein, fat, vitamins, and minerals. These powers are defined as Food Energetics, which cool or warm the metabolism and Organ Systems, moisturize or dry the Organ Systems, and increase or decrease the flow of Qi, Jing, and Xue.

A healthy diet harnesses Food Energetics by combining foods that balance each other, so no one energetic influence becomes too strong.

**Balance your Food Energetics.** If your diet contains an imbalance of Food Energetics, your various Organ Systems and your Qi, Jing, Shen, and Xue are subjected to more of a drying than a moisturizing influence, or more of a cooling than a warming influence. This can cause Stagnation or Depletion of your Qi, Jing, and Xue and disharmony of Shen. You then become vulnerable to diseases and to emotional and spiritual discontent.

**Don't eat too many raw foods.** To balance Food Energetics, eat warm foods to keep the digestive process working well. Despite common beliefs, raw foods are not closer to nature, and they do not contain better nutrition. Chinese medicine sees raw foods as depleting. They may cause a Cold Damp condition because your body has to expend extra energy and heat to "cook" the food in your Stomach.

In my practice, I see the wreckage caused by overconsumption of raw foods. These people have no energy and a constant chill, yet they can't figure out why they don't feel good. It may take aggressive dietary therapy to rebalance the body after a diet of too many raw foods. The only people who should eat raw foods in higher than the recommended amounts are those who are very Hot.

**Avoid iced and frozen foods.** It takes warmth and Qi to digest foods that are cold, and this uses up the digestive Fire. Therefore all foods should be warmed up and cooked if they are cold or frozen, such as frozen vegetables. You should only rarely eat ice cream or frozen yogurt. When you do, I often recommend drinking ginger tea first to warm up the digestion.

**Chew each bite of food carefully.** This makes the digestive process easier and conserves the digestive Fire. This Fire is produced by the Central Qi, which warms the central Organ Systems so they have the power to digest food. Cold food cools that inner warmth, and that's why it's not good to eat too many cold or raw foods.

**Don't stuff yourself.** Overeating overwhelms the digestive Fire and causes stagnation and disease.

**Drink scant liquid during meals.** If you drink too much liquid during meals, you'll drown the digestive Fires.

**Eat organic foods as much as possible.** The elimination of pesticides, hormones, antibiotics, and other chemical residues in vegetables, meats, and dairy increases available Qi, removes antagonists to your overall health, and also makes food taste better. Obviously, this is not a component of Chinese medicine because in ancient times all food was organic. But today, with the proliferation of harmful chemical additives to food, we must add it to the top of our list of most important dietary considerations.

If you eat meat, it is best to eat meat from animals that have been fed organic diets. For beef, it is best that the cows have been grass-fed for their entire lives. Researchers at California State University in Chico reviewed three decades of research and found that beef from grass-fed cows is lower in saturated fats, contains more omega-3 fatty acids and antioxidants, and was lower in calories.

**Eat unprocessed foods as much as possible.** Simply put, avoid eating foods that come out of boxes or bags. In particular, do not eat any foods with high fructose corn syrup (HFCS). Read every label because many foods have HFCS. (See page 303 for more information.)

## FOOD FLAVORS

Chinese medicine dietary practice discusses the impact of food in terms of five flavors: sour, bitter, sweet, spicy, and salty. Each flavor has a Hot and Cold quality. For example, there is a Warm Sour and a Cool Sour, a Hot Bitter and a Cold Bitter. A balanced diet is generally composed of mostly sweet, warm foods. Cold, spicy, bitter, salty, and sour foods are best eaten as accents. As a general rule, a little of any flavor tonifies. A salty flavor concentrates. Sour contracts. Bitter descends. Sweet expands, and spicy disperses. No flavors are bad, except in excess or when you are fighting a disharmony.

### THE IMPORTANCE OF BALANCE

"If people pay attention to the five flavors and blend them well, Qi and Xue will circulate freely, and breath and bones will be filled with the essence of life."

—From the *Nei Jing*

You can use your own reactions to flavor as an indicator of what is out of balance in your body. For example, if you have an unusual craving for sweets, your Earth is out of harmony. If you have an aversion to sour, your Wood is affected. Eating too much salty food could negatively impact Water, and an excess of bitter or pungent foods can cause disruption of the Metal and Fire Channels and also Organs.

## FOOD FLAVORS, ENERGETICS, AND TEMPERATURES

A food's flavor, energetics, and temperature were determined in much the same way as herbs were—over centuries of observation of how they affect the body.

| HOT FOODS | WARM FOODS | COOL FOODS | COLD FOODS | NEUTRAL FOODS |
|---|---|---|---|---|
| Cayenne: spicy | Anchovies: sweet | Apples: sweet | Agar: sweet | Adzuki beans: sweet + sour |
| Ginger, dried: spicy | Basil: spicy | Bananas: sweet | Asparagus: sweet + bitter | Alfalfa: bitter |
| Soybean oil: spicy + sweet | Bay leaf: spicy | Barley: sweet + salty | Clams: salty | Almonds: sweet |
| Trout: sour | Black pepper: spicy | Celery: sweet + bitter | Crab: salty | Beef: sweet |
| | | | | Beets: sweet |
| | Brown sugar: sweet | Cucumbers: sweet | Kelp: salty | Cabbages: sweet |
| | Butter: sweet | Eggplants: sweet | Mango: sweet + sour | Carrots: sweet |
| | Capers: spicy | Gluten: sweet | Mulberries: sweet | Cheeses: sweet + sour |
| | Cherries: sweet | Lettuces: sweet + bitter | Mung bean sprouts: sweet | Chicken eggs: sweet |
| | Chestnuts: sweet | Millet: sweet + salty | Nori: sweet + salty | Coconut meat: sweet |
| | Chicken: sweet | Mushrooms: sweet | Octopus: sweet + salty | Corn: sweet |
| | Chicken livers: sweet | Pears: sweet | Persimmons: sweet | Duck: sweet |
| | Coconut milk: sweet | Peppermint: spicy | Plaintains: sweet | Figs: sweet |
| | Coriander: spicy | Radishes: spicy + sweet | Romaine lettuce: bitter | Grapes: sweet + sour |
| | Dill seeds: spicy | Sesame oil: sweet | Salt: salty | Honey: sweet |

*(continued)*

| HOT FOODS | WARM FOODS | COOL FOODS | COLD FOODS | NEUTRAL FOODS |
|---|---|---|---|---|
| | Fennel seeds: spicy | Soybeans: sweet | Seaweed: salty | Kidney beans: sweet |
| | Garlic: spicy | Spinach: sweet | Tomatoes: sweet + sour | Milk: sweet |
| | Ginger, fresh: spicy | Swiss chard: sweet | Watermelons: sweet | Olives: sweet + sour |
| | Leeks: spicy | Tangerines: sweet + sour | | Oysters: sweet + salty |
| | Litchi: sweet + sour | Tofu: sweet | | Papaya: sweet + bitter |
| | Mussels: salty | Watercress: spicy + sweet | | Peanuts: sweet |
| | Mustard greens: spicy | Wheat: sweet | | Peanut oil: sweet |
| | Mutton: sweet | Wheat bran: sweet | | Peas: sweet |
| | Nutmeg: spicy | | | Pineapples: sweet |
| | Onions: spicy | | | Plums: sweet + sour |
| | Peaches: sweet + sour | | | Pork: sweet + salty |
| | Pine nuts: sweet | | | Potatoes: sweet |
| | Rosemary: spicy | | | Pumpkins: sweet |
| | Safflower: spicy | | | Raspberries: sweet |
| | Scallions: spicy + bitter | | | Rice: sweet |
| | Shrimp: sweet | | | Rice bran: spicy + sweet |
| | Sorghum: sweet | | | Rye: bitter |
| | Spearmint: spicy + sweet | | | Sardines: sweet + salty |
| | Squash: sweet | | | Shark: sweet + salty |
| | Strawberries: sweet + sour | | | String beans: sweet |
| | Sweet potatoes: sweet | | | Sugar, refined: sweet |
| | Sweet rice: sweet | | | Turnips: spicy + sweet |
| | Vinegar: sour + bitter | | | Whitefish: sweet |
| | Walnuts: sweet | | | Yams: sweet |

## FOOD FLAVORS AND ENERGETICS: FIVE TASTES

### SWEET

Adzuki beans (also sour)
Almond
Anchovy
Beef
Beet
Brown sugar
Butter
Cabbage
Carrot
Cheese (also sour)
Cherry
Chestnut
Chicken
Chicken livers
Coconut Meat
Coconut Milk
Corn
Cucumber
Duck
Eggplant
Eggs (chicken)
Figs
Gluten
Grapes (also sour)
Honey
Kidney beans
Lettuce (also bitter)
Litchi (also sour)
Mango (also sour)
Milk
Millet (also salty)
Mulberry
Mung bean sprouts
Mushrooms
Mutton
Nori (also salty)
Octopus (also salty)
Olives (also sour)
Oysters (also salty)
Papaya (also bitter)
Peach (also sour)
Peanut oil
Peanuts
Pear
Persimmon
Pineapple
Pine nuts
Plantain
Plum (also sour)
Pork (also salty)
Potato
Pumpkin
Raspberry
Rice
Sardines (also salty)
Sesame oil
Shark (also salty)
Shrimp
Sorghum
Soybean
Spinach
Squash
Strawberry (also sour)
String beans
Sugar (refined)
Sweet potato
Sweet rice
Swiss chard
Tangerine (also sour)
Tofu
Tomato (also sour)
Turnip (also spicy)
Walnut
Watermelon
Wheat
Wheat bran
Whitefish
Yam

### SPICY

Basil
Bay leaf
Black pepper
Capers
Cayenne
Coriander
Dill seed
Fennel seed
Garlic
Ginger, dried
Ginger, fresh
Leek
Mustard greens
Nutmeg
Onion
Peppermint
Radish (also sweet)
Rice bran (also sweet)
Rosemary
Safflower
Scallion (also bitter)
Soybean oil (also sweet)
Spearmint (also sweet)
Watercress (also sweet)

### SOUR

Trout
Vinegar (also bitter)

### SALTY

Clams
Crab
Kelp
Mussels
Salt
Seaweed

### BITTER

Alfalfa
Romaine lettuce
Rye
Shrimp

## Dietary Principle Two: Most of Your Food Should Be Eaten in Season

Your diet should be dictated by the rhythms of the external world. Food gains power to maintain health from its relationship to the external world. Food, the fuel of the mind/body/spirit, should be taken into the body in a pattern that's attuned to the rhythms of the environment. This perspective is based on the Tao, the Chinese philosophy of the unity and interrelationship between the external and internal worlds.

As you look around the outside world, you can see that in the spring, energy moves up. In the summer, it moves out. In the fall, energy moves down, and in the winter, it moves inward. Likewise, green sprouting vegetables, such as lettuce and bean sprouts, move energy up, so enjoy more of them in the spring. Spices, flowers, and leaves, such as basil and edible flowers, have outward-moving energy, so enjoy plenty of them in the summer. Root vegetables, such as burdock and turnips have downward-moving energy, so give in to the natural desire to eat them in the fall. Grains, seeds, and nuts, such as almonds and buckwheat, have inward-moving energy, so eat plenty of them all winter long.

To reap the benefits of food's energetic relationship to the seasons, you may want to eat foods in their own season when their power is strongest or in the season before to prepare your body for the coming season.

## Dietary Principle Three: Moderation and Variety in Diet Are Essential for a Balanced Mind/Body/Spirit

**Understand the spirit of a balanced diet.** A balanced diet results from a combination of the foods you eat and the way you prepare, eat, and think about your food. You could not create the perfect diet pill that combined all the Food Energetics needed to achieve wholeness and harmony. Food Energetics is not simply the result of chemistry. It is also a result of spiritual forces. The power of food—positive and negative—to influence your mind/body/spirit is affected by how it is prepared, served, and eaten.

There is no list of good foods and bad foods. Eating too much of a healthy food is unhealthy. For example, you can overdo broccoli and whole grains. Small amounts of unrefined sugars are not necessarily unhealthy. However, too much sugar or highly processed refined sugar or high fructose corn syrup are. Organic meats in small quantities may be useful in some people's diets. Eating too much meat or meat that is processed or containing chemicals is not healthy.

Balance comes from eating a wide variety of food, including vegetables, grains (especially low glycemic—see page 100), fish, meats, fruits, and dairy, each in moderation. If you do that, you can pretty much eat most foods. The percentages of each type of food that you should eat depend upon your constitution and your specific Chinese medicine patterns.

The modern American diet notion that you should only eat from a roster of mildly unappealing, healthy foods and avoid all "bad" foods is not doable for many people. For example, if you have a little bit of chocolate, it is not a sin. In fact, we now know it may have good anti-inflammatory effects.

As important as moderation is in achieving balance, it is also vital to strive for the proper attitude toward food. Food prepared as a gift, served calmly, eaten with respect, and digested in a harmonious atmosphere bestows positive benefits. Food slapped together without regard or with resentment, served as quickly as possible, gobbled down, or eaten while driving, watching TV, or even reading cannot be assimilated healthfully. If you eat fast food or if you eat food fast, you're better off fasting than feasting.

To achieve the spirit of a balanced diet, consider the following:

- Eat in a peaceful setting.

- Relax before you begin to eat. Take a deep breath. Appreciate the food: its existence, its aroma, and its appearance.

- Eat slowly enough to chew adequately.

- Eat with others whose company you enjoy.

- Eat at regular times.

## BODY SIGNS

The first step to improving harmony and balance through diet is to become aware of your current eating patterns. Think about which of the following foods you eat most often.

- Red meat: How many times a week?

- Chicken: How many times a week?

- Fish: How many times a week?

- Vegetables: How many times a day?

- Beans: How many times a week?

- Grains: How many times a day?

- Dairy: How many times a day?

**Be flexible.** It's so easy to get fanatic about diet. But rigidity about how you eat is itself a disease-producing behavior, even if you're being rigid about eating healthy foods. Health depends on a graceful adaptability to your surroundings and your ability to nourish yourself, even if perfect foods aren't available.

In our food-obsessed, food-unhealthy culture, it's easy to misinterpret the Chinese medicine perspective on diet. For example, people sometimes use the Five Flavors in combination with the Five Phases and create artificial rules, such as: Sour is associated with Wood and spring is associated with Wood, so you should (only) eat sour things in the spring.

Chinese medicine doesn't work that way: That's too pat. Dietary Therapy is a guide to help you find balance and moderation. It does not establish rigid dos and don'ts, rights and wrongs.

**Apply a balanced meal plan.** The number of times a day you eat is highly individual. Some people do better grazing on small meals through the day, especially if they have trouble maintaining their blood sugar levels. Other people are happy with the traditional three meals a day. Some people find their bodies run best with two meals. You want to follow what works for you. However, as you begin to practice Chinese medicine dietary principles as well as receive acupuncture and herbal therapy from a Chinese medicine practitioner, you may find that your body becomes more balanced and needs fuel less frequently.

If you follow the traditional three squares a day, here's a plan to help guide you.

- Meal one: Eat a moderate amount of food within two hours of waking up. In our practice, we recommend protein in the morning along with low glycemic (see page 100) grains, vegetables, and small amounts of fruit. This meal should be made up of cooked, warming foods that stimulate your Qi.

- Meal two: This is your largest meal of the day. You can combine a moderate amount of high-grade protein, such as fish, soy foods (if you can tolerate them), beans, or a small amount of meat. A great variety of foods is the best. If indicated by your constitution or your practitioner's diagnosis, raw cool foods, such as salads or fruits, can be eaten now.

- Meal three: This is your smallest meal of the day. It is best if it does not contain stimulating animal protein or spicy foods. Eat more than three hours before going to bed so that you can fully digest your food before retiring as well as to reduce the damage from having too much blood sugar during sleep.

**Consider the composition of your meals.** No matter how many times a day you eat, or what adjustments you have to make to circumstances, you want to follow a basic balance of foods. Traditionally, the Chinese medicine perspective recommends the following:

- 60 to 75 percent of your calories from grains, vegetables, and legumes (grains should account for two-thirds of this, and vegetables and legumes/beans for the other third)
- 10 percent of your calories from fruits
- 20 percent of your calories from protein, including meats, dairy, seafood, fish, and eggs

However, modern diets may need to be adjusted for living in modern cultures with more sedentary lifestyles, new food choices, and new understandings of health and longevity.

**Understand the glycemic index (GI).** In our practice, we recommend that people—especially those who are overweight or obese or who have prediabetes, metabolic syndrome, insulin resistance, and/or fatty liver—pay attention to the glycemic index and glycemic loads of foods.

The GI was developed in the past twenty years at the Human Nutrition Unit, School of Molecular Bioscience at the University of Sydney. The following description from their website explains the glycemic index:

*The glycemic index (GI) is a ranking of carbohydrates on a scale from 0 to 100, according to the extent to which they raise blood sugar levels after eating. Foods with a high GI are those that are rapidly digested and absorbed and result in marked fluctuations in blood sugar levels.*

*Low GI foods, by virtue of their slow digestion and absorption, produce gradual rises in blood sugar and insulin levels, and they have proven benefits for health. Low GI diets have been shown to improve both glucose and lipid levels in people with diabetes (type 1 and type 2). They have benefits for weight control because they help control appetite and delay hunger. Low GI diets also reduce insulin levels and insulin resistance.*

*Recent studies from Harvard School of Public Health indicate that the risks of diseases such as type 2 diabetes and coronary heart disease are strongly related to the GI of the overall diet. In 1999, the World Health Organization (WHO) and Food and Agriculture Organization (FAO) recommended that people in industrialized countries base their diets on low-GI foods to prevent the most common diseases of affluence, such as coronary heart disease, diabetes, and obesity.*

GI values are not necessarily intuitive. The best way to determine the GI of various foods is continually being tested in laboratories. The ones we use in our clinic are:

- The University of Sydney GI site at www.glycemicindex.com/index.php is very helpful.

- The Nutrition Data site at www.nutritiondata.com is extremely user friendly.

On those sites, you can look up the glycemic values of foods as well find which foods contain which nutrients.

The amount of food you eat is also important. Even if a food is high on the glycemic index, it may still have a low glycemic *load*. According to the Glycemic Research Institute, glycemic load is a function of both GI and carbohydrate intake. Glycemic load is calculated as the GI multiplied by the amount of carbohydrate in a serving.[1] Therefore, if you eat very small amounts of high-GI food, you may still have a low GI load. You may look up the GI and glycemic load of foods on reputable websites. New quantities and levels are always being researched. You can also balance high-glycemic foods with low-glycemic foods or no glycemic foods at one meal to keep the overall glycemic index low.

## METABOLIC SYNDROME

The National Institute of Diabetes and Digestive and Kidney Diseases, part of the National Institutes of Health (NIH), defines metabolic syndrome as a group of conditions that put you at risk for heart disease and diabetes. We also now know that the development of fatty liver is associated with metabolic syndrome. Metabolic syndrome is a group of conditions that includes the following:

- High blood pressure
- High blood glucose, or blood sugar, levels
- High levels of triglycerides in your blood
- Low levels of HDL, the good cholesterol, in your blood
- Too much fat around your waist

Not all doctors agree on the definition or on the cause of metabolic syndrome. For example, the cause might be insulin resistance. Insulin is a hormone your body produces to help you turn sugar from food into energy for your body. If you are insulin resistant, too much sugar builds up in your blood, setting the stage for disease.

BODY SIGNS

To help you take control of your dietary habits, try writing down everything you eat and drink for a full day. Include all meals and snacks, sodas, juices, water, and coffee. What is your percentage of grains, and how much is low glycemic? How many servings of vegetable and legumes did you eat?

There are variations among organizations that provide measurements of the GI values of foods. Also, the preparation of food can change its GI. One thing that is important as well is that the GI only refers to carbohydrates in foods, so you still must eat the correct quantity and balances of other foods, including proteins and fats.

Many other aspects of modern food science relate to good health and longevity. (See the appendix on page 332 for references.)

Also, if you have dietary preferences, such as vegetarianism, veganism, or eating only fish or vegetable proteins, this must be taken into consideration. You must create your balanced diet accordingly.

The main thing to remember from a Chinese medicine perspective is to always remain moderate in your consumption. Balance your intake according to your constitution and disharmonies.

## EATING LEGUMES AND GRAINS

Within Dietary Principle Three, let's talk for a moment about the importance of eating legumes and grains. In Chinese medicine, one way that Qi enters the body is through Gu (Grain) Qi, which indicates how important grains are to the health of the mind/body/spirit. Our modern diet has moved away from a focus on grains. Traditionally, grains form the basis for many indigenous cuisines. They provide building blocks for protein and many of the essential vitamins and minerals. In China, it is no different. Rice is the predominant grain found in China, although wheat is a staple in some parts of China.

Traditionally, grains form the center of the diet. So, if you would like to follow a traditional diet, you may want to expand your diet to include additional grains, such as millet, kasha, oats, rye, couscous, barley, wild rice, and brown rice. If you take the time to discover the many varieties that are available, you'll find it is much easier to make whole grains an important feature of your diet.

Grains are enhanced—both in nutrition and in flavor—when combined with legumes, such as limas, kidney beans, black beans, garbanzos, fava beans, white beans, pinto beans,

## GLUTEN IN GRAINS

If you want to try a completely gluten-free diet, the following lists will assist you with this process:

- Grains *with* gluten: wheat, including varieties such as spelt, kamut, farro, and durum, also products such as bulgur, couscous, semolina, barley, rye, triticale, and oats[2]
- Gluten *free* grains: amaranth, buckwheat, corn, millet, montina (Indian rice grass), oats,[3] quinoa, rice, sorghum, and teff

navy beans, lentils, adzuki beans, soybeans, and split peas. In Western nutritional terms, the combination of grains and beans forms complete proteins. Also, beans are generally low glycemic, and when beans are combined with grains, it balances the GI of foods.

In the past couple of decades, a new understanding has developed about carbohydrates in general. There are two recent developments. First is the development of the glycemic index for carbohydrates as discussed earlier. Second is the increased awareness of gluten intolerance in a certain portion of the population.[4]

Many of the people who come into my clinic don't know how to cook. They are frustrated in their attempts to improve their diet because they eat out or get take-out food all the time. The following basic recipes will help you prepare legumes or grains at home.

### BARLEY *(*contains gluten)*                                           SERVES 3 OR 4

Barley is good in soups and casseroles or for breakfast.

1 cup (185 g) barley

3 cups (700 ml) cold water

1 tablespoon (15 ml) oil

1 pinch sea salt

In a large bowl, cover the barley with water and let it soak for 10 to 15 minutes. After soaking, in a colander, drain the barley and rinse it twice with clear water.

In a large saucepan, boil the water and the add oil and salt. Add the barley to the boiling water. Cook for 1 minute. Reduce the heat to a slow simmer and cook for 1¼ to 1½ hours, stirring occasionally.

## MILLET (HULLED) *(*gluten-free)*                SERVES 2 OR 3

Millet is good in casseroles and loafs and mixed with rice or vegetables.

  1 cup (200 g) millet

  1 cup (235 ml) water

  1 pinch sea salt

In a colander, rinse the millet 3 times under cold water.

In a large saucepan, boil the water and add the salt. Add the millet. Boil the millet for 1 minute. Reduce the heat to a slow simmer and cook for at least 45 minutes.

## QUINOA *(*gluten-free)*                SERVES 2 OR 3

Quinoa is great in casseroles and desserts or for breakfast.

  1 cup (175 g) quinoa

  1¼ cups (295 ml) cooking liquid (water or soup stock, depending on final use)

In a bowl, soak the quinoa in water for 15 to 60 minutes, and then rinse it in a fine metal strainer.

Put the quinoa into a pot with the cooking liquid. Bring it to a simmer and reduce the heat to low. Cover and cook for 15 to 35 minutes, and then remove it from the heat, cover, and let stand for 5 minutes.

## COUSCOUS (CRACKED WHEAT) *(*contains gluten)*                SERVES 2 OR 3

Couscous is good for casseroles, baking, and desserts.

  1 cup (155 g) couscous

  2½ cups (590 ml) water

  1 pinch sea salt

In a colander, rinse the couscous 2 or 3 times.

In a large saucepan, bring the water to a boil. Add the salt. Add the couscous to the boiling water. Cover the saucepan. Reduce the heat to low and slowly simmer it for 15 minutes.

## A SIMPLE GUIDE TO COOKING BEANS

Often, canned beans are high in fat, salt, and sugar and low in vitamins. However, a number of companies, such as Trader Joe's and Costco, package and sell canned plain, organic cooked beans. One caveat: If you are reducing sodium, pay attention to how much is added. Eden Organics makes BPA-free canned beans without added sodium.

Cooking dried beans is a great alternative to canned beans. The following table provides a simple guide to a wide variety of freshly cooked beans.

### ADZUKI BEANS

Cooking: Soak beans overnight in enough water to cover. Boil in 3 to 4 cups (700 to 940 ml) water for 1½ to 2 hours.

Description: These beans have a delicate flavor, which combines well with rice, quinoa, or millet.

Serving Suggestion: Add squash, garlic, or onion for additional flavor.

### BLACK BEANS

Cooking: Soak beans overnight in enough water to cover. Boil in 3 to 4 cups (700 to 940 ml) water for 1½ to 2 hours.

Description: These beans have a rich, earthy flavor that's good with grains and in soups.

Serving Suggestion: Traditional Latin American dishes often include black beans cooked with onions, garlic, and perhaps a whole orange, and then served with rice.

### GARBANZO BEANS (CHICKPEAS)

Cooking: Soak beans overnight in enough water to cover. Boil in 3 to 4 cups (700 to 940 ml) water for 1 to 2 hours.

Description: They have a nutty flavor.

Serving Suggestion: They work well with curry, and they are good in soups and salads.

### KIDNEY BEANS

Cooking: Soak beans overnight in enough water to cover. Boil in 3 to 4 cups (700 to 940 ml) of water for 1½ to 2 hours.

Description: These beans are relatively bland.

Serving Suggestion: They work well in soups, stews, and salads.

(continued)

## LENTILS

Cooking: These do not need soaking. Boil in 2 cups (470 ml) water for 30 to 45 minutes.

Description: These are mild tasting.

Serving Suggestion: They are good in soups and salads and with grains.

## LIMA BEANS

Cooking: Soak beans overnight in enough water to cover. Boil in 2 cups (470 ml) water for 45 minutes to 1½ hours.

Description: Rich, sometimes nutty flavor.

Serving Suggestion: Good in soups and casseroles.

## PINTO BEANS

Cooking: Soak beans overnight in enough water to cover. Boil in 3 to 4 cups (700 to 940 ml) water for 1½ to 2 hours.

Description: Mild, earthy flavor.

Serving Suggestion: Traditionally, they are used in Mexican food, sometimes whole and often refried.

## SOYBEANS (ONLY USE ORGANIC BECAUSE OTHERS ARE GENETICALLY MODIFIED)

Cooking: Soak beans overnight in enough water to cover. Boil in 3 to 4 cups (700 to 940 ml) water for 3+ hours.

Description: They have a bland flavor.

Serving Suggestion: They are best in casseroles, salads, and bean burgers. Adding onion and garlic gives a good flavor. Often people make bean burgers with soybeans and grated vegetables. Soybeans are high in protein.

## SPLIT PEAS

Cooking: No soaking time is needed. Boil in 2 cups (470 ml) water for 30 to 45 minutes.

Description: Sweet, earthy flavor.

Serving Suggestion: Onions are often added to split peas, along with spices. Split pea soup is a favorite in many part of the United States.

## Dietary Principle Four: Food Is Powerful Medicine

Chinese medicine's dietary practices form the basis for effective preventive medicine. When you eat foods that maintain the flow of Qi and the harmonious functioning of the Organ Systems, the immune system remains strong, bones and muscles remain flexible and supportive, digestion is good, the skin is healthy, the mind and spirit remain clear, and stress and anger dissipate.

However, as with so many Chinese medicine concepts, the effect of diet on bodily functions is not linear, and it cannot be viewed as a process of cause and effect. Instead, the association between food, Qi, Jing, Shen, Xue, the Organ Systems, and digestion depends on each element's influence over and reaction to the other elements.

This feedback mechanism is reflected in the role of the Spleen and Stomach Systems, which govern digestion and the assimilation of food. The Stomach System releases the energy stored in food, and the Spleen System distributes the food energy through the body. This maintains a harmonious flow of Qi, which in turn helps nourish the Spleen and Stomach Systems with an ample supply of Essential Substances, keeping them in balance. Without a well-balanced diet, the entire network of interdependence is interrupted.

You can also see the delicate yet powerful interdependence of diet and healthy (or unhealthy) Organ Systems when you look at the relationship between diet and the Triple Burner System—particularly the Middle Burner.

Food keeps the Middle Burner balanced so it maintains a strong Middle Burner Fire. This Fire warms the center and allows for proper digestion. If the Fire becomes weak through lack of proper foods, the Middle Burner is forced to supplement its Fire with energy drawn from the Lower Burner. When that happens, Kidney Fire, which the Lower Burner fuels, may become depleted. That, in turn, can cause anxiety, imbalance, or agitation in the mind and spirit. Agitation in the mind and spirit can interfere with proper digestion. Before you know it, you've become trapped in a cycle of depletion and disharmony affecting mind/body/spirit—all because your diet was not balanced and couldn't support the Middle Burner's Fire.

### STAGES AND AGES OF DIETARY GUIDES

To reap the preventive benefits of Chinese medicine's dietary practices, you want to adjust your eating habits—and your family's—to the stages and ages of life. Infancy and childhood, adolescence, maturity, and old age each have unique dietary requirements.

**Infants and children:** Infants and children are immature energetically, although they do have Excess Qi and usually are Warm to Hot. In this stage, the Middle Burner is very sensitive, and the Triple Burner is not very strong. Because the Middle Burner Qi (Central Qi) is not strong, Spleen Qi weakness can develop, leading to Dampness. As a result, infants are likely to produce phlegm.

Before six months of age, feed only breast milk. From six to twelve months, breast milk is still the most healthful food. If you use other milks, don't give any dairy before one year of age. If you use soy milk, make sure it is made of whole soybeans that were grown organically. Soy milk may be too cooling for children, and it may produce a Damp condition—loose stools—that can aggravate allergies and runny noses and trigger croup and diaper rashes. The first solid food to give a child—while still breastfeeding—is organic, whole-grain rice. Cook 1 cup (195 g) of rice in 5 cups (1175 ml) of water to make a very watery gruel. Other foods, such as sweet potatoes, can then be added when breastfeeding stops.

Young children's diet should contain easy-to-digest, warming foods, such as cooked vegetables, a modicum of well-cooked rice, and only a little meat or meat broth. Young children need to eat foods that strengthen the Spleen, such as warming and neutral foods: carrots, string beans, yams, and potatoes. (See "Food Flavors, Energetics, and Temperatures" on page 94 for more examples.)

Young children should not be fed too much meat or grains because they may not completely digest them, and that produces phlegm. Wheat, corn, and dairy foods can create congestion and Dampness.

Fruits, raw foods, and cold drinks from the refrigerator are too cooling. Serve foods warm and offer beverages at room temperature.

**Teens:** Adolescents need lots of food to thrive. This is when the fire of sex, Kidney Fire, is surging. Adolescents should stay away from hot, spicy, or excessively sweet or oily foods, which force heat to rise from the Stomach. This may be associated with acne and emotional ups and downs, which are the plague of so many teenagers. Although for a healthy Spleen, everyone has to eat warming foods, teens do well to increase slightly the amount of cool and neutral foods they consume.

**Maturity:** Mature adults should eat a diverse diet, with a full range of Food Energetics to maintain their vigor. Over age forty, the Jing becomes depleted.

**Old age:** In old age, the Kidney Fire declines. Yin is consumed. As the Kidney Fire becomes exhausted, the Middle Burner Fire also becomes weak. The diet should return to the simple, easy-to-digest foods of the very young. Foods that are cool or cold are to be avoided, and moderation becomes ever more important to maintain energy.

For adults and especially the elderly, avoid eating more than two or three types of food at any one meal. That taxes the digestive Fire. It is especially important not to overeat. Stagnation and disharmony follow. Also, as we age, it's harder and harder to restore balance. New animal and human studies suggest that having limited food intake decreases disease development. For seniors especially, food should be eaten in a relaxed atmosphere and never when you're upset.

These are the basics of healthful, well-balanced dietary practices. They provide protection against disease and help maintain vigor at all ages. But Chinese medicine's dietary guides can do far more than maintain health and prevent disease. They are also used to treat diseases and disorders (see chapter 7, page 112).

A CUP OF TEA

Tea is both a medicine and a beverage. It's also an excuse for socializing and for solitary contemplation. Since the twelfth century BCE, tea has occupied a special place in Chinese culture. It was so valuable that it was used as money in business transactions well into this century.

As a folk medicine, tea has been used to help heal cuts and infections, soothe the stomach, clarify the skin, and energize the mind and spirit. An ancient Chinese proverb could be translated:

> *Drinking a daily cup of tea*
> *will surely starve the apothecary.*[5]

The healing properties of tea have been confirmed by modern research. Tea is known to contain polyphenols, which stimulate digestion. Research in China and the West also indicates polyphenols may work as anticancer agents and enhance immune strength.[6] Green tea may be the most efficacious; however, according to recent research, black tea is highly beneficial and contains important antioxidant properties. Tea also contains essential oils that may reduce circulating lipids and ease digestion. In small quantities, tea's caffeine can help circulate Xue and invigorate the mind.

A particular type of tea called *pu-erh*, which is a tea that is the most oxidized and usually aged, is a form of black tea renowned in China for its medicinal properties. Chinese people credit pu-erh with many health benefits, especially promoting weight loss, helping digestion, easing diarrhea, reducing serum cholesterol, and protecting the cardiovascular system. Animal studies indicate that tea reduces cholesterol and/or triglycerides.

## COMPARATIVE CAFFEINE LEVELS

| BEVERAGE | CAFFEINE (MILLIGRAMS) |
| --- | --- |
| 2 ounces (28 ml) espresso | 60 to 69 |
| 6 ounces (175 ml) drip coffee | 60 to 180 |
| 6 ounces (175 ml) black tea | 25 to 110 |
| 6 ounces (175 ml) oolong | 12 to 55 |
| 6 ounces (175 ml) green tea | 6 to 18 |

Tea contains caffeine, and too much caffeine is not healthy. Tea has less caffeine than coffee. Because the caffeine steeps out of the tea leaves after the color and flavor, cutting the brewing time can reduce that further. Black tea that is steeped for five minutes contains twice the caffeine of a tea that has steeped for three minutes.

**Recognize the types of tea.** There are three types of Chinese tea: green, oolong, and black. They are all made from the same types of leaves. It's the processing that makes them taste, smell, and look so different. Green, oolong, and black teas are differentiated by how "fermented" they are. The word *fermented*, however, is a misnomer, because the tea is not processed using a fermenting organism, but rather is oxidized by a process of breaking down the structure of the leaves and exposing it to the air. Green tea is not oxidized, and rather incorrectly called not fermented; oolong tea is oxidized for a short period of time, rather incorrectly called semi-fermented; and black tea is oxidized, rather incorrectly called fully fermented.

The most popular Chinese teas include green teas such as gunpowder, hyson, and dragonwell; oolongs such as Formosa oolong, Ti Kuan Yin, and Wuyi; and black teas such as lapsang ouchong, Yunnan, and pu-erh. Blended Chinese black teas include the familiar English and Irish breakfast teas. Scented teas include jasmine, which is made with green tea, and Earl Grey, which combines China black tea with oil of bergamot.

## HOW TO MAKE A PERFECT CUP OF TEA

A perfect cup of tea is made with boiling water and loose tea, steeped for the proper length of time, and then consumed immediately. (If you prefer, you can use tea bags, but only buy organic tea in unbleached tea bags.) Here's how to make it.

1. Rinse the teapot with clean water, without using soaps or cleaning products.

2. Boil filtered or spring water.

3. **To make green tea:** Allow the water to just barely reach boiling. Place 1 teaspoon green leaf tea in the bottom of the teapot per 1 cup (235 ml) of water. Pour the boiling water directly onto the leaves. Steep for 3 minutes.

   **To make oolong tea:** Allow the water to come to a full boil. Place 1 teaspoon oolong leaf tea in the bottom of the pot per 1 cup (235 ml) of water. Pour the boiling water directly onto the leaves. You can steep oolong tea for up to 10 minutes without it becoming acrid or bitter.

   **To make black tea:** Allow the water to come to a full boil. Place 1 teaspoon black leaf tea in the bottom of the pot per 1 cup (235 ml) of water. Pour the boiling water directly onto the leaves. Steep for 4 to 5 minutes.

4. The tea leaves can be strained or not, as you wish. To strain, pour the leaves and water through a strainer. Some teapots have built-in strainers.

5. If you prefer to sweeten your tea, add a little sugar, honey, lemon, or cream.

*Note:* In general, black tea can only be steeped once. Good-quality oolong teas can be reused several times. Some green teas will produce additional cups if water is poured over the damp leaves and steeped for 1 minute.

# 7

# REBUILDING ESSENTIAL SUBSTANCES AND ORGAN SYSTEMS

## Treating Disharmony with Chinese Medicine Dietary Therapy

Treating disharmony with Chinese Dietary Therapy is the first step in reclaiming wholeness and balance. That's why I call it the First-Step Dietary Therapy Program. In some instances, it is the lead medicine in a treatment plan. At other times, it serves as an adjunct to acupuncture and herbal remedies and/or Western therapies, helping the other treatments work more effectively.

Anyone suffering from imbalances can benefit from a program of general purification—unless you are extremely weak. Dietary Therapy gives your body a break—a time to calm down, gather its forces, and clear out foods that are causing disharmony or discomfort. This allows for restoration of normal bowel function so your body can harmoniously absorb and use food and harmonize the Qi and the other Essential Substances.

The First-Step Dietary Therapy Program is especially helpful for people with digestive troubles, such as colitis, lactose intolerance, or irritable bowel syndrome; immune system difficulties such as allergies, hepatitis, HIV, or chronic fatigue; chronic gynecological disturbances; chronic sore throats or colds; and skin disturbances.

# GENERAL DIETARY GUIDELINES

Before beginning the First-Step Dietary Therapy Program, understand the following simple guidelines.

- The First-Step Dietary Therapy Program should be followed within the context of a total healing program under the supervision of a licensed practitioner.
- Each Phase may run from one-half day to one week. You and your practitioner can determine the duration.
- If a Phase seems inappropriate for your specific situation, skip it and go on to the next one.
- If you are already losing weight due to disease, do not use any Phase that may cause weight loss.
- If you feel weak or unable to do a Phase, you may skip it or shorten it. The Phases are intended to help you cleanse as well as rebuild your energy and health.

# THE FIRST-STEP DIETARY THERAPY PROGRAM PHASES

The First-Step Dietary Therapy Program is divided into five phases.

## Phase One

To tonify the Spleen and Stomach, limit your diet to the following foods for one to seven days.

**Miso broth:** Miso is a fermented paste made from grains and beans, originating in Japan. It contains good bacteria that replenish the flora that may have been depleted or destroyed in the digestive tract through antibiotic or hormone use, poor diet, alcohol intake, or stress. In general, I recommend rice-based miso. If you are not gluten sensitive, try using mugi (barley) miso with some mellow yellow (light yellow miso) if it is summertime. Avoid hatcho (dark) except when it is very cold. I especially like natto miso.

If you are on a low-sodium diet, it may be better to skip using miso because it contains a lot of sodium. If you are lactose-intolerant or do not eat dairy products, a good nondairy alternative is nondairy kefir. Because miso contains soybeans, make sure that you use organic miso as all other soybeans are genetically modified.

**Vegetable broth and juices:** You can drink fresh organic vegetable broth and juices during this Phase. These could include carrot, beet, celery, daikon, and watercress juices.

Avoid adding onion or garlic at this stage. When vegetables are juiced, they increase in Yang qualities, and they may become more warming than just the raw vegetable. It is also much easier to digest raw juice than raw vegetables. I recommend that you cook the juice into a warm broth as well. You may add an unsalted pure vegetable powder used for vegetable stock to the fresh vegetable broth. This increases the nutrients as well as the flavor.

Lentil broth (cook lentils, strain off the water, and drink as a soup) may also be used in addition to the vegetable broths.

If you have an immune system disorder, I recommend that you wash all vegetables thoroughly to avoid parasites and bacteria, even organically grown ones. Remember that organic vegetables are grown in manure, which is filled with microorganisms. Wash the vegetables in a diluted bleach solution (½ teaspoon bleach in 1 quart [946 ml] water) to kill microorganisms. Use only plain bleach that contains no additives. (Many bleaches sold are not pure bleach.) Rinse off the bleach completely after washing. An alternative to this are vegetable and fruit washes found in your local natural foods store.

**Brown rice cereal:** Organic brown rice cereal provides added protein and energy. You may find this in any natural foods store.

## Phase Two

After you have comfortably tried—or skipped—Phase One, you may want to move on to Phase Two for no more than seven days. You also may choose to skip it and go directly to Phase Three.

To the foods in Phase One, add steamed fresh organic vegetables, especially root vegetables (carrots, daikon root, burdock, turnips, and beets) and green vegetables (cruciferous such as broccoli, kale, and chard). Again, make sure all your vegetables are washed thoroughly in a diluted bleach solution.

## Phase Three

Begin this Phase only if you feel strong. Follow Phase Three for no more than seven days.

To the foods in Phases One and Two, add organic cooked grains, including brown rice, millet, barley, and buckwheat. If you have a very Hot condition, avoid buckwheat. Check with your practitioner for advice. You may also add unbleached white rice or white basmati rice for diarrhea. Avoid wheat, corn, and oats. Do not eat any bread products in Phase Three.

## Phase Four

To the foods in Phases One, Two, and Three, add other organic foods and fish or high-quality plant-based proteins. Watch for any unfavorable reactions to foods and eliminate them from your diet. Make sure that you do not sacrifice moderation, balance, and sound nutrition. At this point, it is great to establish a balance of low- to moderate-glycemic carbohydrates along with good organic protein sources.

## Phase Five

Once you establish a moderate natural foods diet that is unrestricted, except by your health considerations, you will have entered Phase Five, which is a dietary regime for lifelong good health and harmony.

# THE FIRST-STEP DIETARY THERAPY PROGRAM
# THERAPEUTIC RECIPES

To augment your dietary program, the following delicious, but medicinal, foods will provide you with well-balanced energy and nutrition.

## To Purify Xue

### KICHAREE                                                          MAKES 4 SERVINGS

Kicharee is a well-balanced Ayurvedic medicine healing dish, and it is high in easily assimilated protein.

- ½ cup (80 g) cooked mung beans or lentils
- ½ cup (85 g) steamed brown rice
- Sesame oil or clarified butter (ghee)
- Pinch cumin seed
- ⅓ teaspoon turmeric
- 1 teaspoon ground coriander
- 4 cups (940 ml) water
- Yogurt, such as goat's milk yogurt (optional)

In a pan, sauté the mung beans or lentils and rice in the oil or ghee for 5 minutes with the cumin seed, turmeric, and coriander. Add the water and simmer for 20 to 25 minutes.

To serve, top the mixture with the yogurt, if using.

*(From Abigail Surasky, L.Ac., Berkeley, California)*

## To Regain Strength

### CONGEE

MAKES 4 TO 6 SERVINGS

Rice is often used for healing in Chinese medicine. Congee is a porridge made from rice or other grains that is an extremely therapeutic food that strengthens the constitution of people who suffer from chronic disease or are convalescing. Many Chinese families eat congee at least once a week to help prevent disharmony.

The many varieties of congees are suitable for different conditions. Your Chinese medicine practitioner can give you recipes using herbs and/or protein sources and vegetables that are specific for your constitution or diagnosis.

1 cup (195 g) rice (see Note on following page)

7 to 9 cups (1.6 to 2.1 L) filtered water

Health-giving ingredients (optional, see below)

Cook the rice in the water for 6 to 8 hours. A slow cooker is extremely useful for simmering congee while you are off doing other things. Once the rice is cooked, add health-giving ingredients from the list below, if using.

To add health-giving properties to congee, add the following ingredients to your congee, to taste.

- Herbs, such as ginseng, Dang Gui, Codonopsis, red dates, and ginger: Traditional Chinese families serve congee made with herbs on a weekly basis.

- Astragalus: This is often used in immune tonic congee.

- Wheat congee is soothing to the spirit and cooling to fevers.

- Sweet rice congee strengthens the Stomach, tonifies Qi, and is a tonic for diarrhea and vomiting.

- Mung bean congee cools fevers and aids in detoxification.

- Adzuki bean congee removes Dampness, helps ease swelling and edema, and aids in the treatment of Urinary Bladder-Kidney diagnoses.

- Carrot congee eases indigestion and dysentery.

- Leek or garlic congee warms and tonifies.

(continued)

- Kidney congee is used to tonify the Kidney and is traditionally recommended for impotence, premature ejaculation, and lumbago.

- Liver congee helps fight general Yin Deficiencies and strengthens the Liver.

- Lamb congee helps rebalance poor circulation and coldness. It is often recommended for women in general, with the addition of ginger and Dang Gui (see page 148).

- Beef congee bolsters a weak Spleen.

- Chicken congee is also good for women who do not have stagnant Qi, with ginger and Dang Gui added.

- Ginger, garlic, and scallion congee is good for staving off the External Pernicious Influence Wind-Cold.

*Note: In the clinic, we recommend alternative grains other than rice to make congee, such as barley (if you can eat gluten) or quinoa (if you can't eat gluten) along with other grains, depending on the Chinese diagnosis as well as to reduce the glycemic load and index.*

## AMERICAN BREAKFAST CONGEE    MAKES 2 GENEROUS PORTIONS

½ cup (100 g) white rice, well rinsed

1 tablespoon (8 g) grated ginger

1 clove garlic, finely chopped

3 cups (700 ml) chicken stock

1 cup (235 ml) water

Mushrooms

Bell pepper

Green onions, white parts separated and chopped

Cooked chopped chicken or leftover vegetables (optional)

Red Boat fish sauce

Sesame oil

*(continued)*

Chopped cilantro

Soy sauce

Chopped peanuts

In a pan, place the rice, ginger, garlic, stock, and water. Bring the mixture to a boil, cover, and simmer for 1 hour, stirring occasionally to prevent the rice from sticking. Prepare and use as much of the mushrooms, bell pepper, onion, cooked chicken, leftover vegetables, fish sauce, oil, cilantro, soy sauce, and peanuts as you wish.

In a sauté pan, 10 minutes before the congee is ready, sauté some mushrooms, bell pepper, and the white parts of the green onions. At this point you can add cooked chopped chicken or leftover cooked vegetables to the congee too, if using. Taste the congee and add Red Boat fish sauce and sesame oil to season it. Add in the sautéed vegetables and some chopped cilantro along with the remaining green parts of the green onions.

Serve the congee with soy sauce, hot sauce, and chopped peanuts to be added at the table.

*(From Jill Blakeway, M.S., L.Ac, founder of the YinOva Center in New York)*

## To Tonify Qi and Xue

### GRAMMY ETHEL'S CHICKEN BROTH
MAKES 6 TO 8 SERVINGS

Chicken broth is the base of many soups that are used as Xue and Qi tonics in Chinese medicine. Taken plain, it serves as a Xue tonic. When chicken meat is added, however, it can create Stagnation and Dampness. When possible, use free-range, antibiotic-, and hormone-free chicken to make your broth. This is a secret family recipe. My grandmother always said to use a "plump" chicken! My Aunt Jane's recipe adds a clove of garlic.

Plump 3-pound (1.4 kg) chicken

1 parsnip

1 carrot

1 onion

Unbleached cheesecloth bag

Rice, vegetables, herbs, or a matzo ball (optional)

*(continued)*

Place the chicken in an 8- to 10-quart (8 to 10 L) pot. Cover the chicken with water, bring to a boil, reduce the heat, and simmer for 1 hour.

Place the parsnip, carrot, and onion in the bag, tie it closed, and immerse it in the broth. Cover and cook for another hour.

Remove the bag and the whole chicken. Take the boiled chicken off of the bones, eat it separately, or add it back to the broth when appropriate.

Cover the pot of broth and refrigerate it overnight. The next day, skim the fat from the top of the broth.

Reheat the broth and serve it alone or add rice, vegetables, herbs, or a matzo ball, if using. This nearly fat-free broth can be used alone or as a base for soup or congee.

## CHINESE GINGER CHICKEN SOUP
MAKES 6 TO 8 SERVINGS

3-pound (1.4 kg) whole chicken, skin removed

5 green onions, sliced lengthwise and then in half

1 fresh ginger root, halved and sliced into slivers about ½-inch (1.3 cm) long and 1/16-inch (2 mm) wide

Salt (optional)

Place the chicken in a 10-quart (10 L) pot and cover it with water. Bring the water to a boil, reduce the heat to low, and simmer for about 5 minutes.

Add the green onion and ginger. Cover the pot and simmer for 1½ hours.

When finished, remove the chicken from the pot and debone. Return the chicken chunks to the pot. Add salt to taste if you wish.

## DANG GUI CHICKEN

MAKES 6 TO 8 SERVINGS

This chicken soup, made with Dang Gui, is good for keeping the Essential Substances and Organ Systems in harmony. If you have one serving a week or month, you'll find you are stronger and less vulnerable to disease.

Traditionally, this recipe uses a special covered Chinese clay pot—available in Chinatowns and kitchen specialty stores—that has an opening in the bottom that resembles an angel food cake or Bundt pan. If you cannot find one, you can use a regular double-boiler.

2 yards (1.8 m) unbleached cheesecloth

1 medium chicken, cut up into about 10 pieces

20 grams Dang Gui

Ginger (optional)

Root vegetables, such as carrots, turnips, potatoes, onions, and parsnips (optional)

Salt

Fill a 3-quart (3 L) saucepan with water. Roll the cheesecloth lengthwise into a long sausage shape and place it like a collar along the rim of the saucepan. (When done, rinse for reuse.) Place the clay pot on top of the cheesecloth ring, as the top of a double boiler.

Place the chicken into the clay pot. Add the Dang Gui.

Add the ginger and root vegetables if you like. Cook over low heat for 1 to 2 hours, until the chicken is completely cooked and there is ample broth accumulated in the upper pot.

Add salt to taste.


## For Vitalizing Xue


## SAN QI CHICKEN

MAKES 6 TO 8 SERVINGS

Prepare this herb recipe in exactly the same way as Dang Gui Chicken above. Substitute 20 grams of San Qi for the Dang Gui. To improve your circulation, eat one to two servings each week.

## To Aid Digestion

### BASIC MISO SOUP
MAKES 4 SERVINGS

Miso soup, which rebuilds intestinal flora, is used to rebalance digestion. Its salty flavor can also stimulate the Kidney Organ System.

1 strip kombu, arame, or other sea vegetables (available at many natural food stores and Japanese groceries)

5 cups (1.2 L) water

½ cup (65 g) sliced carrots

5 teaspoons miso

1 cup (67 g) chard, kale, or other greens

Rinse the kombu in cold water for 10 minutes. (If using arame, do not soak.) Wipe the kombu with dry towels. Cut the kombu into small strips and add them to a pot. Cover the kombu with the 5 cups (1.2 L) water and bring the water to a boil. Add the carrots. Cover the pot and reduce the heat to medium-low. Simmer for about 10 minutes.

Place the miso in a small bowl. Take a little of the broth out of the pot and mix it with the miso to form a puree. (Miso should not be boiled because it will kill the beneficial bacteria.) Return the miso to the pot and simmer for 2 or 3 minutes. Add the chard, kale, or greens. Simmer for 2 minutes.

### HEARTY MISO VEGETABLE SOUP
MAKES 4 SERVINGS

1 cup (30 g) arame

6 cups (1.4 L) water

1 teaspoon sesame oil

½ cup (65 g) sliced carrots

½ cup (55 g) diced daikon

½ cup (85 g) cooked brown rice, barley, quinoa, or beans

1 teaspoon grated ginger or garlic

6 fresh medium-size shiitake mushrooms, stemmed and sliced (If the shiitake are dried, soak them overnight and then drain them and throw out the water.)

(continued)

1 cup (67 g) greens, such as kale, chard, or beet tops

2 tablespoons (32 g) pureed miso

½ cup (50 g) thinly sliced green onions, for garnish

Soak and rinse the arame to remove excess salt.

Place the arame in a pot and cover it with the 6 cups (1.4 L) water. Add the oil. Adjust the heat to medium-low and simmer for 10 minutes. Add the carrots and daikon and simmer for 3 minutes. Add the rice or beans and ginger or garlic and simmer for 3 minutes. Add the mushrooms and greens and simmer for 3 minutes. Add the miso at the end and simmer for 1 minute. Garnish with the green onions.

## THERAPEUTIC VEGETABLES

MAKES 4 SERVINGS

Eating several vegetables in every meal provides a sound nutritional remedy for many disharmonies. Remember to eat vegetables according to the season and to take advantage of fresh, local produce. For example, root vegetables are recommended primarily in the winter. At each meal, try to include one root vegetable, one sea vegetable, one ground vegetable, and one leafy vegetable. For example, daikon, arame, broccoli, and chard; carrot, wakame, snow peas, and kale; beets, wakame, acorn squash, and bok choy; or onions, arame, cauliflower, and mustard greens.

1 sea vegetable, such as wakame

1 root vegetable, such as turnip

1 ground vegetable, such as acorn squash

1 leafy vegetable, such as chard

In a bowl, soak the sea vegetable in water for 10 to 15 minutes to be soft enough to steam. Rinse and drain it to reduce the sodium level up to 50 percent.

In a pot, combine the vegetables and steam the vegetables until cooked but crisp.

## WARNING

Esteemed doctor Lyn Patrick, N.D., recommends that the seaweed hijiki be avoided because there are documented high levels of arsenic sequestered in it. It has been removed from the food supply in several countries. Other sea vegetables are safe to eat.[1]

# COMMONLY ASKED DIET QUESTIONS

Here are some of the most common questions I am asked about the First-Step Dietary Therapy Program.

**Q:** Do I have to change how I eat today?

**A:** No. I would never say you should or shouldn't eat this or that.

For people who have chronic sinusitis, general fatigue, or digestive problems, diet therapy is used immediately. But for others, dietary changes can be more gradual.

The guiding principle is that slower adjustment is more important than radical change. Embracing Chinese Dietary Therapy is a process of expanding what you eat, not constricting your diet. You may give up some foods. However, you will find there's a whole world of varied foods you may have never tried before. To make a shift in your diet—from out of balance to balanced—you must find the place in your heart and consciousness that makes the transition comfortable and unforced.

Discovering the best way for you to improve your diet is a very personal process. You can't rush it. You must give yourself the time to learn about how your body functions and adjust to what it tells you.

**Q:** Is it better to eat Asian foods than an American diet?

**A:** Becoming healthy is not about growing up in Pennsylvania and eating like someone from Beijing. Chinese Dietary Therapy philosophy suggests that you generally embrace your native foods and eat foods grown locally and in season. What is unhealthy about "American foods" is not the fact that they are American, but that they are too often commercial inventions instead of natural foods. If you stick to natural, homegrown, and chemical-free products, you'll have a bountiful supply of healthful food choices.

**Q:** Is meat bad for you?

**A:** It depends. The body handles meat protein best in small quantities. You should eat no more than 2 to 3 ounces (55 to 85 g) at a meal. Many physicians recommend that you limit the amount of red meat you eat to no more than 6 ounces (170 g) a week. Begin to think of meat as an accent, rather than as the centerpiece in any meal. All meat should be organic as much as possible and always grass-fed and raised with no hormones or antibiotics.

People with certain diseases, such as cirrhosis, should never eat red meat. Diets such as vegan include only plant-based proteins and no animal products. President Bill Clinton and other prominent people have adopted vegan and vegetarian diets to reverse heart disease. However, a recent meta-analysis shows that diets high in saturated fats, found in meat and dairy,[2] are not associated with heart disease. Other evidence suggests that various forms of cancer may be associated with a diet high in saturated fats from processed meats, such a hot dogs and hams.

**Q:** What about sugar?

**A:** Sugar can be part of a balanced diet when eaten in very small quantities. Refined sugars have the fewest nutrients, but other complex sugars come tucked into nutritionally beneficial foods. Some systems of food healing believe that maple sugars/syrup is a good source. Another natural alternative to sugar is stevia.

Traditionally, Chinese medicine occasionally prescribes small amounts of sugar to tonify the Spleen and improve appetite.

A diet that includes too many high-glycemic foods, which would include refined sugars and certain carbohydrates, can lead to insulin resistance, metabolic syndrome, prediabetes, and fatty liver.

There is a lot of controversy over sugar. However, one thing many people can agree upon is that high fructose corn syrup (HFCS) should never be eaten. (See "The High Fructose Corn Syrup Connection" on page 303.)

**Q:** I'm pregnant. Should I change my diet completely?

**A:** It's not a good idea to make a radical shift in your diet during pregnancy. You want to eliminate coffee, alcohol, drugs, and cigarettes. As for other shifts, simply concentrate on eating as nutrition-packed calories as possible. That will naturally lower your fat intake and increase your consumption of the grains and vegetables.

If you are planning to become pregnant, however, you may want to make a dietary renovation part of your plan. Being at the proper weight and body mass index (BMI) before becoming pregnant should be your goal. Whatever you do, remember the growing embryo requires fuel. Women who eat too few calories in an attempt to control weight gain or follow strict food plans are hurting themselves and their babies.

**Q:** What will happen when I change my diet?

**A:** Suddenly changing to a diet rich in whole grains, legumes, vegetables, fruits, and high-quality protein can come as a surprise to your body. It will free the Qi to move throughout your system, and that can evoke all kinds of transitory negative feelings until the flow is established. That's why you want to go through the process gradually and comfortably. Also, you may want to work simultaneously with other aspects of healing, such as herbs and acupuncture, because they all reinforce one another.

If you feel you need to help your body purify itself, which is more of a Western natural medicine concept, you may want to eat Liver-supporting foods such as beets, carrots, and burdock.

**Q:** Are all grains good for healing?

**A:** Yes. All of the grains can be used to make healing congees—Chinese therapeutic rice soups. (See the recipes on page 117.) However, some grains are not for everyone. For example, many Westerners are already too Damp and have Phlegm; therefore, I would not recommend oatmeal in damp conditions, especially in damp climates. Oatmeal is beneficial, however, for Lung Yin, Dryness, or Yin Deficiency. If you like, put a little honey, milk, and butter on it because this helps increase Yin and Jin-Ye. (See the information on gluten intolerance and glycemic index on page 306.)

**Q:** What can you do to grains to make them appropriate for treating Deficiency or Cold conditions?

**A:** Add spicy or warm foods, such as scallions, ginger, and cinnamon. For some of the Spleen Deficiency conditions, a small amount of sweet foods are good. However, honey is contraindicated if you have diarrhea.

**Q:** What is the most life-extending diet?

**A:** Chinese medicine has long advocated moderately flavored, unprocessed food for a long, healthy life.

This diet can be pure, subtle, and sweet. Grains, beans, meat, and most root vegetables are sweet. But we've become used to heavy, over-flavored, impure foods that promote Dampness, Heat, Phlegm, and a cloudy pallor.

# APPLYING CHINESE DIETARY THERAPY

Chinese Dietary Therapy provides a powerful tool for correcting disharmonies, and it is used in conjunction with acupuncture, herbal therapy, and Qi Gong to restore balance to the Essential Substances, Organ Systems, and Twelve Channels. Generally, Diet Therapy can help sedate Excess, tonify Deficiency, cool Heat problems, warm Cold problems, moisten Dry problems, and dry Excess Dampness. *Symptoms* describe what you feel when you are not well. *Signs* are the manifestations of disharmony that Chinese medicine practitioners look to guide them in identifying and diagnosing particular imbalances.

## To Treat Deficient Qi

**Symptoms** include lethargy, loose stools, fatigue, weakness, decreased appetite, shortness of breath, and occasionally cold extremities and frequent urination.

**Signs** that your Chinese medicine practitioner will look for include a thin, weak pulse and a tongue that is pale, possibly swollen with tooth marks.

**Western** diagnoses include chronic fatigue, asthma, and urinary incontinence.

**Your diet should contain:** Traditional Chinese theory says that half of total calories should come from grains and legumes, a third from vegetables, and about 15 percent from fish or meats. With meats, you don't want to tax your digestion or build Phlegm—so eat only about 2 to 3 ounces (55 to 85 g) of animal protein per serving. Five percent of total calories can come from dairy. Recommended foods include rice or barley, broth, garlic, leeks, string beans, sunflower seeds, sesame seeds, and carrots. However, modern understanding of the glycemic index as well as protein intake gives us the ability to modify this diet. In this case, when one eats carbohydrates, it is best to eat low- to moderate-glycemic carbohydrates with a low glycemic load. It is important to eat these carbohydrates along with sufficient protein to balance the glycemic index and load.

**Your diet should not contain:** Raw food, salads, fruits, and juices in excess.

**To treat cold symptoms with Deficient Qi:** Add dried ginger, cinnamon bark, and chicken's eggs.

## To Treat Deficient Spleen Qi

**Symptoms** include lack of appetite, bloating, mild abdominal pain better with pressure, loose stools, and fatigue.

**Signs** that your Chinese medicine practitioner will look for include a weak pulse and pale, soft tongue with tooth marks and thin white fur.

## DIETARY GUIDELINES FOR LOOSE STOOLS

Follow these guidelines for Spleen/Stomach and Qi and Yang Deficiencies.

**Foods to tonify digestion:** Warm and cooked foods, moderate-size meals, congees and soups (no cream), white rice, black tea, cinnamon tea, barley (has gluten), ginger tea, and add herbs to congee (ask your practitioner first)

**Foods to enhance flora:** Miso soups and sauces, *Lactobacillus acidophilus* (and other probiotics as recommended by practitioner), sauerkraut (without vinegar), kefir (try nondairy), pickled vegetables (without vinegar), and kimchi

**Foods to avoid:** Raw and cold foods, spicy foods, coffee, dairy, and excessive fats and oils

For food poisoning, eat goat's or sheep's milk yogurt after the sickness has subsided.

**Western diagnoses** include diarrhea, gastric or duodenal ulcers, anemia, and even chronic hepatitis.

**Your diet should contain:** Cooked, warming foods, such as squash, carrots, potatoes, yams, rutabagas, turnips, leeks, onions, rice, oats, butter, small amounts of chicken, turkey, mutton or beef, cooked peaches, cherries, strawberries, figs, cardamom, ginger, cinnamon, nutmeg, black pepper, custards, and small amounts of honey, molasses, maple syrup, and sugar.

Food should be well chewed and eaten in moderate amounts.

**Your diet should not contain:** Salsa, citrus, too much salt, tofu, millet, buckwheat, milk, cheese, seaweed, and excess sugar.

## To Treat Deficient Spleen Qi Leading to Deficient Yang

If Deficient Spleen Qi is not treated early, the body becomes ever more depleted. The Qi cannot be replenished through what you eat and drink. Eventually, a more serious Yang Deficiency develops.

**Symptoms** include aversion to the cold, craving warm drinks, and chilled fingers, toes, ears, and nose tip.

**Signs** that your Chinese medicine practitioner will look for include a slow, thready pulse and tongue that is moist and pale with indentations/tooth marks on the sides.

**Western diagnoses** include swelling, gastritis, enteritis, kidney disease, and colitis.

**Your diet should contain:** Foods as noted for Deficient Spleen Qi (see page 127).

**Your diet should not contain:** Raw or chilled foods or foods that are difficult to digest, such as fatty foods, raw cruciferous vegetables, and milk. They exhaust the digestive fire.

## To Treat Dampness Associated with Deficient Spleen Qi Deficiency

This is a complicated case of Excess and Deficiency.

**Symptoms** include headaches, watery stools, and queasy stomach.

**Signs** that your Chinese medicine practitioner will look for include a slippery pulse, tongue fur that is thick and greasy, and a tongue body that is swollen with tooth marks along the sides.

**Western diagnoses** include hepatitis, dysentery, gastroenteritis, parasites, and severe diarrhea.

**Your diet should contain:** Foods as denoted for Deficient Spleen Qi (see page 127) along with foods that drain Excess Dampness, such as barley, corn, adzuki beans, garlic, mushrooms, mustard greens, chicken, alfalfa, shrimp, scallions, and rye.

**Your diet should not contain:** Too much red meat, salt, or sugar and food that produces Damp, including dairy products, pork, shark meat, eggs, sardines, octopus, coconut milk, cucumber, duck, goose, seaweed, olives, soybeans, tofu, spinach, pine nuts, and alcohol.

## To Treat Spleen Qi Deficiency with Damp Cold

**Symptoms** include water retention, puffiness, feeling cold, mild nausea, trouble breathing, watery stools, and clear, frequent urine.

**Signs** that your Chinese medicine practitioner will look for include a pulse that is weak and slippery or soft and slow and a pale tongue with tooth marks on the sides.

**Western diagnoses** include edema, parasites, ulcers, and Crohn's disease.

**Your diet should contain:** The traditional recommendation of about 65 percent of total calorie intake from grains or legumes. Around 25 percent of your diet should be vegetables. Eat 10 percent red and white meat, with no more than 25 ounces (700 g) a week. Modern recommendations would lower the intake of carbohydrates to closer to 30 percent. Also, the wisdom is to eat low-glycemic carbohydrates in balance with high-quality proteins to lower the glycemic index as well as the glycemic load.

**Your diet should not contain:** Raw food, fruits, sugar, and dairy products.

## To Treat Spleen Deficiency with Damp Heat

**Symptoms** include a hot and heavy feeling, fever, nausea, costal or abdominal pain, labored breathing, and diarrhea.

**Signs** that your Chinese medicine practitioner will look for include a weak and slippery or soft pulse that's rapid and a tongue that's swollen and reddish, possibly with yellow fur.

**Western diagnoses** include colitis, acute hepatitis, and Crohn's disease.

**Your diet should contain:** The traditional diet of 65 to 70 percent of calories from grains and legumes, 25 to 30 percent from cooked vegetables, 5 percent from white meats with not more than 6 to 12 ounces (170 to 335 g) in a week. An occasional salad is suggested.

**Your diet should not contain:** Red meat, raw vegetables (other than the occasional suggested salad), fruit juices, and dairy.

## To Treat Upward Movement of Qi and Phlegm

This condition is the result of several underlying disharmonies that, only when added together, create symptoms. First, the stresses and strains of daily life coincide with a stressful diet of sugar, caffeine, and alcohol or drugs. This exhausts the Kidney Fire (in the Lower Burner), and digestion (Middle Burner) becomes sluggish. Phlegm builds up. Simultaneously, stress triggers an elevation in Liver Yang. Negative emotions make the Liver energy rise upward. Qi and fluids from the Lung rise and becomes rebellious, uncontrolled, and erratic. This combines with the Excess Phlegm production.

**Symptoms** include sexual problems, cold extremities, low back pain, susceptibility to every passing cold or flu, joint pain, fear, anxiety, and impatience.

**Signs** that your Chinese medicine practitioner will look for vary, but whatever else is present, there are all the signs of weak Spleen, Kidney, and Stomach Systems.

**Western diagnoses** include sinus allergies, watery eyes, skin rashes, sinus headaches, and chronic cough.

**Your diet should contain:** Cooked foods, rice, barley, mung beans, sweet rice congee, adzuki beans, mustard greens, and broth-based vegetable soups.

**Your diet should not contain:** Sugar, coffee, alcohol, citrus, dairy, soy, and all raw, iced, or chilled foods and all energetically Cool and Cold food.

## DIETARY GUIDELINES FOR FATIGUE AND LETHARGY

Fatigue and lethargy can stem from Deficiency, Xue Deficiency, Yang Deficiency, Dampness, and Qi Stagnation.

To remedy fatigue caused by Qi Deficiency, eat foods that tonify Qi and improve energy levels, including:

- Cooked and warm foods

- Frequent, small meals

- Sweet foods (See "Food Flavors, Energetics, and Temperatures" on page 94.)

- Cooked, yellow vegetables

- Small amount of chicken and turkey, especially in soups

- Warming spices, such as dried ginger and cinnamon (except with Xue Deficiency)

- Avoid Cold or Cooling foods and tofu, milk, cheese, liquids with meals, and excess sweet foods

To remedy fatigue caused by Stagnant Liver Qi, eat foods that move Stagnant Qi, including:

- Chicken livers

- Kelp

- Nori

- Eggplant

- Saffron

- Avoid alcohol, fatty foods, food additives, unnecessary medicines, and overindulgence in sugary foods

- Avoid chicken and turkey.

- Spicy food in small amounts move Qi (see page 92); excessive use of spices creates more Stagnation

## DIETARY GUIDE FOR CONSTIPATION CAUSED BY DRYNESS

**Foods that lubricate bowels:** Alfalfa sprouts, apples, apricots, bananas, beets, carrots, cauliflower, honey, oil, okra, peaches, pears, pine nuts, prunes, seaweed, sesame seeds, soy products, spinach, walnuts, and wheat (has gluten)

**Foods that promote bowel movement:** Asparagus, bran, cabbage, coconut, fig, papaya, peas, and potato

**Flora-enhancing foods:** Kefir (try nondairy), miso, sauerkraut (without vinegar), pickled vegetables (without vinegar), *Lactobacillus acidophilus*, kimchi, and natto

## To Treat Excess Heat

**Symptoms** include warm or hot extremities, sweatiness, acne or boils, decreased bowel movements, a loud voice, irritability, and feeling hot.

**Signs** that your Chinese medicine practitioner will look for include a rapid, full pulse and a red tongue that may have a yellow coating.

**Western diagnoses** include skin disorders along with redness, digestive difficulties, chronic constipation, manic behavior, and/or headaches.

**Your diet should contain:** Almost half of total calories should be grains and legumes. A third should be cooked and raw vegetables. About 20 percent could be juices and fruits.

**Your diet should not contain:** Frozen or icy foods or chicken. Eat only minimal amounts of meat, sugar, and dairy products.

## To Treat Stagnant Liver Qi

**Symptoms** include tenderness in the rib cage, nausea, premenstrual lability, irritability, and swollen breasts and abdomen.

**Signs** that your Chinese medicine practitioner will look for include a wiry pulse and a tongue that is dusky or purplish.

**Western diagnoses** include alcohol abuse, type A personality, fibrocystic breasts, swelling or lumps in groin or breasts, goiter, PMS, menstrual irregularities, hepatitis, and headaches.

**Your diet should contain:** Liver-sedating foods, such as beef, chicken livers, celery, kelp, mussels, nori, plum, and amazake (a fermented rice drink). Also recommended are foods that regulate or move Qi, including basil, bay leaves, beets, black pepper, cabbages, coconut milk, garlic, ginger, leeks, peaches, scallions, and rosemary.

**Your diet should not contain:** Alcohol, coffee, fatty foods, fried foods, excessively spicy foods, excessive red meat, sugar, and sweets.

## To Treat Fluid Dryness

**Symptoms** include dry throat, dizziness, emaciation, spontaneous sweating, and shortness of breath. Other symptoms vary, depending on whether the underlying syndrome is Deficient Xue or Deficient Yin.

**Signs** that your Chinese medicine practitioner will look for include a pulse that is fine, halting, or hollow and weak and a tongue that is uncoated and pink.

**Western diagnoses** include type 2 diabetes and chronic constipation.

**Your diet should contain:** Dairy products, most noncitrus fruits, honey, pork, liver congee, tofu, olive oil, peanut oil, and sesame oil. For Deficient Kidney Yin, eat kidney congee and liver congee. (See "Deficient Xue" below for additional guidelines.)

**Your diet should not contain:** Raw fruits and vegetables, cold foods, caffeine, purgative herbs and medicines, and alcohol.

**Special note:** If you have type 2 diabetes, combining a Chinese medicine diet along with incorporating an understanding of the glycemic index is incredibly important. (See "The Glycemic Index" on page 306 for more information.)

## To Treat Deficient Xue

**Symptoms** include dizziness, low weight, blurred vision, tingling in toes or fingers, dry skin or hair, and a pale, lusterless face. The symptoms vary, depending on the relative Deficient Xue.

**Signs** that your Chinese medicine practitioner will look for include a thready or hollow pulse and a pale tongue.

**Western diagnoses** include anemia; headaches; anxiety; nervousness; lack of, painful, or possibly heavy periods; dry skin; and dry constipation with difficult stools.

**Your diet should contain:** Oysters, sweet rice, liver, chicken soup, Dang Gui Chicken (see the recipe on page 121), eggs, and green beans.

**Your diet should not contain:** Raw fruit and vegetables, cold liquids, and ice.

## HOW FIVE PHASES PRACTITIONERS USE DIET THERAPY

Five Phases practitioners put an emphasis on the flavors associated with the Phases. When the diet becomes unbalanced, the flavors may become Excess or Deficient. That can trigger disharmony in associated Organ Systems. To remedy the imbalance, Five Phases Diet Therapy advocates the addition of counterbalancing flavors. Each flavor has special powers to restore balance.

**Wood is associated with sour.** Sour is astringent and gathering. A diet that has an excess of sour flavor is associated with weakening of the Spleen, overproduction of saliva by the Liver, and injury to the muscles. It can be counteracted by the addition of metal-pungent food.

**Fire is associated with bitter.** Bitter is drying and strengthening. A diet that has an excess of bitter is associated with Spleen Dryness, congestion of Stomach Qi, and a withering of the skin. It can be counteracted by the addition of salty flavor.

**Earth is associated with sweet.** Sweet is harmonizing and retarding. A diet that has an excess of sweet is associated with achy bones, unbalanced Kidney, full Heart energy, and hair loss. It can be counteracted by the addition of sour foods.

**Metal is associated with hot, pungent, and aromatic.** Metal is dispersing. A diet that has an excess of pungent is associated with muscle knots, slack pulse, a damaged Shen, and unhealthy finger- and toenails. It can be counteracted by the addition of bitter foods.

**Water is associated with salty.** Salty is softening. A diet that has an excess of salty is associated with deficient muscles and flesh, lack of strength in the large bones, and depression. It can be counteracted by the addition of sweet foods.[3]

## To Treat Stagnant Xue

Stagnant Xue results from a traumatic injury, as a manifestation of gynecological imbalances, and the outcome of long-term Stagnant Qi or Deficient Xue.

**Symptoms** include missed periods, excessive clotting with period, fixed painful lumps, dry skin and lips, thirst, susceptibility to cold extremities and constipation, and liver (or other organ) fibrosis.

**Signs** that your Chinese medicine practitioner will look for include a choppy pulse and a tongue that is purple and may have purple spots on the sides or on other parts, along with purple or blue sublingual veins.

**Western diagnoses** include endometriosis, menstrual cramps, pelvic inflammatory disease (PID), uterine fibroids, fibrosis/cirrhosis, bruising, and fixed pain.

**Your diet should contain:** A small amount of chives, cayenne, eggplant, saffron, safflower, basil, brown sugar, and chestnuts to improve circulation of the Xue.

Foods and spices that disperse Stagnant Xue include turmeric, adzuki beans, rice, spearmint, chives, garlic, vinegar, basil, scallions, leeks, ginger, chestnuts, rosemary, cayenne, nutmeg, kohlrabi, eggplant, and white pepper.

Foods that strengthen the Stomach and Spleen Organ Systems to promote sufficient production of Xue include rice, trout, and small amounts of chicken and chicken liver.

Foods that build Yin, which strengthens Xue, include mussels, wheat germ, and millet.

**Your diet should not contain:** Duck, alcohol, fatty foods, and sweets. If you are cold, avoid citrus fruits and tomatoes.

# NUTRITIONAL SUPPLEMENTS

Chinese Dietary Therapy, based on the ancient texts, does not contain suggestions for nutritional supplements. In a perfect world, we wouldn't need supplements, but food contaminated with pesticides, drugs, and hormones, a sedentary lifestyle, and constant stress make it unlikely most of us receive sufficient nutrition through diet alone.

Using nutritional supplements within the context of Chinese Dietary Therapy means that you really can't substitute vitamin pills for a balanced diet. Popping a pill won't undo the damage done by a poor diet. Furthermore, vitamins and minerals are meant to work together, and taking too much of one or not enough of another may have a negative impact on how your body can use many supplements. That's why I believe that nutritional supplements should be taken only after a consultation with a well-informed practitioner or nutritionist.

The following nutritional supplements are those we recommend to most clients at Chicken Soup Chinese Medicine.

## *Lactobacillus Acidophilus*

*Lactobacillus acidophilus* is found naturally in the human gut. Antibiotics, other drugs, a sugar-laden diet, and other imbalances can create a lack of this normal growth. *Lactobacillus* produces vitamin K and lactase, which is an enzyme that digests milk sugar lactose. It is used to promote beneficial bacterial growth in the digestive tract and to suppress yeast.[4] It alleviates Dampness, especially the nondairy forms. Recommended dose is ¼ to ½ teaspoon of powdered *Lactobacillus acidophilus* one or two times a day in unchilled water away from meals. In our clinic, we like to use the Natren brand.

## Vitamin D$_3$

Vitamin D is often found to be deficient, especially in the northern part of the United States and Canada, as well as in older people. Your body can make vitamin D from exposure to the sun, but many people cover up with sunblock creams that block vitamin D production. Vitamin D is found in small amounts in fatty fish, such as herring, mackerel, sardines, and tuna. To get the proper amount of vitamin D, I recommend starting supplemention with vitamin D$_3$ (cholecalciferol) in the range from 2000 IU to 4000 IU per day and then lower or raise the dose as needed. The best way to determine deficiency is through lab testing. The lab test you want to get is known as the 25(OH)D or 25-hydroxyvitamin D test. Labs vary in their normal reference ranges. We consider the best range to be between 50 and 70 ng/mL for disease prevention.

## Omega-3 and Essential Fatty Acids

Essential fatty acids—particularly the omega-3s eicosapentaenoic acid (EPA), docosahexaenoic acid (DHA), and alpha-linolenic acid (ALA)—are critical to your health. They support joint health, decrease inflammation, are essential to cognitive functions and visual acuity, reduce cardiovascular risk, and may help ease depression. EPA and DHA have much higher efficacy for most of these functions than does ALA. EPA and DHA are found in certain types of fish, including anchovies, herring, mackerel, bluefish, wild salmon, sardines, sturgeon, wild trout, and tuna. Omega-3 ALA comes from plant sources—flaxseed, walnuts, evening primrose, canola oil, and soybean oil; however, they are either low in or lacking EPA and DHA. ALA converts to DHA in the body, but at a very low rate.[5]

Vegetarians can get omega-3s from plant sources; however, the intake needs to be quite high. My recommendation is to use krill oil, rather than fish oil or plant sources, whenever possible. Krill oil typically has more EPA than fish oil. It reduces arthritis pain, inflammation, and stiffness, and it is reported to be more successful for PMS symptoms and lowering blood lipids.[6] It contains astaxanthins that have anti-inflammatory properties. Krill oil is also considered to be more tolerated digestively, and it does not cause burping like fish oil does. It is also a more sustainable product.

The suggested daily intake of EPA and DHA is from 500 milligrams to 1,000 milligrams. Ask your practitioner what is best for you. Because omega-3 supplements may thin the blood, people taking blood thinners should talk with their doctors before ingesting omega-3 supplements.

## Calcium/Magnesium

Supplementation of these two minerals in one balanced pill is a good idea for women, people with night leg cramps, people who have bone fractures, and anyone who drinks a lot of caffeine in coffee or colas. The National Institutes of Health (NIH) recommends 1,000 milligrams of calcium for men and women and 1,200 milligrams a day for postmenopausal women and all people over age seventy-one. Magnesium is recommended at 420 milligrams per day. Therefore, a 2:1 calcium/magnesium supplement can give you close to the correct dosing. Or you can take them separately.

Because it is difficult for most people to eat enough calcium in a day, supplements are important. Calcium calms the Shen and decreases Stagnant Qi. Magnesium has a tendency to move Qi downward, causing loose stools, and so it should not be taken as a supplement if you have Deficient Spleen Qi. This is an important area to discuss with your practitioner.

In addition to taking a supplement, to help maintain sufficient calcium levels, you should avoid foods that produce calcium loss. The main culprits are foods that contain caffeine (including sodas), alcohol, excessive sodium, and meats, which contain phosphoric acid.

## Other Supplements to Consider

With a qualified practitioner guiding you, you may also want to consider a multivitamin/mineral, vitamin C, vitamin E, coenzyme $Q_{10}$, glutamine, B-complex, and others according to your medical conditions and diet.

# DANCING WITH DANG GUI AND FRIENDS

## A Survey of Chinese Herbal Therapy

Wholeness = Dietary Guidelines + **Herbs** + Acupuncture + Qi Gong

In 3,500 BCE, Shen Nung, the god of husbandry, founded Chinese herbal medicine. According to a tale passed down through the ages, he had a hole in his stomach through which he watched his internal processes. Because of this remarkable ability, he became curious about what happened to his body when he ate various plants, minerals, and animals. This led him to take 365 types of herbs to determine their healing effects. But even a god could not dodge the perils of experimentation with unknown herbs. After cataloging hundreds of them, he died of poisoning.

Besides this being a good story, it offers an important take-home message—and one that I hope you'll take to heart. You should never take any herbs not included in the Medicine Cabinet section (see page 230) without consulting a trained herbalist.

## CHARACTERISTICS OF CHINESE HERBAL MEDICINE

Herbs have the power to restore balance to the Twelve Channels, Organ Systems, and Essential Substances. The art and science of using these powerful botanicals, minerals, and animal products comes in knowing how to prescribe the right herb or mixture of herbs to do the job.

The process usually begins with a diagnosis of the disharmonies. Then the herbalist will prescribe an herb or a combination of herbs to remedy the problem. Herbs wield their curative powers in four ways: through temperature, taste, direction, and organs entered.

**Temperature** is broken down into Hot, Cold, Warm, Cool, and Neutral. If a disease is considered Hot, then an herb with Cooling properties is selected. If the disease is considered Cold, then a Warming herb is used. The degree of Warming and Cooling needed will direct the practitioner toward various herbs and combinations of herbs.

**Tastes** are characterized as Acrid, Sweet, Bitter, Sour, and Salty. Taste has an important influence on the therapeutic effect of any herb or combination of herbs. Acrid substances disperse and move; sweet substances tonify and harmonize; bitter substances drain and dry. Sour substances are astringent and prevent or reverse the normal leakage of Jin-Ye and Qi. Salty substances purge. Bland substances—foods that have no recognized flavor quality—remove Dampness and promote urination.

**Direction** means that the energy of herbs rises and floats (moves upward and outward) or falls and sinks (moves downward and inward). The direction of an herb is employed to move Qi and other Essential Substances as required to reestablish harmony. For example, if you suffer from Stagnant Stomach Qi and have a diagnosis of Stagnant Food in the Stomach, you might use an herb that moves Qi downward. Or for sinus blockage, you might use an herb with energy that moves upward and helps direct the other herbs in the formula toward the problem.

**Organs entered** indicates which specific Organ System(s) the herb is able to affect.

## FORMS OF HERBAL MEDICINES

Chinese herbs come in many forms, such as bulk herbs, decoctions, powders, pills, syrups, plasters, pellets, medicinal wines, tinctures, and enemas. Two common forms are bulk herbs and pills.

**Bulk herbs** are generally processed before they are used in herbal therapy. They may be altered to detoxify components that would otherwise be harmful. Bulk herbs can be processed to change the way the herb works, such as to make the herb more Yang or more Cooling or change its energetics so that its tonifying effects come to the forefront. Some examples of these processes are baking, dipping in honey, boiling, soaking, or frying the substance before it is turned into powders and decoctions.

**Decoctions** are made by cooking a combination of prepared bulk herbs in water to make an herb soup, which is sometimes called a tea. They are useful because, unlike pills, they can be individualized with each prescription. Every time a person comes in for an evaluation, the practitioner may be able to adjust the formula by adding or subtracting herbs or keeping it the same.

Decoctions are particularly effective against acute problems, such as the External Pernicious Influences like Wind-Cold. They are usually only prescribed for a few days. If the herbs are required for chronic conditions, many practitioners will provide pills or powders, although bulk herbs may be used as well. In our clinic, people who are undergoing cancer support or who have complex gynecological conditions often are prescribed bulk herb formulas.

Decoctions are also used for steaming, making poultices, and other external applications. Not all herbs should be made into decoctions, however. Some Fu Zheng herbs, such as Ganoderma, which is in many immune modulating formulas, are more effective in other forms.

**Powders** are created in two different ways. The first way is by pulverizing the bulk individual herbs or herb formula. The second way is by decocting, concentrating, and spray-drying the individual herb or formula and creating dry granules.[1] Different companies use different patented processes. Powders or granules are commonly swallowed with warm water either as a powder or in capsules. Sometimes the powders or granules are placed into boiling water in a Thermos and steeped overnight to create a tea. Practitioners may either put together individual formulas from single granulated herbs, or they may order and prescribe granules of prepared formulas. Often, a prepared formula is used as a base and individualized with single herbs.

**Pills** in the form of Chinese herbal tablets and capsules almost always contain herbal formulas rather than individual herbs, and they are targeted to treat specific disharmonies. There are different types of herbal pills. Some are made from powders, and others are made from concentrates. Practitioners and clients often favor pills over bulk herbs for the following reasons:

- The cost is lower. Many of the herbs in the formulas are expensive to buy individually, but when herbs are purchased in large quantities by the manufacturers of the tablets or capsules, the cost goes down.

- They're easier to use. This means that people are more apt to follow the recommended therapeutic routine.

- They are formulated for specific disharmonies. Some herbal formulas on the market have been devised to address extremely specific problems. They offer the practitioner and patient the assurance of high-quality therapy.

TIP

You can tell what form an herb will come in by its name. If it includes the word *tang*, it will be a decoction. *San* means it is a powder. *Wan* or *pian* indicates it is a pill.

- They may have a more concentrated pharmacological effect. It is important that you buy your herbal pills from companies that prepare the herbs in the traditional way, such as frying them in honey or cooking them in rice wine, before manufacturing the pills. Your Chinese medicine practitioner should be aware of the process the herb company uses to prepare the herb pills they provide to you or prescribe from an herbal pharmacy.
- They provide access to rare or very expensive herbs not carried by most herbal stores, practitioners, or pharmacies.

**Syrups** are prepared by reducing herbs to a thick concentrate. Granulated sugar or honey is added, and the syrups are then ingested orally.

**Plasters** are made by preparing herbs in oil along with other substances. The resulting salve is spread over a cloth that is used as a compress or plaster or directly applied to the skin or orifice.

**Pellets or special pills** are usually made from extremely rare medicinals. They are super-refined into a fine powder that is mixed with a gluey substance. Pellets are used internally and externally.

**Medicinal wines** are therapeutic beverages made by soaking or simmering herbs in wine.

**Tinctures or extracts** are drinks or topical formulas made by steeping herbs in alcohol or glycerin.

**Enemas** are made from easily dissolved herbs or cooked teas and used to remedy digestive problems along with other internal medicine conditions.

With the advent of modern manufacturing processes in China, in the tradition that everything always changes, new processes for manufacturing are continually being developed and used.

# HOW TO PREPARE BULK HERBS AT HOME

If you are given bulk herbs to prepare as a decoction at home, there are several steps to follow. *Note: These directions are general, and they are meant only to familiarize you with the process of cooking herbs. If an herbalist gives you herbs, follow her or his exact instructions because they might be different than this description.*

1. Obtain a clay pot. You can buy a special clay pot specifically for cooking herbs in a Chinese kitchen or herb store or from your herbalist. Using metal cookware may reduce the effectiveness of the herbs.

2. Prepare your clay pot by immersing it in warm water for 20 to 30 minutes. Allow it to dry completely. Rub all unglazed surfaces with organic cooking oil. Allow the pot to stand overnight. The next morning, wash the pot with warm water; don't ever use soaps or household cleansers on the clay. Re-oil the pot periodically.

3. Place the herbs in the pot and soak them as prescribed by the herbalist.

4. Add the amount of water prescribed by your herbalist, and then briefly bring the water to a boil. Reduce the heat to a simmer. Reduce the liquid as directed by your practitioner.

5. Strain the liquid into a glass container with a lid and leave the herbs in the pot. Take the decoction as prescribed. Store the remaining decoction in the covered glass container in the refrigerator.

6. The next day, add more water as directed by your practitioner. Repeat steps 4 and 5. Discard the herbs after two days.[2]

If you are interested in more detailed information regarding Chinese herbal medicine, practitioners use many books for studying herbs. The following are three of the most common books:

- *Chinese Herbal Medicine: Materia Medica*, 3rd Edition[3]
- *Chinese Herbal Medicine: Formulas and Strategies*, 2nd Edition[4]
- *Chinese Medical Herbology and Pharmacology*[5]

## COMBINING HERBS

Whatever form the herbs come in, they are often assembled into formulas that combine two or more herbs to produce a targeted effect. The herbs each have one or more roles within the formula. The basic roles are the following:

**Chief herb** is the main herb and provides the predominant actions in the formula.

**Deputy herb** augments or promotes the action of the chief herb or addresses a different pattern of disharmony.

**Assistant herb** reduces side effects or potential toxicity of the chief herb or reinforces the chief herb.

**Envoy herb** harmonizes the herbs, allowing them to work together as a unit. (Licorice is often used in this capacity.)

The herbs in a formula interact with one another in several ways. They are:

**Additive:** When two or more herbs with the same effect are used together, their action may be amplified. No herbalist would ever add herbs together without knowing the additive effects.

**Synergistic:** Sometimes adding two or more herbs together produces an effect that is greater than the sum of its parts. When this happens, the herbs are said to potentiate each other.

**Mutually restraining:** Sometimes two or more herbs are used together to weaken or neutralize some aspect of another herb. This is particularly useful if an herb causes several physiological reactions, only one or some of which are appropriate for the diagnosis.

**Inhibitive:** One herb's effect inhibits the action of another herb.

**Destructive:** The combination of two herbs decreases the toxicity of one.

**Oppositional:** Opposing herbs are two or more botanicals that are harmful when taken together.

## CHOOSING A QUALIFIED HERBALIST

Only a competent, trained herbalist should prescribe Chinese herbal remedies.

Taking recommendations from untrained personnel at health food stores, through mail-order catalogs, or from untutored practitioners is foolish at best and dangerous at worst.

In my clinic, I try to buy from herbal companies that sell only to licensed, primary health care providers or licensed pharmacies. Consumers should beware of herb suppliers who make claims for formulas and then sell them to anyone who asks for them.

Chinese herbal medicine is not a separately licensed profession; therefore, licensing is not required unless they also practice acupuncture in a state that licenses acupuncture. Most states do not require herbal training or examination for acupuncture licensure.

However, the National Certification Commission for Acupuncture and Oriental Medicine (NCCAOM) does provide certification through a national examination for Chinese herbal medicine. (See General Resources and References on page 344.) As of this writing, only nine states require the NCCAOM herbal examination for acupuncture licensure. You can check on the NCCAOM website for specific details on the current requirement.[6]

While herbal examination is often not required for licensure, nonetheless many Chinese medicine practitioners are nationally certified in Chinese herbal medicine. You can check the NCCAOM website for national certification.[7] As of this writing, California, which licenses a bit more than one-third of all licensed acupuncturists in the United States, does not use the NCCAOM examination. The California board requires herbal training and examination to become licensed.

Some well-trained and qualified practitioners are not nationally certified. You should ask them what training and testing process they received. If you go to a Chinese herbalist who has been prescribing and/or dispensing herbs for years, of course it is best for you rely on personal recommendations and reputation as well as asking how he or she was trained in herbal medicine.

Regarding herbal quality assurance, to know the quality and testing of the herbs, practitioners can ask their herbal supplier for a certificate of analysis (COA) for the herbs that are sold to them. You can ask herbalists to provide you with the quality assurance policies of the herb companies they use.

SIDE EFFECTS OF HERBS

Some herbs and formulas, especially pills or granules, may cause undesirable side effects. The most common are digestive problems. This may result from the fact that pills and granules contain the natural plant fiber. People who do not get much fiber in their diets before taking herbs, herb pills, or granules find that the herbs may increase their fiber intakes dramatically. These people might experience digestive side effects, such as gas and bloating. These effects usually pass after two to three days, as the body adjusts to increased fiber intake and begins to rebalance itself.

If side effects persist, often changing the time of day the herbs are ingested and/or their dosage can control them. Sometimes a digestive formula needs to be added to the herbal regimen to restore balance. A practitioner can tell the difference between the presence of a disease that causes digestive upset and herbal side effects.

# AN HERBAL SAMPLER

The following list is a sample of the individual herbs that I prescribe extensively in my clinic as part of herbal formulas. They are listed in alphabetical order. These herbs are commonly used in many Chinese medicine practices. At the end of each section are examples of a variety of formulas that contain these individual herbs.

I have had the good fortune to be able to design herbal formulas that are used widely in the Chinese medicine community. Some of these include Enhance, Tremella American Ginseng, Source Qi, Clear Heat, Marrow Plus Channel Flow, and Cold Away. These Chinese herbal formulas are available to your licensed practitioner from a supplier called Health Concerns. (See General Resources and References on page 344.)

## Astragalus

*Astragalus membranaceus* (*Huang Qi*) is one of the most important tonifying herbs, and it is a major ingredient in many formulas to strengthen Qi. It tonifies Spleen and Lung Qi, increases overall energy, aids in digestion and absorption of food, stops spontaneous sweating, promotes urination, and helps heal injured tissue.

According to Western research, astragalus has immune restoration capabilities. Several Chinese studies found it increases the red blood cell count and also claimed increased survival rates in people with lung and liver cancer from 28 to 71 percent.[8] In another Chinese study of chronic active hepatitis, liver functions returned to normal in 18 of 31 participants.[9] Animal studies have shown its effectiveness in lowering blood pressure.[10]

FORMULA EXAMPLES CONTAINING ASTRAGALUS
- Central Chi Tea (*Bu Zhong Yi Qi Tang*)
- Enhance

## Atractylodes

*Atractylodes alba* or white atractylodes (*Bai Zhu*) is also a Qi tonic. It tonifies the Spleen and Stomach, removes Spleen Dampness, helps with digestion, relieves edema, and helps increase body weight and muscle strength.

Many reports from China profess the ability of atractylodes to increase white blood cell counts, and it is used regularly in formulas to support the immune system.[11] Studies show it also lowers blood sugar and prevents concentration of glycogen in the liver.[12]

FORMULA EXAMPLES CONTAINING ATRACTYLODES
- Central Chi Tea (*Bu Zhong Yi Qi Tang*)
- Four Gentleman Decoction (*Si Jun Zi Tang*)
- Enhance
- Source Qi

## Buplerum

Bupleurum root (*Chai Hu*) is what is called a Release Exterior herb. It is used to treat diseases that cannot be categorized as either interior or exterior, but that are in the process of moving inward. This stage of illness is called Shao Yang, and it is associated with pain in the rib cage, alternating chills and fever, a bitter taste in the mouth, and vomiting.

Bupleurum is also used to spread the Liver Qi, allowing the Qi to move more smoothly throughout the body, and to raise the Spleen Qi in order to harmonize Spleen and Stomach Deficiency patterns, reduce fever, and calm the mind.

Research has revealed that bupleurum has anti-inflammatory, antiviral, antibacterial,[13] and liver-protective effects.[14] Bupleurum is often used to lower fevers associated with upper respiratory infections. In Asia, it's used to treat malaria.

FORMULA EXAMPLES CONTAINING BUPLEURUM

- Minor Bupleurum Decoction (*Xiao Chai Hu Tang*)
- Ease Plus (modified bupleurum and dragon bone)

## Codonopsis

Codonopsis (*Dang Shen*) strengthens and harmonizes the functions of the Spleen and Stomach. It is often used in formulas in the place of ginseng to tonify Qi.

In Chinese and Japanese studies, codonopsis has been shown to increase red blood cells and to enhance T-cell activity.[15] In combination with other herbs, it has been shown to increase white blood cell counts in people undergoing chemotherapy and radiation. In China, chronic kidney disease and anemia are also treated with codonopsis. It is used to overcome fatigue, reverse appetite loss, strengthen tired limbs, stop diarrhea, ease phlegmy cough, and support digestive functions.

FORMULA EXAMPLES CONTAINING CODONOPSIS

- Women's Precious Pills (*Ba Zhen Wan*)
- *Shen Ling Qi Bai Zhu Tang*
- Source Qi

## Cordyceps

Cordyceps (*Dong Chong Xia Cao*) is an ancient Chinese tonic food and herbal medicine. Traditionally, cordyceps, a fungus, has been used for extreme fatigue, tuberculosis, impotence, post-disease weakness, and spontaneous sweating. It supports the Kidney and Lung Qi.

Today it is known as a Fu Zheng herb. Fu Zheng means "restore the normal" in Chinese. The Fu Zheng herbs encompass a number of herbs, such as ganoderma and astragalus. The Fu Zheng concept was fully developed in China during the 1970s to provide support for people undergoing Western cancer treatments, especially to support the immune system and strengthen Qi. More recently, in the 1980s, our group at Quan Yin Healing Arts Center in San Francisco, along with a few other Western practitioners, specifically adapted this approach to working with people with immune deficiency diseases, including people with HIV/AIDS.

We created formulas to support people, along with Western medicine, who have viral hepatitis, HIV, and other diseases that have viral and immune components. These formulas include Fu Zheng herbs, such as cordyceps, ganoderma, astragalus, ginseng, and atractylodes, along with additional Clear Heat Clean Toxin herbs[16] (these are herbs that clear Toxic Heat, which is often associated today with viral and bacterial infections), herbs that tonify Xue and Jing, and herbs that vitalize Xue and move Qi.

A wealth of cell and animal studies and the early development of clinical trials support its use. Studies of cordyceps include research into liver fibrosis,[17] for enhancement of chemotherapy in small-cell lung cancer through specific polysaccharides in cordyceps,[18] along with compounds shown to kill human leukemia cells.[19] In China alone, more than 100 institutes are devoted to the development of medicinal uses of fungi, including this ancient herb.

FORMULA EXAMPLES CONTAINING CORDYCEPS

- Cordyceps PS
- Cordyseng
- Enhance

## Dang Gui

Dang Gui (*Angelica sinensis*) tonifies and moves Xue, and it is used for menstrual disorders. It disperses cold, alleviates pain, and moistens dry stools. The literal translation means "state of return."

FORMULA EXAMPLES CONTAINING DANG GUI

- Woman's Balance
- Relaxed Wanderer (*Xiao Yao San*)

## Eclipta

*Eclipta prostrata* (*Mo Han Lian*) nourishes and tonifies the Liver and Kidney Yin. It also cools Xue. Historically, it was used to treat ringing in the ears, blurred vision, premature graying of the hair, night sweats, and excess bleeding. In modern times, eclipta is used as a liver-protecting compound for people with hepatitis and liver disease caused by exposure to chemical toxins, including environmental illness.[20, 21]

FORMULA EXAMPLE CONTAINING ECLIPTA

- Ecliptex

## Ganoderma

Ganoderma (*Ling Zhi*) is a Qi tonic that also tonifies the Xue and calms the Spirit. It is used in asthma, insomnia, anxiety, and immune modulation,[22] especially cancer support.[23] Like cordyceps, it is a Fu Zheng herb (see page 147). There are six types of ganoderma mushrooms, each a different color. The red Ling Zhi is considered to be the most powerful.[24] Polysaccharides, found mostly in the spores, are the active ingredients, and they have a regulatory effect on the immune system.[25]

FORMULA EXAMPLES CONTAINING GANODERMA

- Enhance
- Tremella American Ginseng
- Cordyseng

## Ginseng

Ginseng (*Ren Shen*), species *Panax ginseng*, is a slightly bitter root that is used because it tonifies the Spleen and Lung, calms Spirit, and revitalizes Qi. It promotes secretion of bodily fluids and stops diarrhea. It is used for insomnia, palpitations, and forgetfulness, and it is prescribed for extreme weakness and fatigue. It should not be used by someone with Excess Heat. Myriad research has been conducted on ginseng. It has immuno-modulatory effects,[26] exerts an effect on the central nervous system, acts as an antihistamine, impacts the endocrine system, affects the metabolism—including reduction of blood sugar[27] and blood cholesterol—and is cardioprotective.[28]

FORMULA EXAMPLES CONTAINING GINSENG

- *Bu Zhong Yi Qi Wan*
- Source Qi

## Ginseng, American

American ginseng (*Xi Yang Shen*), species *Panax quinquefolium*, is quite distinct from ginseng (*Ren Shen*), species *Panax ginseng*. American ginseng primarily replenishes the Yin and Qi, cools Fire from Deficient Yin, and tonifies the Lung Yin. It promotes the secretion of bodily fluids, reduces irritability, stops cough due to Deficient Lung Yin, stops night sweats, and improves overall energy. It has been demonstrated to have a sedative effect on the brains of animals in lab experiments, it creates an excitatory action on the central nervous system, and it is a cardiotonic.

FORMULA EXAMPLES CONTAINING AMERICAN GINSENG

- Tremella American Ginseng
- Cordyseng

## Isatis

Isatis leaf (*Da Qing Ye*) and isatis root (*Ban Lan Gen*) are what Chinese medicine calls Clear Heat Clean Toxin herbs. Many Clear Heat Clean Toxin herbs are known for their antiviral and antibacterial properties. In China, isatis is used in many anticancer formulas. Isatis is also used in China for viral meningitis,[29] pneumonia, and bacterial infections, such as shigella, salmonella, streptococcus, and staphylococcus. The two herbs, which are really different parts of the same plant, are often combined in formulas with other herbs.

FORMULA EXAMPLES CONTAINING ISATIS

- Enhance
- Tremella American Ginseng
- Clear Heat
- Isatis Gold

## Licorice Root

Licorice root (*Gan Cao*), also *glycyrrhiza*, is included in many Chinese herbal formulas to harmonize the formulas, which mean it enters all Twelve Primary Channels and directs various herbs to enter the Channels. For this reason, it is one of the most commonly used herbs in formulas, usually in very small quantities. In addition, it tonifies the Spleen Qi,

WARNING

In prolonged high doses, licorice root may have a steroidal effect, causing high blood pressure and water retention, reduction in thyroid function, and decrease in the basal metabolic rate. However, when properly prescribed in an herbal formula, usually very small amounts are used. Always take *glycyrrhiza*, especially in its extracted forms, under the care of a qualified, licensed health care provider.

moistens the Lung, removes toxins, and drains Fire. By itself, licorice is a Spleen Qi tonic, and it is traditionally used for fatigue and loose stools, to help remedy weak digestion, and to decrease effects of toxic substances. Licorice root is used to stop pain and spasms, and it is often used for inflammation, arthritis, and gastric ulcers.

Japanese and Chinese researchers have explored licorice's anticancer, anti-HIV,[30] antiviral, antihepatitis,[31] and antifungal properties. In Germany, a multicenter study with licorice extract showed a success rate of 30 to 40 percent against chronic viral hepatitis B.[32]

## FORMULA EXAMPLES CONTAINING LICORICE

- Four Gentlemen Decoction (*Si Jun Zi Tang*)
- Enhance
- Tremella American Ginseng
- Source Qi

## San Qi

San Qi, which is often given in powder form as a single herb, is used for injuries of all types through its action to disperse Xue and Qi. By itself or in combination with other herbs, it is used for pain relief and to stop bleeding. In China, it has been used for thrombosis as well as postpartum problems associated with stagnant Qi and Xue. If there is profuse bleeding, only use it after a physician sees you and prescribes the herb. It can be used in soups for general health support. It should not be taken during pregnancy because it regulates Xue, and these types of herbs theoretically can cause miscarriage.

## FORMULA EXAMPLES CONTAINING SAN QI

- Resinall E Tabs
- *Zheng Gu Shui*
- San Qi Powder (the individual herb)

## Scutellaria

Scutellaria (*Ban Zhi Lian*), species *Scutellaria barbata*, is traditionally used as a Clear Heat Clean Toxin herb to invigorate Xue, promote urination, and reduce swelling and sores. In China, today *Scutellaria barbata* is used in formulas for specific cancers, such as ovarian, breast, lung, and liver cancer, in conjunction with other herbs, often oldenlandia (*Bai Hua She She Cao*). Recent studies show specific extracts of scutellaria have antitumor activity.[33] Research into other gynecological cancers has also been performed.[34]

## FORMULA EXAMPLES CONTAINING SCUTELLARIA BARBATA

- Used in bulk herb formulas

## Spatholobus

Spatholobus (*Ji Xue Teng*) is a unique herb that both vitalizes and tonifies Xue. Traditionally, it is used for menstrual pain, lack of menses, irregular menstruation, abdominal pain, numbness in the extremities, lower back pain, and knee pain. In China, since the 1970s, it has been used extensively during cancer chemotherapy and radiation treatment to support the bone marrow. Research suggests that spatholobus ameliorates the side effects of lowered white blood cell count and aplastic anemia.[35]

## FORMULA EXAMPLES CONTAINING SPATHOLOBUS

- Marrow Plus
- Enhance
- Tremella American Ginseng

### WARNING

Spatholobus increases contractions in the uterus, so it's contraindicated during pregnancy unless specifically prescribed by a Chinese herbalist and your Western doctor.

## COMMON HERB FORMULAS

The following table includes some of the most common herb formulas we use.

| FORMULA | CHINESE FUNCTION | INDICATIONS |
|---|---|---|
| Bu Zhong Yi Qi Tang (Central Chi Tea) | Tonify Spleen Qi, strengthen Middle Jiao, raise Yang, and counter prolapse | Fatigue, weak limbs, headache, loose stools, spontaneous sweating, and shortness of breath |
| Cordyceps PS | Tonify Kidney Yang, nourish Lung Yin, strengthen Wei Qi, stop cough, and transform Phlegm | Fatigue, immune weakness, post-illness weakness, chronic cough, health maintenance, general tonic, and support athletic performance |
| Cordyseng | Tonify Qi and Yin through Fu Zheng action and strengthen Lung, Spleen, Stomach, and Kidney | Fatigue, recovery from serious illness or operation, support immune function, support lungs, and improve athletic performance |
| Enhance | Tonify Qi, Xue, Yin, Yang, and Jing; Clear Heat Clean Toxin; clear Phlegm; and strengthen Spleen, Stomach, Kidney, and Wei Qi | Fatigue, immune dysfunction, frequent colds and flus, and chronic viral illness |
| Marrow Plus | Vitalize and tonify Xue, tonify Qi, and strengthen Spleen and Kidney | Marrow suppression, offset side effects of medications, and chronic pain and numbness |
| Si Jun Zi Tang (Four Gentlemen Decoction) | Tonify Qi and strengthen Spleen | Improve gastrointestinal system, support immune function, and fatigue |
| Tremella American Ginseng | Tonify Yin, Qi, Xue, and Jing; Clear Heat Clean Toxin; strengthen Wei Qi; and strengthen Spleen, Stomach, Lung, and Kidney | Fatigue, immune dysfunction, frequent colds and flus, chronic viral illness, afternoon night sweats and fever, and chronic dry cough |
| Xiao Yao San (Relaxed Wanderer) | Spread Liver Qi, relieve stagnation, tonify Spleen, and nourish Xue | Irritability, depression, moodiness, fatigue, headache, dizziness, breast distention, irregular menstruation, and menstrual pain |
| Xiao Chai Hu Tang (Minor Bupleurum Decoction) | Harmonize Shao Yang Stage Disorders and harmonize and tonify Middle Jiao | Alternating chills and fever, dry mouth and throat, bitter taste, irritability, dizziness, fullness and discomfort in the rib cage and chest, loss of appetite, nausea, vomiting, and heartburn |

# 9

# METAL AND FIRE
## The Arts of Acupuncture and Moxibustion

Wholeness = Dietary Guidelines + Herbs + **Acupuncture** + Qi Gong

Acupuncture, as described traditionally, is the art and science of manipulating the flow of Qi and Xue through the body's Twelve Channels—the invisible aqueduct system that transports the Essential Substances to the Organ Systems, tissues, and bones. Manipulation of the Qi and Xue is accomplished by the stimulation of specific acupuncture points along the Channels where the Essential Substances flow close to the skin's surface.

Present-day practitioners use many different methods for stimulating acupuncture points, including electrostimulation and lasers as well as the traditional fine metal needles. Whatever the technique, acupuncture is relatively painless. It is often accompanied by feelings of heaviness or warmth and sensations of movement. These sensations occur because acupuncture points are like gates in an aqueduct system. When the points are stimulated, they may open a gate, so that Excess or Stagnant Qi or Xue can disperse. Or if Qi and Xue are Deficient, stimulation of certain acupuncture points may close a gate, so the Essential Substances can collect as needed. When this is done, the distribution of Essential Substances throughout the whole system of Channels becomes more evenly balanced, allowing for a smoother flow into all areas of the body.

This adjustment of the body's Qi and Xue can be used to maintain or restore balance between Yin and Yang, alleviate emotional disorders, protect the Organ Systems, moisten tendons, and keep the joints healthy. Acupuncture works on a spiritual level and on a physical, energetic level.

## GEORGE'S STORY

In 1987, George came to me for treatment for alcoholism.

"Once I had the acupuncture treatments, I stopped, and I never drank again," George said. "I had no craving whatsoever."

But George's medical problems were not over. Two years later, he had to go on dialysis. By 1994, he had suffered two serious episodes of high blood pressure.

"I almost had a stroke and was taking Procardia—a high blood pressure medicine—when I went for more acupuncture treatments. It was amazing. After two or three visits, my pressure was normal, and I had to stop the medicine. Now I go [for acupuncture] once every two weeks, and my pressure has stayed normal for several months."

You may experience the same beneficial effects of acupuncture, but never stop taking high blood pressure or other medication without consulting both your Western and your Chinese medicine doctors—and, if possible, having them talk with each other directly.

# TYPES OF ACUPUNCTURE

When it comes time to select an acupuncturist, you may be surprised to find out that there are many different types of practitioners. Some are Traditional Chinese Medicine acupuncturists—as I primarily practice. Other systems include Japanese, Classical Chinese Medicine, Korean Constitutional, Five Phases, Worsley, Richard Tan, Van Nghi, and other style practitioners. Each approach has a tradition and a practice that has been refined and shaped so that it provides effective therapy. There is no one way that is correct.

As Charles Chace, a noted Chinese medicine scholar, pointed out in an article on the diversity of Chinese medicine, "While specific people throughout history may have believed they had a lock on the truth, the Chinese as a people never took this very seriously and never really strove toward a single truth. Chinese society as a whole never cared about a single truth. They just cared about what is useful, about what makes logical sense. . . . A concept of absolute knowledge is not Chinese, and also the concept of either/ or is not Chinese. Chinese medicine has historically allowed opposing points of view to exist simultaneously."[1]

In the following sections, I will briefly review four of these systems: Traditional Chinese Medicine Acupuncture, Japanese Acupuncture, Traditional Acupuncture, and Korean Acupuncture. (For more information on how to find practitioners, see the appendix on page 332.)

## Traditional Chinese Medicine Acupuncture

After the Chinese Revolution, Traditional Chinese Medicine (TCM) was consolidated to unify diverse ancient practices into one coherent theoretical framework. My practice is based on TCM, and I predominately use the style of acupuncture that corresponds to that system of thought. It is based on the Eight Fundamental Patterns, Seven Emotions, Essential Substances, Organ Systems, and Channels.

In TCM, there are 365 basic acupuncture points located along Twelve Primary Channels, Eight Extraordinary Channels, and Fifteen Collaterals. (Over the centuries, more than 2,500 points have been identified, but the average practitioner uses about 150.)

## Japanese Acupuncture

Japanese acupuncture focuses on clinical symptoms, and it is pragmatic. To Miki Shima, O.M.D., L.Ac., one of the leading proponents, Japanese acupuncture is a "healing art, based on the direct, nonconceptual, and intuitive observations of the patient."

This system uses meridian (Channel) therapy based on a diagnostic process that includes looking, listening, questioning, pulse diagnosis, palpation of meridians, and most importantly, abdominal diagnosis. Although there are several schools of abdominal diagnosis, they all focus on the belly as the area of the body where toxins become stagnant and as the source of illness. Organs and meridians are associated with sections of the abdomen, and the texture, density, tenderness, appearance, and responses to touch of each section indicate specific disharmonies.

Other diagnostic techniques used by some Japanese acupuncturists include Akabane and the O-ring test. Akabane is the practice of using a lit incense stick to test reaction to heat at the acupuncture points on the fingertips. The length of time it takes for a person to react to the heat indicates the nature of disharmony in the meridians. The O-ring test, designed by Yoshiaka Omura, M.D., a teacher of acupuncture, is a subtle system of testing muscle strength that is used in conjunction with herbal therapy and acupuncture.

When the practitioner uses acupuncture, he or she determines which acupuncture points to needle by palpation of the meridians. The Japanese school believes that the points are not found at fixed anatomical sites, but rather that they move along the meridians, depending on the disharmony that's present.

In addition to the Japanese practitioner's own system of acupuncture, they use an herbal system called Kampo, which is based on the original Chinese herbal text, *The Shang Han Lun*. Herbal formulas are prescribed based on symptoms without discussion of herbal properties. They rarely modify or add to formulas.

## Traditional Acupuncture

This school of thought was developed in England and the United States by professor J. R. Worsley, founder of the College of Traditional Acupuncture in the United Kingdom. This system is also known as Five Element Worsley Acupuncture. This school uses the Five Phases—Metal, Fire, Water, Earth, and Wood—and the Channels associated with them for diagnosis and treatment. Traditional Acupuncture's main emphasis is on the emotional and spiritual basis of disharmony.

Traditional Acupuncture emphasizes observation of facial color, interpretation of a person's vocal quality, and reading pulses, using distinctly different pulse patterns than those used in TCM.

## Korean Acupuncture

Korean, or Constitutional, acupuncture is based on system of identifying Qi imbalances through pulse diagnosis (modified from the Chinese) and determining which one of eight constitutional types a person falls into. Each constitutional type is linked with one Organ System that is overactive and another Organ System that is depleted. For example, if your constitution is identified as Hespera, that could mean you have Large Intestine Excess with Small Intestine Deficiency.

Identification of constitutional type is then combined with the Five Phases understanding of the Organ Systems. Wood is linked with Gallbladder and Liver, Fire with Heart and Small Intestine, Earth with Spleen and Stomach, Metal with Lung and Large Intestine, and Water with Kidney and Urinary Bladder. This directs the practitioner to which of the Five Phases Channel points to tonify or sedate.

# FUNCTIONS OF ACUPUNCTURE

Whichever type of acupuncture you receive, it will be effective for diagnosis, prevention, and treatment of disharmony. Let's talk about each in turn.

## Diagnosis

When the body is in disharmony, acupuncture points along the Channels become tender to the touch, alerting the practitioner to the location of disturbances in the Channels and in associated Organ Systems. Some points become particularly tender when disease is present, and they offer vivid diagnostic help. For example, when the Lung or Heart

System has disease, the Qi is detained in the crook of the elbow, making that point tender to the touch.

## Prevention

Acupuncture maintains a balanced flow of Qi and Xue. By using it for regular tune-ups, you can keep your mind/body/spirit in harmony. Furthermore, acupuncture can be used to prevent disease from becoming more severe. You may have noticed emotional and spiritual changes or disturbances often appear as the first sign of illness and imbalance: You don't quite feel right, you might have dream-disturbed sleep, or you might become easily irritated. These early clues to the onset of disease can be present in the body, and they can be identified through careful diagnosis before symptoms emerge. Acupuncture can then be used to rebalance the Qi and prevent the developing disharmony from turning into a full-blown illness or disorder.

## Treatment

In the TCM system of acupuncture, we adjust the flow of Essential Substances so that Excesses are dispersed, Deficiencies are overcome, Dampness is dispelled, Dryness is eased, Cold is warmed, and Heat is cooled. It reestablishes balance and promotes a self-healing response by stimulating communication pathways within the body that promote tissue repair and natural pain control.

Acupuncture—used alone or in conjunction with dietary therapy, herbal remedies, bodywork, and Qi Gong—is a powerful force for promoting health and well-being.

### ALICIA'S STORY

Alicia was suffering from chronic sciatica that had developed from an old sports injury. Painkillers only dulled her pain, physical therapy had not helped, and massage, although refreshing, had not offered lasting relief.

Alicia came to my clinic after she has been forced to postpone a much-needed vacation because she couldn't possibly sit on an airplane for five hours straight.

Her treatment included acupuncture with electrostimulation, ear acupuncture, moxibustion and self-moxa, herbal therapy, and massage. After eight treatments, she had no more debilitating flare-ups, and she could sleep through the night.

"You can stick a needle anywhere you like," she said with a laugh. "I don't question how it works. I just know this has given me my life back."

# THE TAO OF ACUPUNCTURE

When a Chinese medicine practitioner uses acupuncture for diagnosis and treatment, he or she does not view the person's health as a phenomenon that is isolated from what is going on in the world outside or the general stages of life. Climate, geographic location, and age and individual conditions all impact the harmony of the mind/body/spirit. Consequentially, they must be taken into consideration in evaluation and in the development of a treatment plan. We'll discuss each here.

## Climate

According to the ancient Chinese text *Ling Shu*, "In spring, the pathogenic factors are most likely to attack the superficial layer; in summer, they are most likely to attack the skin; in autumn, they are most likely to attack the muscles; and in winter, they are most likely to attack the bones and tendons." In treatment of such disorders, the *Ling Shu* also says that techniques should remain consistent with the seasons, "that's why in the spring and summer, shallow acupuncture is generally used, and in winter and autumn, deep acupuncture is preferred."

## Geographic Location

Geographic location has an impact on acupuncture treatment because climate affects diet and lifestyle, which in turn affects the way Essential Substances and Organ Systems function. People who live in desert areas, such as eastern Washington state or southern Arizona, or who live in cold damp areas, such as San Francisco or London, need to have acupuncture treatments that are appropriate to such geographic conditions and help the mind/body/spirit maintain balance in the presence of the External Influences.

## Age and Individual Conditions

Acupuncture treatment is also tailored to the age, gender, and the general constitution of the recipient. People of different ages and genders have different physiologies. Sensitivity to acupuncture can vary widely. The *Ling Shu* explains these distinctions: "A middle-aged strong person with sufficient Qi and Xue and hard skin may, if being attacked by pathogenic factors, be treated by a deep needling with a needle retained for some time. . . . An infant has weak muscles and less volume of Qi and Xue, [so] acupuncture treatment is given twice a day with shallow needling and weak stimulation." The text also suggests deep needling for people engaged in physical labor and shallow needling for people who perform mental work.

## HOW DOES ACUPUNCTURE WORK?

While it is important scientifically to research the mechanisms of acupuncture, the science of how acupuncture works is not the primary basis on which a practitioner develops a treatment plan and uses acupuncture. For example, what Chinese medicine practitioners and the many surgical patients in China who have used acupuncture for anesthesia and postoperative pain care about are the effects of acupuncture.

TCM describes acupuncture's impact on the mind/body/spirit in the following six ways:

**Reinforcing** is used when there are no strong pathogenic forces at work in the body. It bolsters the Organ Systems, and it replenishes Yin, Yang, Qi, and Xue.

**Reducing** dispels pathogenic factors and breaks up Stagnation. Reducing is used for Excess conditions.

**Warming** removes blockages in the Channels, nourishes Qi, dispels Cold, and restores Yang.

**Clearing** dispels Heat and remedies Heat syndromes with swift needling.

**Ascending** raises Qi, prevents Sinking Qi, and prevents Organ prolapse.

**Descending** sends Upward Rebellious Qi downward and subdues Yang. It is not generally used when Deficiency is present. (Note: The difference between Sinking and Descending Qi is that Sinking indicates what happens to Qi when it is not being supported or helped up. Descending indicates what happens to Qi when it is being pushed down.)

## THE SCIENCE OF ACUPUNCTURE

Clinical and basic science research have been conducted on acupuncture. The National Institutes of Health (NIH) funds both clinical and basic acupuncture research, most often through the National Center for Complementary and Integrative Health (NCCIH),[2] formerly known as the National Center for Complementary and Alternative Medicine (NCCAM).

The leading acupuncture research organization in the United States is the Society for Acupuncture Research (SAR). SAR's mission is "to promote, advance, and disseminate scientific inquiry into Oriental medicine systems, which include acupuncture, herbal therapy, and other modalities. SAR's leadership and members value quantitative and qualitative research addressing clinical efficacy, physiological mechanisms, patterns of use, and theoretical foundations."[3]

SAR provides a library of evidence-based assessments to SAR members. SAR's members include researchers, educators, students, acupuncturists, health care practitioners, and members of the public. Being able to use this evidence to inform their practices benefits practitioners.

## Mechanisms Research

Since the middle of the past century, the mechanisms of acupuncture have been studied. Although there are many theories on how acupuncture works and several mechanisms have been proposed, much more work remains to be done. Here are some selected possible mechanisms.

**Connective tissue theory:** Helene Langevin, M.D., a professor in the department of neurological sciences at the University of Vermont and a professor in residence of medicine at Harvard Medical School, Brigham and Women's Hospital, has been doing seminal work in the area of connective tissue for fifteen years. Dr. Langevin has shown that a twisted acupuncture needle creates a localized stretch by gripping the underlying connective tissue. She proposes this may be one way in which acupuncture works.

**Gate theory:** The gate theory posits the idea that the nerves that transmit pain impulses from the body through the spinal cord to the brain have gates that can be switched open or closed. The theory is that acupuncture may add an electronic message to neural pathways that causes the gate to open, interrupting the flow of information, such as pain. This way, the pain impulses never make it to the brain.[4]

**Endorphins theory:** The endorphins theory, documented in animal and human trials since the 1970s, attributes acupuncture's pain-blocking effects to stimulation of the body's own painkillers, which are neurotransmitters called endorphins.[5] Other researchers have investigated the impact of stimulation of the endorphin system on the immune system. They suggest that acupuncture's curative powers may involve immunomodulation of prostaglandin hormones and interleukin-2.[6]

Research has been conducted into other areas as well. However, none of these theories considers the interaction of acupuncture and Qi and Xue. Western science has not yet developed a quantitative measure for these Essential Substances. Chinese medicine, however, does quantitate it—in Chinese medicine terms.

## Neuroimaging Research

Since the mid-1990s, a number of researchers have been using neuroimaging to study acupuncture's effects. Neuroimaging allows scientists to explore brain function as a mechanism of acupuncture efficacy. A main imaging technique used in acupuncture research is the functional MRI (fMRI), which can estimate activity anywhere in the brain every few seconds. In 2012, a systematic review on fMRI and acupuncture was published in *PLOS One*, a premier journal of the Public Library of Science.

The study concluded, "Brain response to acupuncture stimuli encompasses a broad network of regions consistent with not just somatosensory, but also affective and cognitive processing. While published results on acupuncture and fMRI were heterogeneous, from a descriptive perspective most studies suggest that acupuncture can modulate the brain activity within specific brain areas, and the evidence based on meta-analyses confirmed part of these results."[7]

Images can be found online in the journal article.

## Clinical Research

The primary clinical research into acupuncture has been in the area of pain, although there are currently other areas of inquiry. One reason this is important is that insurance companies often look to published evidence to cover acupuncture treatments. As of December 2014, if you do a Google Scholar search for "acupuncture clinical research" you can find 197,000 returns, mostly scientific articles.

A 2012 meta-analysis from the *Archives of Internal Medicine* concluded the "... study provides the most robust evidence to date that acupuncture is more than just placebo and a reasonable referral option for patients with chronic pain."[8]

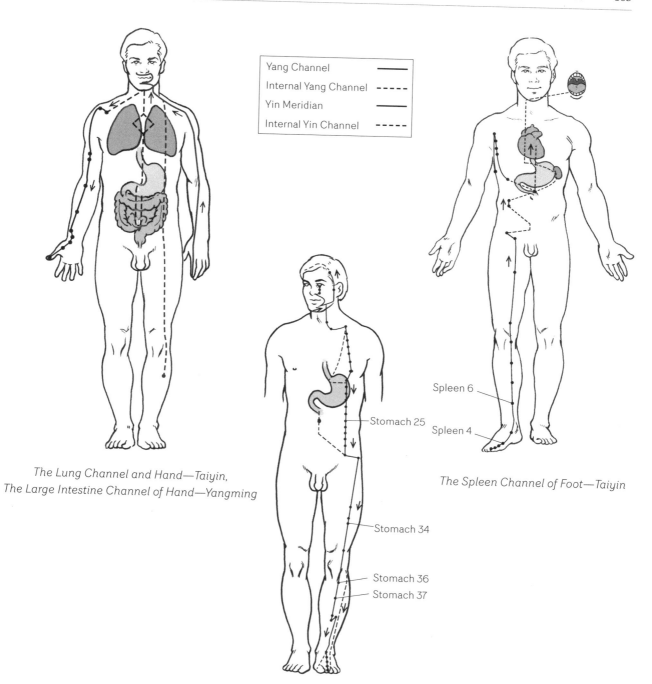

| | |
|---|---|
| Yang Channel | ——— |
| Internal Yang Channel | - - - - |
| Yin Meridian | ——— |
| Internal Yin Channel | - - - - |

Spleen 6

Spleen 4

Stomach 25

Stomach 34

Stomach 36
Stomach 37

*The Lung Channel and Hand—Taiyin,
The Large Intestine Channel of Hand—Yangming*

*The Spleen Channel of Foot—Taiyin*

*The Stomach Channel of Foot—Yangming*

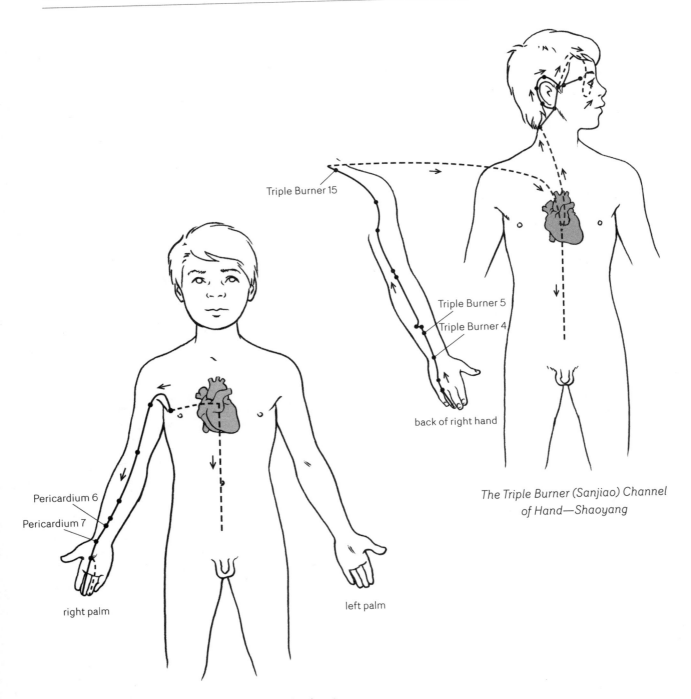

Triple Burner 15

Triple Burner 5

Triple Burner 4

back of right hand

*The Triple Burner (Sanjiao) Channel
of Hand—Shaoyang*

Pericardium 6

Pericardium 7

right palm

left palm

*The Pericardium Channel of Hand—Jueyin*

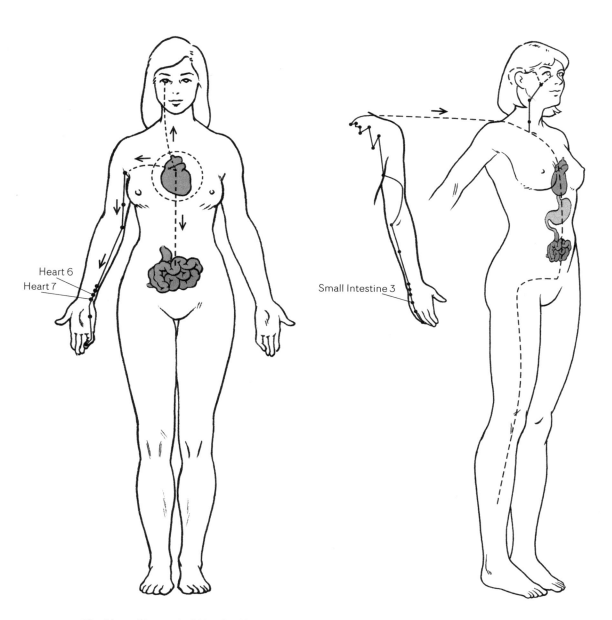

Heart 6
Heart 7

Small Intestine 3

*The Heart Channel of Hand—Shaoyin*

*The Small Intestine Channel of Hand—Taiyang*

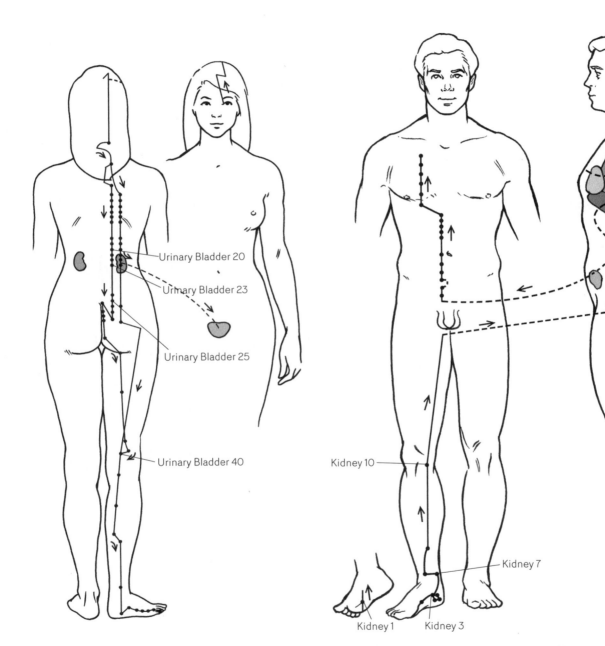

Urinary Bladder 20

Urinary Bladder 23

Urinary Bladder 25

Urinary Bladder 40

Kidney 10

Kidney 7

Kidney 1

Kidney 3

*The Urinary Bladder Channel of Foot—Taiyang*

*The Kidney Channel of Foot—Shaoyin*

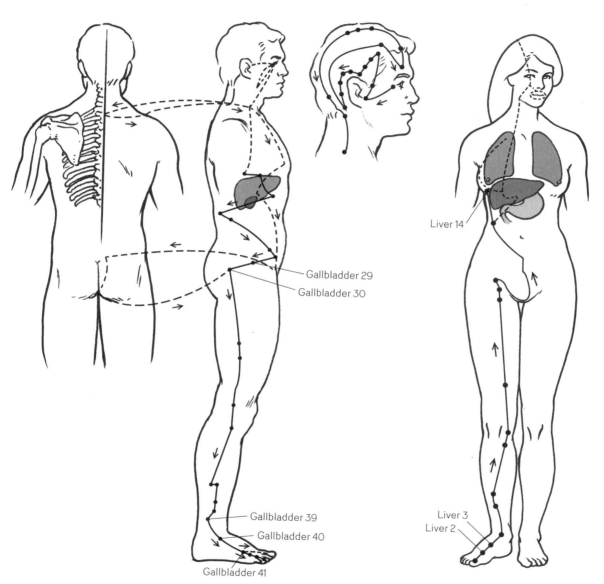

*The Gallbladder Channel of Foot—Shaoyang*

Gallbladder 29
Gallbladder 30
Gallbladder 39
Gallbladder 40
Gallbladder 41

*The Liver Channel of Foot—Jueyin*

Liver 14
Liver 3
Liver 2

## ACUPUNCTURE TREATMENT

Acupuncture, whether done using traditional needles or by more modern techniques, such as electrostimulation or laser, requires extensive training. It should only be done by a qualified practitioner. You can however, use acupressure and massage of acupuncture points, and there are complete instructions and explanations for you to follow (see chapter 11, page 190).

In the hands of a skilled practitioner, acupuncture is particularly effective for recovery from drug and alcohol dependency, for pain control, and for relief from depression, obsessive compulsive disorders, phobias, and anxiety attacks. Acupuncture has been used for immune regulation and to treat allergies, gynecological disorders, infertility, and digestive tract disturbances, as well as to aid postoperative healing and to ease the side effects of Western cancer treatments.

### CHARLES'S STORY

Charles, age sixty-six, came to the clinic with severe shingles with intense pain. He was taking massive doses of painkillers, hadn't slept through the night in months, and had taken a disability leave from work. He had already tried acupuncture with a Western physician to no avail.

At my clinic, we used electrostimulation in addition to a treatment called Surrounding the Dragon, which is designed specifically to remedy syndromes producing symptoms such as shingles.

"The needling feels good, like someone rocking you," Charles reported.

After the first treatment, Charles was pain-free for six hours—the first relief he'd had in two months. After three treatments, he cut his use of painkillers dramatically, and he was able to sleep through the night. After one month of daily treatments, he was able to come every other day, then twice a week, and finally once a week. Charles went off painkillers completely.

Acupuncture and Clear Heat Chinese herbs, in conjunction with topical applications of vitamin E and white flower oil, reduced Charles's skin and nerve irritation and pain.

"I'm considering going back to work now," Charles said.

# COMMONLY ASKED QUESTIONS

Here are some of the most common questions I'm asked about acupuncture.

**Q:** Does acupuncture hurt?

**A:** It shouldn't hurt to have the needles inserted, but there can be a slight pricking sensation when the needle first goes in. When there is a great deal of muscle tightness, spasm, or Qi Stagnation, the sensation may be more intense.

Once the needles are in place, the sensations range from none to tingling or a sense of wavy, pulsing turbulence. Again, there should never be any pain that feels wounding.

On occasion, the sensation of Qi moving can seem overwhelming, and some people request that a treatment be abbreviated, but even that is unusual. Most commonly, there is a sense of deep relaxation and a kind of floating quality.

**Q:** How do you know where the points are?

**A:** The acupuncturist can determine where to place the needles through a combination of several factors. Years of study and practice make the knowledge second nature. Each point also has identifiable anatomical landmarks or measurements. Acupuncturists can also sense the points, which is experienced by practitioners in different ways. Some feel an emanation of energy while others feels indentations or little mounds. Each point is different in its character. For example, on the back of your hand at the crook between your thumb and first finger, about ½ inch (1.3 cm) from the edge, is Large Intestine 4 (L.I.4). If you take your index finger from your right hand and circle slowly about ¼ inch (6 mm) above the skin near the crook of your thumb, you will be able to feel the energy center for that point.

**Q:** Is there blood?

**A:** Bleeding is infrequent with acupuncture, although if someone has lots of small veins and capillaries close to the surface of the skin, it is more likely.

**Q:** Is there any risk of disease transmission?

**A:** There is no more risk of transmission of disease through acupuncture than there is through getting a flu shot with a sterile hypodermic needle. The use of sterile disposable needles in a sanitary environment makes acupuncture a completely safe procedure. Just like other medical procedures, the standard of practice is that needles are sterile before being inserted.

**Q:** What are the risks?

**A:** The risks are minor. According to the Mayo Clinic's website:

*The risks of acupuncture are low if you have a competent, certified acupuncture practitioner. Possible side effects and complications include:*

- *Soreness: After acupuncture, you might have soreness, minor bleeding, or bruising at the needle sites.*

- *Organ injury: If the needles are pushed in too deeply, they could puncture an internal organ—particularly the lungs. This is an extremely rare complication in the hands of an experienced practitioner.*

- *Infections: Licensed acupuncturists are required to use sterile, disposable needles. A reused needle could expose you to diseases, such as hepatitis.[9]*

The important point is that you want to use a licensed qualified practitioner who is in compliance with all rules and regulations and has common sense to understand any risk involved. The reality is there are extremely few organ punctures and no instances of verified infection transmission reported in the United States.

Unlike Western medicine procedures, there have been no verified deaths from acupuncture reported in the United States. Broken needles are rarely reported. For people who worry, in my forty years of practice, I have never had a needle break.

## World Health Organization's Recognized Applications for Acupuncture

In a report in 2002 from the World Health Organization (WHO), *Acupuncture: Review and Analysis of Reports on Controlled Clinical Trials,*[10] WHO analyzed all controlled clinical trials through 1998. It has listed the following symptoms, diseases, and conditions that have been shown to be treated effectively by acupuncture.

There have been a number of controlled clinical trials that have tested the effectiveness of acupuncture therapy in specific diseases or disorders, and the report classifies these results into four categories:

- Diseases, symptoms or conditions for which acupuncture has been proved to be an effective treatment (such as hay fever, headache, and hypertension)

- Diseases, symptoms, or conditions for which the therapeutic effect of acupuncture has been shown but for which further proof is needed (such as insomnia, obesity, and cancer pain)

- Diseases, symptoms, or conditions for which there are only individual controlled trials reporting some therapeutic effects, but for which acupuncture is worth trying because treatment by conventional and other therapies is difficult (such as color blindness and deafness)

- Diseases, symptoms, or conditions for which acupuncture may be tried—provided the practitioner has special modern medical knowledge and adequate monitoring equipment (such as coma, coronary heart disease, and paralysis)

The full report, including a complete list of diseases and disorders, can be found on-line at http://apps.who.int/iris/bitstream/10665/42414/1/9241545437.pdf.

# MOXIBUSTION

Moxibustion uses burning herbs, from the mugwort plant, placed on or near the body, to stimulate specific acupuncture points. This warms the Channels and expels Cold and Dampness, creates a smooth flow of Qi and Xue, strengthens Yang Qi, prevents disease, and maintains health.

For hundreds of years, moxibustion has been partnered with acupuncture or used alone as a modality. According to the Chinese text *Introduction to Medicine*, "When a disease fails to respond to medication and acupuncture, moxibustion is suggested."

There are many forms moxibustion. A great modern book that describes all types of Chinese moxibustion treatment is *Moxibustion: A Modern Clinical Handbook*.[11] The two basic forms of moxibustion we use in my clinic are the cone and the stick. If directed by your practitioner, you can use both of them for self-care at home. Your practitioner can supply you with loose moxa or moxa sticks.

You make a moxa cone by compressing the herb mixture, known as moxa wool, into a cone about the size of the upper part of your thumb. The cone is then burned on the body. One of the most common applications is to the navel, where it is effective in relieving abdominal pain and diarrhea and in easing excessive sweating, cold limbs, and a flagging pulse. When moxa cones are burned on other parts of the body, the effect is to ease disharmonies in Channels and Organ Systems associated with those points.

## Using Moxa Cones

Before using moxa at home, discuss this treatment with your practitioner to make sure it is the correct treatment for you.

At home, never place the moxa cone directly on your skin!

Make three cones. Place each one firmly on a slice of dry aconite about ⅛ inch (2 mm) thick and set it within arm's reach. Aconite is a special herb your practitioner can give you or you can buy from an herbalist. It may be toxic if ingested, but perfectly safe when used with the moxa cone. Instead of aconite, you may use a slice of fresh ginger about ⅛ inch (2 mm) thick that you have pierced with four or five small holes. *Note:* The ginger tends to spread the heat more than the aconite, and because it is damp, it doesn't offer as much insulation, so if you are using ginger, be especially careful not to burn your skin.

Lie down. Place a piece of clean cotton somewhere on your torso so you can retrieve it quickly if need be.

Put 2 tablespoons (30 g) of salt in your navel and tamp down until smooth and flat. (If you have an "outie," the Chinese texts suggest taking a long, wet noodle and forming a circle around the navel to contain the salt.)

Pick up the aconite (or ginger) with the cone on top. Light the cone—from the top if you want it to burn cooler and more slowly; from the bottom (don't light the aconite or ginger) if you want it to burn hotter and more rapidly. In my clinic, we light both the top and the bottom for even warmth. Place the aconite (or ginger) with the moxa on top of it over the salt.

If, as the moxa burns, it becomes too hot, gently lift the moxa and aconite (or ginger), slip the piece of cotton cloth over the salt, and set the aconite (or ginger) and moxa back in place.

Let the moxa burn down. If it still feels too hot, remove the aconite (or ginger) and cotton. Let the salt cool. Repeat three times. When you're done, save the aconite; brush off the salt. Throw away the ginger and cotton.

To place moxa cones on other points, skip the salt and use a piece of cotton topped with a slice of ginger or aconite.

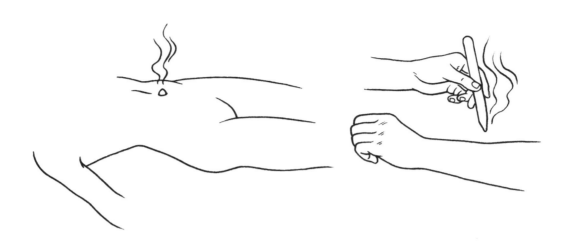

## Using Moxa Sticks

Moxa sticks, which are the size of a big cigar, are available pre-rolled from your practitioner or an herbalist. When lit, they are used like wands by circling their burning ends over various acupuncture points. This method is particularly effective in treating painful joints and chronic problems, such as painful periods, hernias, and abdominal pain.

To use a moxa stick, mark the acupuncture points you want to heat with a small dot. Light the stick with a match and let it burn until it begins to smoke. Holding it in the middle, bring the burning tip 1 inch (2.5 cm) from the skin. Hold your other hand next to the skin so you can feel if it gets too hot. (This is especially important if you are performing moxa on a partner.) Move it slowly in a clockwise circle over the point. If it feels too hot or the skin becomes too red, pull back in ½-inch (1.3 cm) intervals until it feels warming but not burning. Repeat until the area feels bathed in warmth, you can sense the Qi flowing from that spot, and you feel relaxed.

### WARNING

To extinguish moxa sticks, don't use water or try to smash out the fire because if you do, they burn down and can't be reused. The best method is to cut off the supply of oxygen by wrapping the moxa in a piece of aluminum foil or placing it in a small glass container or bottle and completely closing the top. You can also ask you practitioner for a moxa snuffer, which is a special tool we use in the clinic to hold moxa sticks.

## When to Avoid Moxibustion

Moxa is contraindicated for Heat and Excess disharmonies or when there is a fever. Furthermore, at home pregnant women should avoid moxa on the abdominal and lumbo-sacral areas, although practitioners may use moxa in a clinic during pregnancy. Those with numbness in their arms, legs, feet, or toes or who suffers from narcolepsy should not do moxa on themselves. No one should do moxa in bed.

## Where to Apply Moxibustion

Moxa is performed over acupuncture points or areas of the body that need warmth or tonification. The following acupuncture points can be used for moxibustion treatment.

**Ren 6:** Located three fingers below the navel, tonifies Deficiency, tonifies Qi, strengthens the Kidney, and is good for gynecological disorders.

**Ren 8:** Located in the navel, tonifies Yang, warms the abdomen, strengthens Qi, and is good for all types of diarrhea and Coldness.

**Stomach 36:** Located four fingers below the knee, near the bone on the outer side of the leg. This is a major Qi point on the body, and it tonifies and regulates Qi, harmonizes the Stomach and the Spleen, and is good for digestive disorders and lack of energy.

**Spleen 6:** Located four fingers above the bone that sticks out of the inner ankle, known as the Three Yin Meeting Point, it tonifies the Spleen, Kidney, and Liver and is good for gynecologic and digestive disorders.

**Ren 12:** Located halfway between the navel and the tip of the sternum, effective in dispelling Dampness and treating digestive problems associated with Cold.

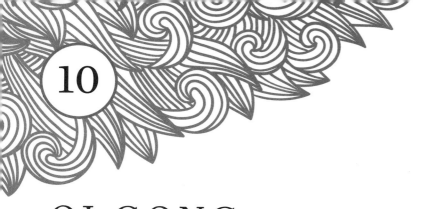

# 10

# QI GONG
## Chinese Exercise and Meditation

Wholeness = Dietary Guidelines + Herbs + Acupuncture + **Qi Gong**

Exercise/meditation is the fourth pillar of Chinese medicine therapy. Without its Qi-balancing effects and benefits to mind/body/spirit, wholeness cannot be achieved.

I recommend Qi Gong to many of my clients as part of a total program. (Some of my clients prefer Yoga or other forms of exercise instead.) Qi Gong can be very important to the process of restoring harmony. For people who are not particularly interested in exercising, it offers you immediate gratification—you feel good right away—without having to go through a painful aerobics routine, joining an overcrowded health club, or spending money on equipment. If you are an exercise enthusiast, Qi Gong offers you many of the health benefits of running or weight training—without the risks. Also, Qi Gong does what other forms of exercise cannot do: It strengthens and harmonizes the flow of Qi.

Many people come into my clinic suffering from the fanatic pursuit of Western exercise: sore muscles, bruised bones, twisted ankles, sore backs, tension, and stress. These frequent injuries occur in part because the concept of exercise has become distorted. Feel the burn. Bop 'til you drop. No pain, no gain. We battle to make our bodies look like the modern ideal—which has little or nothing to do with genuine healthfulness. We compete with one another for glory, prestige, and ego gratification. This notion of exercise often injures the mind/body/spirit; it makes us sore and exhausted instead of agile and refreshed. For some people, it damages the Qi by reducing energy. They end up feeling generally fatigued overall. For other people, exercise has become a kind of poison to the system instead of an expression of the joyous unity of mind/body/spirit.

In contrast, Qi Gong exercise/meditation is a unified process dedicated to creating balance, strength, agility, and grace that assures vitality through old age. Qi Gong and its relatives, Tai Chi and some martial arts, have evolved as the logical outcome of the Tao and recognition that the body is infused with Qi, which must be nurtured and tended to if wholeness is to prevail.

Historically, many different groups have used Qi Gong. The pragmatic followers of Confucius found the manipulation of Qi to be an aid in managing the demands of the world at large. Taoists thought of Qi Gong as a way to empower their pursuit of immortality and self-improvement. Buddhist monks, relying heavily on meditative/breathing techniques, used Qi Gong to help them escape the confines of earthly woes and to increase strength. A Shaolin monk developed the first text of muscle-training routines in the sixth century, when he became alarmed by the physical weakness of his fellow monks. His *Yi Jin Ching* (Muscle Development Classic) laid out ways to use concentration to develop Qi and increase circulated Qi—and Kung Fu was born.

Eventually, many Chinese schools of thought and practice embraced the concept of working with Qi to increase mental, spiritual, and physical powers. Today, millions of people practice various forms of Qi Gong throughout China and the world.

Following is an introduction to several of the basic techniques, in hopes that you will integrate them into your exercise routines, expanding your definition of physical fitness and experimenting with ways of combining Eastern exercise with Western sports activities. Your expert guide is Larry Wong,[1] an accomplished practitioner and teacher.

# QI GONG 101: UNDERSTANDING THE CHINESE CONCEPT OF EXERCISE/MEDITATION

### by Larry Wong

Welcome. I am Larry Wong, and I am going to introduce you to what I know of the arts of Qi Gong. I urge you to keep in mind that there are many approaches to Qi Gong. Each one provides far-reaching health benefits. I will share only a few of those with you. But that doesn't mean that one method is inherently better than another. With Qi Gong, you may learn the principles and gain the benefits from any number of approaches.

## What Is Qi Gong?

Qi Gong, which combines meditative and physically active elements, is the basic exercise system within Chinese medicine. Qi Gong practice is designed to help you preserve your Jing, strengthen and balance the flow of Qi, and enlighten your Shen. Its dynamic exercises and meditations have Yin and Yang aspects: The Yin is *being* it; the Yang is *doing* it. Yin exercises are expressed through relaxed stretching, visualization, and breathing.

Yang exercises are expressed in a more aerobic or dynamic way. They are particularly effective for supporting the immune system. In China, Qi Gong is used extensively for people with cancer.

Qi Gong's physical and spiritual routines move Qi energy through the Twelve Primary Channels and Eight Extra Channels, balancing it, smoothing the flow, and strengthening it. Chinese medicine uses Qi Gong to maintain health, prevent illness, and extend longevity because it is a powerful tool for maintaining and restoring harmony to the Organ Systems, Essential Substances, and Channels. Qi Gong is also used for nonmedical purposes, such as for fighting and for pursuing enlightenment.

Anyone of any age or physical condition can do Qi Gong. You don't have to be able to run a marathon or bench press a car to pursue healthfulness and enjoy the benefits. When you design your exercise/meditation practice, you will pick what suits your individual constitution. Some of us are born with one type of constitution; some with another. We each have inherited imbalances that we cannot control but with which we must work. That's why for some people it is easier to achieve balance and strength than it is for others. But whatever your nature, Qi Gong can help you become the most balanced you can be.

Qi Gong is truly a system for a lifetime. That's why so many people over age sixty in China practice Qi Gong and Tai Chi. The effects may be powerful, but the routines themselves are usually gentle. Even the dynamic exercises—some of which explode the Qi—use forcefulness in different ways than in the West. The following are some effects of Qi Gong.

**Maintaining health:** Qi Gong helps maintain health by creating a state of mental and physical calmness, which indicates that Qi is balanced and harmonious. This allows the mind/body/spirit to function most efficiently, with the least amount of stress.

When you start practicing Qi Gong, the primary goal is to concentrate on letting go, letting go, letting go. That's because most imbalance comes from holding on to too much for too long. Most of us are familiar with physical strength of muscles, and when we think about exercising, we think in terms of tensing muscles. Qi is different. Qi strength is revealed by a smooth, calm, concentrated effort that is free of stress and does not pit one part of the body against another.

**Managing illness:** It's harder to remedy an illness than to prevent it, and Qi Gong has powerful preventive effects. However, when disharmony becomes apparent, Qi Gong also can play a crucial role in restoring harmony.

Qi Gong movement and postures are shaped by the principle of Yin/Yang: the complementary interrelationship of qualities such as fast and slow, hard and soft, Excess or Deficiency, and External and Internal. Qi Gong uses these contrasting and complementary qualities to restore harmony to the Essential Substances, Organ Systems, and Channels.

**Extending longevity:** In China, the use of Qi Gong for maintaining health and curing illness did not satisfy those Buddhists and Taoists who engaged in more rigorous self-discipline. They wanted to be able to amplify the power of Qi and make the internal Organ Systems even stronger. This arcane use of Qi Gong was confined mostly to monasteries and the techniques have not been much publicized. One of the most difficult and profoundly effective techniques is called Marrow Washing Qi Gong. Practitioners learn to master the intricate manipulation of Qi—infusing the Eight Extraordinary Channels with Qi, and then guiding the Qi through the Channels to the bone marrow to cleanse and energize it. The result, according to religious tradition, is that monks can extend their life span to 150 years or more. The Taoists have a saying, "One hundred and twenty years means dying young."

Although few if any of us can devote our lives to the stern practices of the monks, the health benefits of Qi Gong certainly do improve the quality of life of everyone who practices it.

**Waging combat:** Around 500 CE, in the Liang Dynasty, Qi Gong was adopted by various martial artists to increase stamina and power. For the most part, the breathing, concentration, and agility were assets to the warriors and improved their well-being.

**Attaining enlightment:** Buddhist monks who use Qi Gong in their pursuit for higher consciousness and enlightenment concentrate on the Qi Gong's ability to influence their Shen. Mastering Marrow Washing allows the practitioner to gain so much control over the flow of Qi that he or she can direct it into the forehead and elevate consciousness. The rest of us can enjoy the influence of Qi Gong on our Shen, but at a lower level.

Whatever reason you use Qi Gong, the practice should raise your Qi to a higher state if you increase concentration, practice controlled breathing, and execute the Qi Gong routines.

## The Basic Techniques

Here are the basic Qi Gong techniques.

**Concentration:** Concentration leads to and results from Qi awareness, breathing techniques, and Qi Gong exercises. It is a process of focusing in and letting go at the same time. Focusing does not mean that you wrinkle up your forehead and strain to pay attention. Instead, through deep relaxation and expanding your consciousness, you are able to create a frame of mind that is large enough to encompass your entire mind/body/spirit's functions, yet focused enough to allow outside distractions, worries, and everyday hassles to drift away.

This inward focus that expands outward to join you with the rhythms of the universe epitomizes Yin/Yang. Yin tends to be more expansive, and Yang more concentrated. You discover your Yin/Yang balance by treating Yin and Yang as ingredients in a recipe: Add a bit more Yin, toss in a dash of Yang to make the mixture suit your constitution or circumstances. Some people need more or less Yin or Yang, depending upon the situation. Extending the Qi exercise on page 183 provides a clear demonstration of how you can practice establishing your balanced blend of Yin and Yang.

You will find that as you do exercise/meditation you become more adept at this form of concentration, because it is the natural expression of the practice. As you learn to concentrate more effectively, you will find you have greater power to affect Qi through the various Qi Gong exercises in this chapter or through the use of other focused meditations and Tai Chi.

**Breathing:** In the sixth century BCE, Lao Tzu first described breathing techniques as a way to stimulate Qi. From there, two types of breathing evolved: Buddha's Breath and Taoist's Breath. Both methods infuse the body with Qi and help focus meditation.

- Buddha's Breath: When you inhale, extend your abdomen, filling it with air. When you exhale, contract you abdomen, expelling the air from the bottom of your lungs first and then pushing it up and out until your abdomen and chest are deflated. You may want to practice inhaling for a slow count of eight and exhaling for a count of sixteen. As you breathe in and out, imagine inviting your Qi to flow through the Channels. Use your mind to invite the Qi to flow; you want to guide the flow, not tug at it or push it.

- Taoist's Breath: The pattern is the opposite of above. When you breathe in, you contract your abdominal muscles. When you exhale, you relax the torso and lungs.

## Qi Gong Routines

There are two basic types of Qi Gong activities: Wei Dan (external elixir) and Nei Dan (internal elixir). Both focus on strengthening and balancing the Qi by using dynamic routines and still postures, but they approach the tasks in two different ways.

## WEI DAN

This practice focuses exercises on the muscles to build up your Qi until it becomes so concentrated that it overflows and runs out from where it has collected, through the Channels, and into all parts of your body.

In dynamic, moving Wei Dan exercises, muscles are tensed and released over and over again with complete concentration. The tension should be as light as possible because tension causes Stagnant Qi, which is the very antithesis of what you want to accomplish. In fact, it is often suggested that you simply *imagine* that you are tensing the muscles. After several minutes, the generated Qi warms the muscles.

Typical routines that use dynamic, moving Wei Dan exercises include the Dan Mo or Muscle/Tendon Changing Classic. In this routine, you slightly tense or imagine you are tensing isolated limb muscles, such as your forearm, your palm, your wrist, your biceps, your shoulder, and then relax completely. Concentration and breath control are vital components of the process.

There are other moving Wei Dan routines that call for moving legs, torso, and arms into specific positions to relax or massage the Organ Systems. For example, you may extend and stretch your arms over your head, hold and relax, thus massaging the Lung Channel and Lung Organ System more enthusiastically than with the less mobile Dan Mo style.

In the still Wei Dan exercises, muscle groups are targeted but not tensed. For example, hold your arms fully extended, palms down, out to the sides of your body. Don't tighten muscles, but hold that position for at least a minute—building up to longer—until the arms begin to shake or feel warm. When you let your arms fall to your side and relax, shrugging your shoulder muscles and shaking your hands gently, the accumulated Qi is sent coursing out through the Channels. In this manner, Qi is stimulated at various locations in the body by continual muscular exertion combined with concentration.

Wei Dan practice is relatively simple to learn, and it provides immediate benefits. But it is not a lesser form of Qi Gong. Even masters of the more arcane processes use Wei Dan for its Qi strengthening powers.

Qi can also be stimulated to a higher state through acupuncture, acupressure, and massage, which are considered Wei Dan exercises.

NEI DAN

This is a more demanding, less easy to master, and more time-consuming form of Qi Gong. It uses mental powers to direct Qi through the Channels. You must have a teacher to guide you and to help you avoid the potential risks associated with doing the practice incorrectly.

In one Nei Dan exercise, you concentrate Qi on the Dantien (below the navel) and then disperse it through the body using the powers of the mind. Qi may travel in the following three pathways:

- **The Fire Path:** In the Fire Path, you build Qi in the abdomen through breathing and/or thought, and once it accumulates sufficiently, you direct it with your mind along the two Extraordinary Channels known as the Conception Channel and the Governing Channel: This is known as the Small Circulation.

The next level is to move Qi through the remaining six Extraordinary Channels. This is called the Grand Circulation.

- **The Wind Path:** In the Wind Path, Qi moves in the opposite direction as it did on the Fire Path.

- **The Water Path:** In the Water Path, Qi moves through the spine and is used in Marrow Washing to prolong life and increase enlightenment.

## The Qi Gong Class

This is a beginning class, designed to help you become sensitive to the positive benefits of Qi Gong and to prepare you for taking classes with a teacher who can guide you through the learning process. One word about teachers: Make sure you find one who has a watchful eye, is compassionate, can perceive your individual blocks, and can direct you to exercises and routines that release those blocks. Not all great masters make good teachers. A teacher must be able to do Qi Gong well and also communicate effectively.

The first part of class is devoted to improving your awareness of tension and blocks in your body, so you can shed unnecessary stress. If you practice Qi Gong without letting go of blocks and tension, it will impair your practice, and your Qi will not flow evenly or as well as it can.

The next step is to begin to be aware of your internal organs and to tune into the flow of Qi throughout the body. Then you're ready to explore breathing exercises and basic Qi Gong routines.

As you travel through these steps, remember that Qi Gong is a process of building awareness. However you are comfortable doing the routines is what's right for you at that time.

## WARM-UP EXERCISES (10 TO 15 MINUTES)

**Exercise One: Gentle Sway:** For five minutes, move both of your arms from your shoulders in a gentle swinging motion. The motion itself is initiated from your waist: Twist from the waist as though your torso were a washcloth that you were wringing out. Don't twist from the knees or you may harm them. Furthermore, twisting from the waist provides a massage to the internal organs and provides you the full benefits of the exercise.

To get started, move your arms side to side across your torso, and then back to front. Keep your knees slightly bent. Let your hips sway. Allow your mind to clear. At first, focus on the release of unnecessary and unconscious stress. After several weeks, you may shift your focus so that you think only about the swaying of your arms and the motion of Qi.

This introduces you to the concept of being mindful of the present, much the same concept as found in Zen walking.

**Exercise Two: The Bounce:** In the beginning, try this for one to three minutes.

With your feet parallel and about shoulder's width apart, bounce with your knees loose and your arms hanging at the sides like a wet noodle. They should feel empty and neutral. This is the zero position for your arms. When you are bouncing back and forth, your arms in zero should get a nice jiggling effect.

Keep your shoulders natural; neither pull them back or let them slump forward too much. When the zero position is used on the whole body, you should receive a feeling of deep relaxation and your internal organs and skin should hang down. This process brings awareness of internal tension so that you can do something to dispel it, if you choose.

The combination of exercises one and two gently massages and tonifies the Organ Systems, which helps promote longevity.

## QI AWARENESS EXERCISES

**Exercise One: Accordion:** In this, you feel the Qi by using your hands like the bellow of an accordion or a bicycle pump.

Close your eyes halfway. Clear your mind and concentrate your attention on your palms.

Allow your breath to become slow, easy, without force. In a way, you are creating the very lightest trance.

Bring your hands together, palms touching and fingers pointing upward. The palm chakras, called Laogong, located in the center of the palms, should be touching. These chakras are areas where Qi can be felt emanating from the body.

Slowly move your hands, keeping the chakras aligned. When they are about 12 inches (30 cm) apart, slowly move them together using the least amount of physical effort possible. You will be compressing the air between them like an accordion would.

Feel a warm or tingling sensation at the Laogong points on your palms.

Move your hands slowly back and forth, varying the range of the bellows. Repeat the accordion technique in different directions: horizontally, vertically, and diagonally.

This exercise cultivates Qi, builds awareness, and sensitizes yourself. When you feel Qi for the first time, it changes your mind-set.

**Exercise Two: Making the Point:** Using your index finger is a powerful way of directing Qi. If you are right-handed, use you right index finger; if you are left-handed, use your left index finger. Point it directly at the flat palm of your other hand. That hand should be perpendicular to the floor with your fingers pointing straight up.

Use your index finger like a paintbrush to swab back and forth across your palm. Begin with your fingertip about 8 inches (20 cm) from your palm. Slowly move it closer and farther away, swabbing all the time.

You may feel a tickling sensation, a cooling, or a warming of your palm.

**Exercise Three: Extending the Qi:** If you have Deficient Qi, you should perform this exercise with your eyes half closed to cultivate and accumulate Qi.

If you have Stagnant Qi, the exercise may be done with your eyes fully open. You will inhale swiftly through your nostrils with your eyes open or half closed when you exhale.

*Note:* You should exercise caution when practicing Qi exercises at home—without a teacher nearby—because they are powerful, and Qi can leak out your eyes.

Once you can sense the Qi, exercise your intention (which is the mind/spirit part of the exercise) and use your mind to move your Qi out from your body, expanding the zone in which you are comfortable. You may allow the Qi to drift out on the exhalation and then hold it there as you inhale.

First move the Qi into an orbit 1 inch (2.5 cm) from your skin. In increments of 6 inches (15 cm), move it outward, aiming for 3 feet (91 cm), but find the point where you are comfortable with it. Then bring it back in until it returns close to your body.

This exercise allows you to communicate with your Qi. By increasing the distance away from your body that you can feel Qi, you expand your area of comfort—your field of generosity—in the world around you. You will have less fear and greater abilities. By being able to bring your Qi halo in to skin level (or inside your skin) you may become more centered, calm, and self-assured. When you have learned to be comfortable expanding and contracting your Qi, you will feel stronger, healthier, and more in harmony internally and externally.

**Exercise Four: Pumping the Qi:** This is a tricky exercise that moves the Qi along the two connecting Extraordinary Channels: the Du Mai and Ren Mai. You may think of it as evolve, devolve, because your posture goes from a slumped, gorilla-like stance to an upright extended pose. It is adapted from the Wild Goose Qi Gong routine.

The first position pushes the Qi down. As your hands push flat down, your spine and head straighten upward. Then as you allow the Qi to flow back upward, your hands rise, elbows bent and palms parallel to the floor. Your shoulders hunch. Repeat this six or seven times, inhaling as your hands come up and exhaling as your hands go down.

When you are comfortable with this exercise, you may combine it with a slow intentional walk forward: left knee bent and raised in an exaggerated stepping motion. When your knee comes up, your hands go down and back and your spine straightens; when your foot touches the ground, your hands come up and your back hunches. Place your feet very gently on the ground and allow each step to proceed in slow motion, at a tempo that soothes and relaxes. Remember to maintain a breathing pattern, too. Inhale as your hands come up and your shoulders hunch. Exhale slowly, expanding your chest as you straighten your back. If this feels awkward, don't despair. Even in a classroom situation, it takes a while to catch on to what to do.

**Exercise Five: Blending Qi:** This exercise should help you become aware of various resonations of Qi and learn to blend them into a harmonious flow.

Stand with your feet a shoulder's width apart, with your knees slightly bent. Allow your hands and arms to hang at your sides.

Shift your weight slightly to the balls of your feet. Simply be aware of the front side of your body. Concentrate on the Channels that pass along the front of your legs and torso, the top of your hands and arms, and your face.

After one minute, shift your weight to your heels. Become aware of the back of your body: the back of your head, your arms, your spine, and your legs. With practice, you may hold these postures for up to five minutes or longer.

You can also do this for the left and right sides of the body.

In each instance, you may want to become aware of each section of the body. For example, the side of your head, the side of your arm and torso, your outer hip, the side of your leg and ankle, and the length of your foot. This makes the exercise a meditation.

Now, shifting to a more Nei Dan form of Qi Gong, repeat the first three steps, but the motion should not be detectable visually. Use your mind to shift your weight forward and backward, feeling your Qi flowing along the front and back of your body.

Next, try to feel your Qi flowing along your back and front simultaneously.

Students are often bewildered by the idea of feeling two sensations at the same time, but a useful analogy is to think of the color yellow and the color blue. When you blend those two colors together, you produce green. That green then becomes its own entity with its own wavelength. The same is true of blending the Qi from your front and from your back. The blend becomes another entity with its own resonation.

## Breathing Exercises

Breathing can direct Qi through the body like the wind filling the sails of a ship. Breathing exercises can invigorate or sedate, depending on how you use them.

On alternate days, practice the following routine, using Buddha's Breath and Taoist's Breath breathing techniques. (See both "Buddha's Breath" and "Taoist's Breath" on page 179.)

Sit on the floor with your legs crossed in lotus or cross-legged style. This is important so that Qi does not enter and become Stagnant in the lower body, but follows the breathing path through your torso and your head.

**Inhale** to a count of four to eight, depending on what you are comfortable with. For Buddha's Breath, extend your belly, filling it up from the bottom. For Taoist's Breath, inhale, contracting your abdomen, and exhale, letting your abdomen relax outward.

As you inhale, turn your attention to your nose. Guide the Qi downward from your nose toward the Dantien, 1 to 2 inches (2.5 to 5 cm) below the navel. Women should not concentrate on the Dantien during their periods. Concentrate on your solar plexus instead.

**Exhale** to a count of eight to sixteen and move the Qi down the torso, around your pelvic region, and up to your tailbone.

**Inhale** and move the Qi up the back to the top of your shoulders.

**Exhale** and move the Qi up the back of your head and back to your nose.

If you cannot feel the Qi clearly, patience and practice will make it more apparent. Once you are comfortable with this practice, you may increase the pace by completing the cycle in one inhalation and one exhalation. On the inhalation, move Qi from your nose to your tailbone. On the exhalation, move Qi from your tailbone back to your nose.

*Thanks again to Sifu Larry Wong for his generosity in sharing his insight, expertise, and practice of Qi Gong.*

# MEDITATION

In this section are meditations that we recommend at Chicken Soup Chinese Medicine.

As a beginner, you want to allow yourself the time and pleasure of learning to meditate. If it feels awkward or if you have difficulty maintaining concentration, take a step back.

Don't set your standards too high. If you expect too much too soon, you disturb your mind/body/spirit and promote restlessness, frustration, and stress. This may defeat the whole purpose of meditation.

Your first goal should be simply to be quiet, relaxed, and comfortable for a few minutes.

Try to meditate in a comfortable environment. As you progress, distractions will become less of a problem. In the beginning, you want to eliminate as many distractions as possible. Choose a quiet room that is not so warm that you fall asleep nor so cold that you tense up. Wear loose-fitting clothing. Turn on meditation music to help block outside noise if need be.

Find a posture that works for you. Not everyone can sit on the floor in a full or half lotus or cross-legged. You may want to lie down, sit in a straight-backed chair, or stand.

Don't eat heavy foods or drink alcohol or caffeine before meditating.

Don't hold on to disturbing thoughts. One of the goals of meditation is to disconnect from worries. If you've had a tough day at work, a disagreement with your spouse, or worries about money, each exhalation of breath is a chance to let a piece of that tension dissipate.

## Qi Meditation

The following is a meditation/visualization that is designed to help you tune into the motion of Qi throughout the Channels and to help in the body's natural process of self-healing.

The first few times you do this meditation, you can have someone read it to you in a gentle, slow voice, cuing you as to the steps. You can also tape this in your own voice and listen to it as you go through the meditation. Eventually, you will be able to go through the steps silently.

Get into a comfortable position. Allow your body to begin to relax. Close your eyes. Close your mouth and place the tip of your tongue against the roof of your mouth. This connects the Yin and Yang Channels and allows for Qi flow.

With your eyes closed, bring your attention to the area around and below your navel; in Japanese it is called the *hara*; in Chinese it's called the *Dantien*. This is one area where Qi is stored.

Allow yourself to begin to breathe into the area. You may use either breathing technique.

As you breathe into your abdomen, into your belly, into the Dantien, notice a warmth from the center of your abdomen, beginning as a small glow and getting brighter and brighter until there is a ball of light filling your abdomen. Allow yourself to feel this ball of light, any color that you'd like.

Now, as you breathe, notice the energy moving up into the area of your heart and opening up into your chest.

Next feel it move to the area in front of your arm, just below the shoulder bone. This energy moves from the area below your shoulder bone, down the outside of your arm all the way to your thumb, on the inside of your thumb. Feel the warmth and the movement of energy down the Lung Channel.

When it gets to the end of the Lung Channel at the tip of the thumb, move your focus over to your index finger, where the Large Intestine Channel begins.

The Qi then moves through your hand, up the outside of the arm, coming up over your shoulder, up the side of your neck, and up to the outside of your nose. Then move to the Stomach Channel that begins below your eye. It flows down the neck, over the front of your body, through your chest, down outside your navel, around your pubic area, then down the outside of your leg, to a very important point, just below your knee, where the energy of the body becomes very strong. It then moves on down across the front of your foot and into the top of your toes, where it meets the Spleen Channel.

The Spleen Channel allows food energy to move through the body and impacts digestion.

Begin inside your big toe, coming up the arch of your foot, in front of your ankle bone, on the inside of your leg, all the way up by your knee, continuing inside your leg, and up the front of your body, curving around your ribs, and ending in your costal (rib) area.

The Spleen Channel then connects internally with the Heart Channel.

The Heart Channel emerges from your heart into the centers of your armpits, moving down the insides of your arms, all the way to your small fingers, where it attaches to the Small Intestine Channel.

The Small Intestine Channel is a very good Channel to help open up the brain.

This Channel runs up your outsides of the arms, coming all the way back up, across your scapulas, up the back of your neck and around your ears, where it ends in front of your ears.

This connects to the Urinary Bladder Channel, the longest Channel, at the insides of your eyes.

From your eyes, the Channel comes up across the top of your head and down the back of your neck, where it splits into two parallel lines, which then extend down your whole back on either side of your spine, connecting the organs together.

The two rows of the Urinary Bladder Channel are side by side, and they connect again at the back of your buttocks, coming down the backs of the middles of your legs through your knees, all the way down your legs, around your ankle bones, and into your little toes.

The Urinary Bladder Channel connects with the Kidney Channel on the very bottom of your feet. The Kidney Channel moves up from your feet, around the insides of your ankles, all the way up the insides of your legs, and up around your navel. And this Channel comes all the way up to the upper part of your chest, where there are some of the most important points in Chinese medicine for meditation and connection with the Shen.

Here the Kidney Channel connects with the Pericardium Channel, which starts in front of your arms, moves down the very middles of your arms, into the palms of your hands, and to your middle fingers, where it then connects with the Triple Burner Channel, the Channel that helps regulate the temperature of your body. The Triple Burner Channel begins on your fourth fingers, comes up over the top of your hands, all the way up your arms and around your elbows, over your shoulders, and up your neck and around your ears, where it connects with the Gallbladder Channel.

The Gallbladder Channel is the most crooked Channel on the body. It zigzags across the top of your head, comes down the back of your neck, across your shoulders, and down the sides of your body, zigzagging again on the sides of your body, and all the way down over your hips and the deepest point in the muscle of your body in your buttocks, then moves down the side of your legs, all the way down to the top of your toes, to the fourth toes.

You pick up the Liver Channel on the big toes. It comes across the top of your feet, and again toward the insides of your feet and around your ankles, up the middles of the insides of your legs by your knees, and all the way up the insides of your legs. This Channel circles the genital area, coming up into your rib cage near the Liver, yet on both sides of your body. And then we return again to the Lung Channel.

Once you have completed the cycle, sit or lie peacefully, allowing yourself time to make your transition back to your surrounding environment in a graceful manner.

## Lotus Blossom Meditation

This is one of my favorite meditations. It is a brief and simple meditation that can be done almost anywhere, any time you feel the need to ease stress or allow your feelings of affection and connection to expand.

Sit peacefully, breathing evenly.

Half close your eyes.

Inhale slowly, filling your body with air.

At the same time, concentrate your attention on the area of the fourth chakra that is located at your breastbone in the center of your chest.

Imagine a beautiful lotus blossom. Its petals are closed, and its scent is but a promise.

As you exhale, see that blossom unfold. The velvety smooth petals extend, reaching out, releasing a beautiful scent.

Inhale and smell the fragrant aroma.

The petals are opening ever further. And as they open, you feel your heart and chest opening up to the world, expanding, relaxing.

You may extend the opening petals as far as you want. Feel your heart open in the same proportion.

When you have arrived at an openness that is comfortable, hold it there as you enjoy the scent of the flower and breathe in and out slowly.

You may practice this meditation concentrating on a chakra, or energy center. Particularly effective are the third chakra, located at the diaphragm, and the second chakra, located below the navel in the Dantien or hara area.

# THE HEALING TOUCH
## Qi Gong Massage and Other Forms of Body Therapy

Massage, whether done solo, with a partner, or by a professional massage therapist, offers the energy of acupuncture, the serenity of meditation, and the spiritual refreshment that comes through being touched. Massage is an important part of your everyday health care routine. Just as you strive to integrate the dietary guidelines from chapter 8 and the exercise/meditation guidelines from chapter 10 into your daily self-care habits, so should you make room for massage as part of the routine you follow to strengthen your immune system and maintain your balance.

In this chapter, we look at Chinese Qi Gong self-massage, self-acupressure, self-ear acupressure, Shiatsu for partners, and Western Reflexology for the foot and hand to do with a partner or by yourself. There are many other forms of massage—such as deep tissue, lymphatic drainage, and Swedish—each valuable for restoring harmony. Although these forms of massage are not presented in detail in this book, you may want to explore them. They can be integrated into your comprehensive programs for preventive care and/or to treat disharmony.

In addition to massage, this chapter offers soaks, saunas, and compresses, to be used for deep muscle relaxation, stress reduction, and pain relief, in conjunction with massage or by themselves.

## QI GONG MASSAGE

Qi Gong massage is an extension of Qi Gong exercise/meditation. Among the more skilled masters of the art, self-massage can be done with the mind, moving Qi and Xue through the Channels, relaxing muscles, and massaging Organ Systems mentally. For the rest of

## WARNING

It is best if you do not perform self-massage or have a massage done to you on any area where you have a skin eruption, a localized infection, swelling, or localized malignancies, or where you've had very recent surgery. Pregnant women should have massage on the abdomen and torso only from a professional massage therapist.

us, manual Qi Gong massage—done on ourselves or with a partner or practitioner—is an important part of any preventive health care program, because regular massage helps nourish the mind/body/spirit and maintains harmony in all systems.

If you exercise three or more times a week, go through the complete Ten Step Qi-Xue Self-Massage once a week. Use the specific self-massage routines for hand, ear, head, or foot as you feel the need.

If you are sedentary, have an injury that's preventing you from exercising, or simply find you're stuck at a desk and cannot exercise for a given period of time, do the foot and head massage every other day and practice the Ten Step Qi-Xue Self-Massage once or twice a week. You will help prevent the formation of disharmonies in the flow of Essential Substances and consequent problems in the Organ Systems.

The benefits of Qi Gong massage include working on the Channels to improve circulation of Essential Substances, particularly Qi and Xue; dilation of the blood vessels; stimulation of the lymph system and elimination of wastes and toxins; improved muscle tone; relief of stress and promotion of relaxation and sleep—and it just makes you feel good.

## Ten-Step Qi-Xue Self-Massage

Based on the flow of the Essential Substances through the Channels and Organ Systems, this massage series provides you with a complete relaxation and rejuvenation routine. You may use all or any part of it any time you feel the need of a little repair work and a bit of TLC.[1]

Establish a slow, rhythmic pattern of breathing while doing self-massage. Inhale slowly for the count of three and exhale slowly for the count of six. As you become more comfortable with this entire series of exercises, try to inhale every time you change the position of your hands and exhale while you massage yourself. The count will give you an even tempo.

## STEP ONE: GENERAL HEAD MASSAGE

Massage promotes general relaxation and the harmonious flow of Qi and Xue. It is particularly good if you are suffering from chronic sinusitis, respiratory allergies, temporomandibular joint disorder (TMJ), headaches, and anxiety or depression.

Using your middle fingers, massage the bridge of your nose on both sides. Complete five circular rubbing motions, moving from the top to the outside, down toward your nose, and then into the point above the inside corner of your eye.

Move your hands up from the bridge to the top center of your forehead.

Spread your hands apart, with the fingers of your right hand moving down to the right temple and fingers of the left hand moving down to the left temple. Massage the temple in a circular motion five times.

Move your hands up to the top of your head and bring them down to your neck. Rub the back of your neck up and down, along the tendons that extend on either side, five times.

Move your hands to the outside of the neck until you can feel the lower point of your jaw joint. Rub that five times.

Now move your hands back to the bridge of your nose and in a smooth motion trace the outline of your eyebrows to your temple and then move your hand down to the hollow of your cheek. Repeat this motion three times.

Slowly rotate your head around, stretching your neck so your right ear is almost touching your right shoulder. Then slowly shift your head to the front so your chin is touching your chest. Then swing your head to the left so the left ear is almost touching the left shoulder. Now move it slowly toward the back. Look up at the ceiling. Repeat three times, then reverse direction and repeat again.

## STEP TWO: EYE MASSAGE

To improve the circulation of Qi and Xue and improve visual clarity, you want to direct Qi to your eyes.

Place your index and middle fingers on the inside points of your eyebrows. Massage in a circular motion five times.

Move your fingers to the outer corner of your eyes and rub gently.

Move your fingers down from the corners of your eyes to the top of your jawbone. Then move the fingers slowly down the length of your lower jaw until they almost meet at your chin.

Place your palms together and rub them back and forth across each other until they become quite warm. Cup your hands over your eyes to share your hand Qi with them. Do not touch your eyes.

## STEP THREE: GENERAL EAR MASSAGE

Use of general ear massage tonifies the whole body—every Organ System, the joints, and all body parts—and keeps your hearing healthy.

If you are wearing large earrings, take them off. Using your two middle fingers, gently rub around the entire ear several times.

Place your thumbs inside your ears and your fingers along the widest part of the ear flap. Now pull gently outward so the thumb moves from the inside to the outer edge of the ear. Hold for a count of three. Repeat three times.

Take each ear lobe between your thumbs and forefingers and rub gently, pulling downward.

Place your palms over your ears and massage the entire ear. Repeat five times.

Press your palms against your ears and then remove quickly.

Shake out your hands and fingers. Sit quietly for two minutes.

## STEP FOUR: NECK MASSAGE

This moves Qi and Xue along the spine.

Sit with your back straight and your head tipped ever so slightly forward.

Place your hands together in a prayer position. Open your fingers and then curl your fingers, allowing them to interweave. Spread your palms apart so your fingers are lying across the backs of your hands and both palms are parallel to the floor.

Place your hands like a cradle against the back of your skull. Your thumbs should be pointing straight down on either side of your neck.

Massage the tendons beneath your thumbs from top to bottom. Repeat five times.

Raise your thumbs up slightly to catch the point at the base of your skull where the bone meets the neck. Rub back and forth along this ridge. Go very slowly, probing the area, feeling where you want to apply more or less pressure. When you find the spot that is particularly tender to the touch, hold your thumb there for a slow count of six. Exhale while holding the point. Repeat as many times as you like.

## STEP FIVE: TORSO MASSAGE

This step and the following one are important for anyone who wants to keep the Lung System clear and the Heart Xue flowing smoothly. The steps are particularly helpful for digestive problems, asthma symptoms, and congestion.

Open your palms. Place them on the front of your neck. Moving your hands from your neck to the front of your body, glide over your chest with long smooth strokes of your open palms. Repeat several times.

Cross your arms. Using your first and second fingers, massage a point about 2 inches (5 cm) above the center of each nipple. Circle your fingers on the right hand over your left nipple; your left hand over your right nipple. You may feel your lungs open up.

Placing your palms flat on each side of your torso (left hand on left side, right hand on right side), move the Qi (from the point above your nipple that you just massaged) to the side and bottom of your lungs. Massage in a smooth flat motion to the side of your torso and then down to your diaphragm.

## STEP SIX: QI UP, QI DOWN

Place the tips of the fingers of your right hand on the pectoral muscle by the crook of your left arm.

Move your fingers in a circular motion, tracing a 3-inch (7.5 cm) circle from the top of your chest moving inward, down, to the outside and back up to the top. Repeat this, creating a spiral shape vertically down a line through the nipple. As you go in this direction (only!) move your hand down the full length of your torso.

Repeat the massage using the tips of your left-hand fingers on the right side of the torso. Make sure that you move your fingers from the top of your torso, toward your breastbone, then to your toes, and finally toward your arm.

## STEP SEVEN: ABDOMINAL MASSAGE

This technique is helpful for anyone with digestive problems, PMS, or cramps, and it helps harmonize the Large Intestine, Small Intestine, Liver, Spleen, Stomach, and Gallbladder. You may want to use oil infused with cinnamon to warm your belly if it is generally Cold during your period or if you have loose stools and abdominal cramps due to Cold.

Lie on a flat, firm surface. If needed, place a small pillow under your knees to take strain off your lower back.

So there is less distraction, close your eyes halfway. Inhale slowly and deeply.

Place your right palm on your stomach, above your navel, with your thumb lying against the skin pointing toward your chin. Place your left hand so it is on top of the right.

Breath in and out slowly, feeling the warmth under your hands. (If you are left-handed, place your left hand on your stomach first.)

Rub your stomach gently in a clockwise motion. Repeat twenty to forty times.

Raise your hands up to the lower edge of your rib cage on either side of your torso. Smoothly massage down the length of your lower torso into the pelvic area and the groin. Repeat five times.

Now move your hand to the center of your abdomen below your navel. Repeat the motion as above.

Sit facing forward; inhale. Turn your head and neck, but not your torso, and look over your left shoulder. Exhale. Now inhale as you turn your head and neck and look over your right shoulder. Exhale.

Take your right hand and place it along your waist on the left side of your body. Inhale. As you exhale slowly, move your palm forward along your waistline toward your navel. Reverse.

With your palm open and flat, rub the front of your lower torso over your hip bones and down onto the tops of your thighs. Use one long, slow motion.

Return to the first position with your right hand over your stomach and your left hand on top of the right. Slowly, gently, rub in a clockwise motion for the count of six. Breathe in on the count of three and out on the count of six. Keep your eyelids at half-mast.

## STEP EIGHT: CIRCULATING THE LOWER QI AND XUE

To promote harmonious flow of Qi and Xue, a complete massage keeps the motion going from your head through your feet in a complete cycle. (If you aren't going to give yourself complete massage but are stopping after the abdomen, take time to do a couple of leg swings and stretches given in the Qi Gong exercise chapter starting on page 175. If you are going to complete the massage cycle, remain seated with your feet flat on the floor about 8 inches [20 cm] apart.)

Sit on a firm, un-upholstered, but comfortable chair without arms. Sit with good posture, but not stiffly. Rub your inner thighs with the same circular motion that you applied to your torso, always moving in a circle that goes from the top of the thigh (twelve o'clock), down the outside toward nine o'clock, and up through six and three o'clock. Spiral down your thighs to your knees. Repeat three times.

Using your thumbs, press gently but firmly on the top center of your thighs and draw your thumbs down to your knees. If you feel any tender spots, stop at that point and gently vibrate your thumb back and forth. Repeat three times.

When you come down to the top of your knees for the last time, hold your thumbs in place and put your fingers across the center of the kneecaps. Rub gently. Then rub your hands down the outside of your calves, from top to bottom (but not back up) five times.

Cross one leg over the other so your calf is in easy reach and lying parallel with the floor.

Place your fingers in the ridge that is formed between the near side of your shin bone and the calf muscle. Slowly move your fingers down from your knee to your ankle. Press with a firm steady motion. If any point is tender, move your fingers in a circular motion on the point. Go from the top to the bottom. Repeat as desired with your other leg.

STEP NINE: GENERAL FOOT MASSAGE

In Chinese medicine, the feet play a crucial role in the functioning of the Channels. They are also associated with the harmonious balance of the Organ Systems and Essential Substances.

To help promote smooth flow of Qi and Xue and keep the Channels working smoothly, you can give yourself a general foot massage, rubbing each part of the foot, starting with your ankle and ending with your toes. Devote extra effort to rubbing your toes and pay attention to the areas between your toes and between the long, thin bones that run along the top of your foot. Foot massage oil can provide an extra soothing touch. Use peppermint-infused oil if you are Hot, and use cinnamon-infused oil if you are Cold.

As you rub your feet, you may want to target several acupuncture points for acupressure. Particularly important points to rub include:

**Kidney 1:** Directly in the center of each foot right below the ball is an important point to help keep the Kidney System working harmoniously, which impacts the functioning of all the other Organ Systems.

**Spleen 4, Liver 3, and Gallbladder 41** are also important foot points to help harmonize Qi and the Organ Systems. (See the illustration on page 206 for their locations.)

STEP TEN: ARM AND HAND MASSAGE

After your arms and hands have worked hard massaging the rest of your body, it's their turn to be pampered.

An arm massage should be done from your shoulder to the tips of your fingers in long, slow strokes along the inside and the outside of your biceps and forearm. Rub between or along the bones, rather than on top of them.

After you extend the Qi through your arm, return to the acupuncture point, Large Intestine 14, at the outside of the biceps below the armpit, the crook of the elbow, and the back of the wrist. On these points, press slowly and evenly. Breathe deeply.

A general hand massage can be done with your thumb moving in a gentle clockwise motion from your wrist to your fingertips, concentrating on the tissue between the bones and the areas around the knuckles and fingertips.

Once you've covered the entire surface of the hand, pull each finger out gently and rub the last section of your finger at the tip. Shake out your hands.

## ACUPRESSURE MASSAGE

Acupressure massage uses the thumb and hands to stimulate the acupuncture points along the Channels. If you are massaging someone else, to gain maximum effect without hurting yourself or straining your hand, use the following guidelines:

- Work the points with the soft, padded part of your thumb—where your thumbprint is.
- Press down firmly and smoothly.
- Don't jab or stab at a point.
- Always brace your thumb with the rest of your hand and fingers. For example, if you are massaging a point on your thigh, place your hand flat along the skin. Move your thumb into position, leaving the rest of your hand in contact with your leg. Press with your thumb. For more pressure or better leverage, don't pick up your hand. If you are massaging someone else, raise yourself up over her or him and press downward. If you are massaging yourself, lean into the pressure.

### For Alertness

**Stomach 36** is located four finger widths from the hollow made when the knee is bent (below the kneecap) on the outside of the leg and one finger width over from the crest of the shin bone. Stimulating this point is also good for digestive problems, boosts energy, and is said by the Chinese to help strengthen the immune system. Stomach 36 was known in the old days as *Three Miles*, because when people hiked or walked to the point of exhaustion, if they stopped and rubbed that point, they were able to go 3 miles (4.8 km) more.

**Large Intestine 4** is located in the webbing between the thumb and index finger. Press into the hollow against the bone from the index finger that extends down the length of the back of the hand. This point is also good for any problems above the neck, such as sinus problems and headaches. It is also beneficial for general inflammation, constipation, and diarrhea.

## For General Health and Immune System Support

**Stomach 36** is located four finger widths from the hollow made when the knee is bent (below the kneecap) on the outside of the leg and one finger width over from the crest of the shin bone.

**Large Intestine 4** is located between the thumb and forefinger in the middle of the forefinger bone that goes from the knuckle to the wrist.

**Liver 3** is located at the point where the bones of the big toe and the second toe meet and form a V. The point is slightly in front of their junction.

**Lung 7** is located 1½ inches (3.8 cm) above the transverse wrist crease on the back of the hand. It is above the large bump on the outside of the wrist bone.

**Kidney 3** is located on the inside of the ankle in the depression between the tip of the ankle bone and the Achilles tendon.

## For Low Back Pain

**Kidney 3** is located on the inside of the ankle in the depression between the tip of the ankle bone and the Achilles tendon. This is also good for immune support.

**Urinary Bladder 60** is located midway between the ankle bone on the outside of the leg and the Achilles tendon, opposite Kidney 3.

**Urinary Bladder 40** can be found in the center of the back of the knee. Points across the back of the knee correspond to the lumbar (lower back) vertebrae, so massage the entire crease. It is also good to massage down from Urinary Bladder 40 to Urinary Bladder 60.

**Du 26** is located one-third of the distance between the bottom of the nose and the center of the top lip, in the slight indentation. This is known as the emergency point, and it is used if someone loses consciousness. For acute back pain, stand up and hold on to the back of a chair with one hand. With the other, press relatively hard on the point with your fingernail while you move the back gently in and out of the area of pain by swaying your hips and torso.

**Pericardium 7** is in the middle of the wrist crease on the inside of the arm. It is also good for irregular heartbeat and tachycardia.

## For General Pain

**Pericardium 6** is located on the inside of the wrist three finger widths above the wrist crease, between the two bones. Also good for anxiety, nausea, and morning sickness.

**Pericardium 6 with Triple Burner 5.** Triple Burner 5 is located three finger widths above the wrist crease on the top of the arm between the two long arm bones. Press Triple Burner 5 and Pericardium 6 at the same time for extra relief. This is good for carpal tunnel problems. These points are regulating points, and they enhance overall calmness.

**Ren 17** is located between the nipples at the center of the chest. It is used to release grief and improve breath by regulating Zong Qi. It is also the area that holds the Ancestral Qi.

**Yintang** is located between the eyebrows in the center of the bridge of your nose. It is used to ease pain and release tension. It is good for headaches and overall relaxation.

## For the Shoulder

**Triple Burner 4** is found on the top side of the wrist at the midpoint of the wrist crease, between the two arm bones.

**Triple Burner 5** is located three finger widths above the wrist crease on the top of the arm between the two long arm bones.

**Small Intestine 3** is located in the indentation below the little finger knuckle on the outside of the hand. It is good for the neck and shoulders. If you have a stiff neck, rotate your neck in and out of the area of stiffness while pressing the point. It is also good for clearing the mind.

## For the Mid-Back

**Liver 3** is located at the point where the bones of the big toe and the second toe meet and form a V. The point is slightly in front of their junction.

**Gallbladder 40** is in the hollow indentation just to the front of the outside ankle bone.

## For Gynecological Problems

**Spleen 6** is located four finger widths above the tip of the inside ankle bone behind the shin bone.

**Ren 4 and 6:** Divide the line that runs from the navel to the pubic bone into five equal sections. Ren 4 is three sections below the navel. Ren 6 is one and a half sections below the navel.

## Deep Touch Head Massage

To ease tension, calm the Shen, and stimulate the harmonious flow of Xue, you may want to perform a Deep Touch Head Massage. Use your two middle fingers or thumbs. Always move your hands upward and to the outside, down to the low point, and then upward along the inside. This massage is also effective for smoothing out wrinkles produced by tension.

First, wash your face with a mild cleansing solution. If you like, apply a gentle cream or oil that will not irritate your eyes.

Begin on the eyebrows (Point 1) and run your thumbs slowly and evenly the length of the brow from the inside to the outside.

Move to the lower orbit and rub around each eye, along the bone, moving from the outside, underneath to the inside, and then to the top of each eye.

On your cheek, target the four points on the diagram on page 201 and gently move your fingers out from those points to the edge of your ears. Repeat five times.

On your jaw in front of your ear at Stomach 7, rub downward to Stomach 6 and then along the jawline to your chin. Repeat three times.

Massage your ears by starting at the lobe, working your way around the rim, and moving into the center and then back out to the rim.

Move your two middle fingers to the center of your forehead at the hairline. Rub your right hand clockwise and your left hand counterclockwise.

Move to your neck at Gallbladder 20 and Urinary Bladder 10. Press gently and firmly on those points for the count of five. Release. Rub with your fingers flat, moving your hands in a circular motion.

Moving your hands around to the tops of your shoulder blades (Gallbladder 21 and Triple Burner 15), rub smoothly and deeply.

Lie back with eyes closed and keep your breathing slow, steady, and deep.

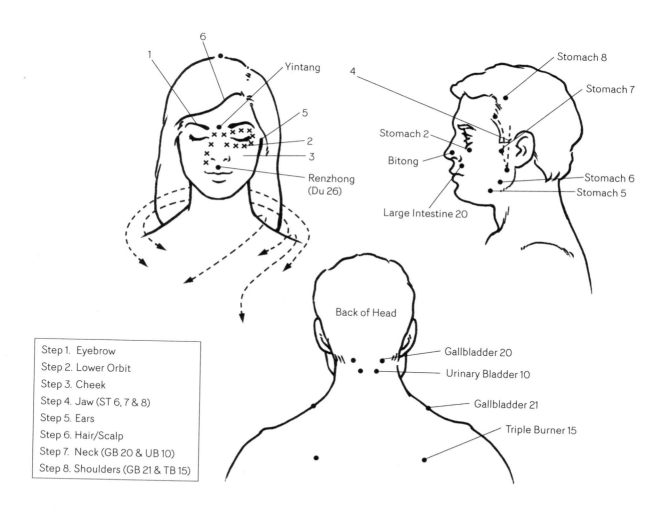

Step 1. Eyebrow
Step 2. Lower Orbit
Step 3. Cheek
Step 4. Jaw (ST 6, 7 & 8)
Step 5. Ears
Step 6. Hair/Scalp
Step 7. Neck (GB 20 & UB 10)
Step 8. Shoulders (GB 21 & TB 15)

## Lower Back Self-Massage

Much low back pain comes from Stagnant Qi and constricted muscles and tendons. This massage allows you to gently stretch them out and ease discomfort.

Sit on a chair with your feet flat on the floor about 6 inches (15 cm) apart.

Inhale. Roll your chin down to your chest as you exhale. Bend your back and drop your shoulders forward as you inhale. Continue downward until your chest is resting on your thighs as you exhale.

Make two fists. Bring your hands up behind your back.

Make circles with your hands all over your lower back.

Press deeply along the spine as far up as you can reach.

With loose fists, pound lightly along your lower back and hips and on either side of your spine. To increase the benefits, use the pounding motion to massage Large Intestine 4, an acupuncture point that is located in the webbing between the thumb and the index finger. Stimulating this point helps invite the low back pain to move downward from the back and disperse.

Let your arms and hands dangle at your sides.

Slowly roll back up, using your arms to help by walking them up your legs. Keep your chin tucked in and upper back rounded until you are sitting upright. Then let the spine straighten from the bottom up.

## Amazing Ear Massage

If the eyes are the windows to the soul, then the ears are the road maps. Located in the external part of those two little organs are acupuncture points that provide a direct route to all of the important functions of the mind/body/spirit.

Ear acupuncture points can be as powerful—or even more so—than points located on the Channels. For example, the three "no smoking points," known as Shenmen, Sympathetic, and Lung, are extremely effective in promoting nicotine detoxification.

To rub ear points, you may use your finger or a cotton swab or you can purchase an ear massage probe online or at a natural health store. Don't worry about touching other points. You'll be able to tell when you're in the right position. Ear points become very sensitive and tender when there is a disharmony in the corresponding part of the body.

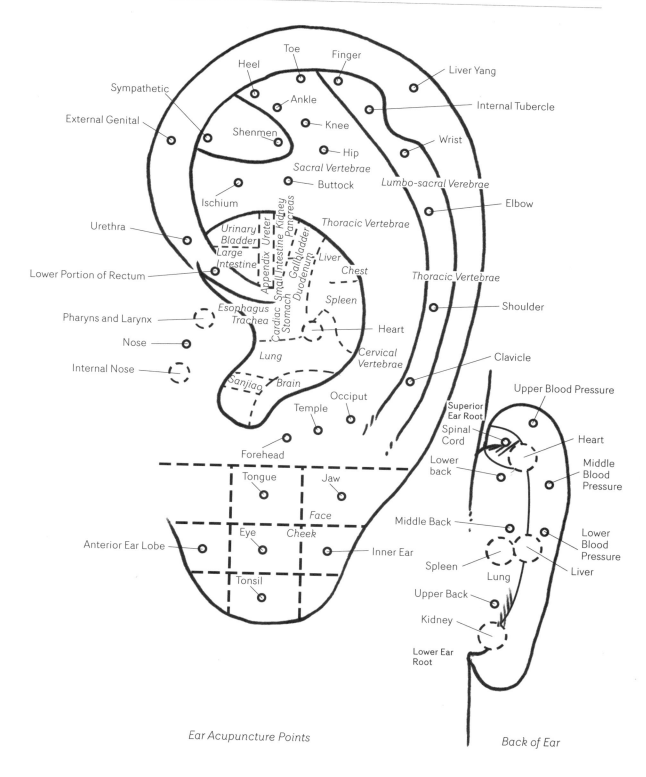

*Ear Acupuncture Points*

*Back of Ear*

### Shiatsu Partnered Massage

Japanese Shiatsu works by exerting deep pressure on the acupuncture points of the body, and it can be used to harmonize the Essential Substances and the Organ Systems and to relieve muscle pain and tension. (Acupressure massage is explained on page 197.)

The Shiatsu massage described here is adapted from the Shiatsu form I was taught by my wonderful teacher, Koichi Nakamura, O.M.D., L.Ac., in New York City in the early 1970s. That is where I began my forty-year practice of Asian medicine. For several years, I taught this form to acupuncture and Shiatsu students as part of their school curriculums. Over the years, I adapted the form to encompass new ways of teaching and new methods.

The following massage cycle provides a complete stimulation of all the Channels. You may extract sections from it to address specific body parts or enjoy the whole. A complete massage should take about fifty minutes. When you're through, you'll discover that it is as beneficial for the person doing the massage as it is for the person receiving it.

Proper breathing is important for both the person giving and for the person receiving the massage. Long, slow breaths with even slower exhalations help tranquilize the mind/body/spirit and assist in the smooth flow of Qi.

#### PREPARE FOR MASSAGE

Have the person receiving the massage lie on his or her stomach on a comfortable but firm surface, such as an exercise mat or plush carpet. Do not do this massage on a bed (which is too soft) or standard massage table.

#### BEGIN MASSAGE

The person who's giving the massage kneels at the person's left side, waist high.

**Spinal stretch:** Place your right hand on the lower back of the person, with your fingers pointing toward her or his toes. Place your left hand on the upper part of the back, with the heel of your hand just below the vertebra that protrudes below the bottom of the neck, at the top of the spine.

Gently rock the person's body from side to side. Then, holding your right hand in place, stretch the spine upward by softly applying an upward pressure to the heel of your left hand. Continue gently rocking the body as you stretch the spine.

Now move your hands so that your right hand is on the person's right hip and your left hand on their left shoulder blade. Stretch and rock. Then reverse sides and repeat.

Move your left hand, palm down, to the area between the shoulder blades and place your extended right hand, palm down, on top of your left hand.

Raise up slightly on your knees for more leverage and begin pushing around—but not directly on—the spine as you move your hand down toward the lower back. Work down to the tailbone and back up.

Leave your left hand between the shoulder blades and place your right hand on the tailbone and do another spinal stretch while gently rocking the body.

**Leg stretch:** Have the person adjust the legs so the toes are pointing slightly inward. Place your left hand on the back of the right leg along the crease between the thigh and the buttock. Cup your right hand over the right heel. Stretch the leg and rock it gently. Repeat on the left leg. Again, raise up on your knees if you need more leverage or to apply more pressure.

**Back to the back:** Now the person giving the massage should stand up and straddle the person receiving the massage, placing his or her feet alongside the person's hips and facing forward. Never sit on the person because it constricts blood flow and tightens muscles. Bending over the person, use both hands to press down on the area just to the right and the left of the spine. Don't press directly on the spine. Work the inner and outer Urinary Bladder Channel (see page 206).

Now slip your hands under the person at the hip bones and gently raise her or him up a little bit off the floor. Release the person and then press down gently on the sides of the back up from the hip bone.

Use your thumbs, supported by your fingers, to press and release as you massage out from the spine over the back above the hip bone.

Move the thumbs to press along the length of the tailbone. Then go to the buttocks and smoothly press along the outside, the middle, and the inner section of each cheek from the lower back to the top of the thigh.

Take a break, shake your hands, and do several shoulder shrugs.

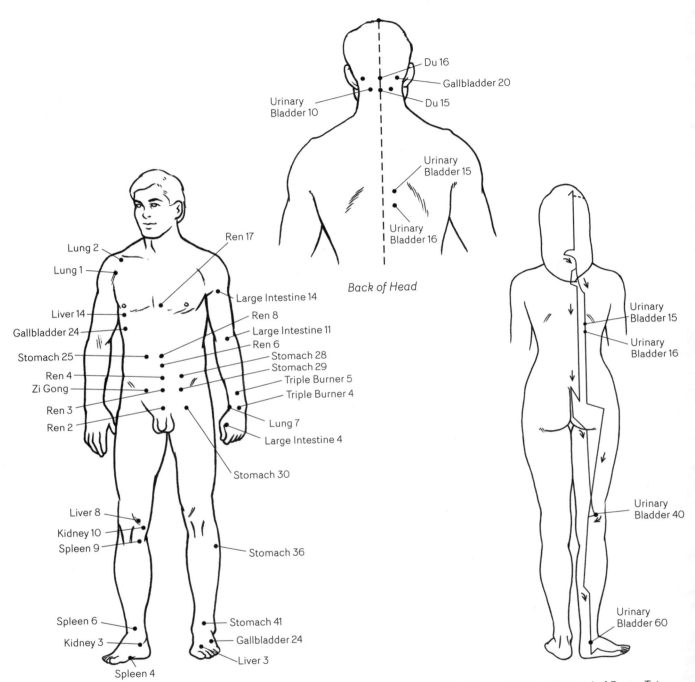

Du 16
Gallbladder 20
Urinary Bladder 10
Du 15
Urinary Bladder 15
Urinary Bladder 16

*Back of Head*

Lung 2
Lung 1
Ren 17
Liver 14
Gallbladder 24
Stomach 25
Ren 4
Zi Gong
Ren 3
Ren 2
Large Intestine 14
Ren 8
Large Intestine 11
Ren 6
Stomach 28
Stomach 29
Triple Burner 5
Triple Burner 4
Lung 7
Large Intestine 4
Stomach 30
Liver 8
Kidney 10
Spleen 9
Stomach 36
Spleen 6
Kidney 3
Stomach 41
Gallbladder 24
Liver 3
Spleen 4

*Acupressure Points in Shiatsu Massage*

Urinary Bladder 15
Urinary Bladder 16
Urinary Bladder 40
Urinary Bladder 60

*The Urinary Bladder Channel of Foot—Taiyang*

ARM MASSAGE

Now move the person's left hand up behind him or her so the back of your hand is resting against the lower back.

Take your thumbs and, beginning with the lower back, press them into the area between the spine and the ribs. Move up toward the left wing bone. Press with your thumb or thumbs in the area below and under the wing bone. Slip the edge of your hand under the bone and pull the wing bone up and out.

Find the point in the middle of the wing bone where there is a slight indentation. Press firmly but gently on that spot.

Move the person's left arm so it is horizontal to the body. Holding his or her wrist in both hands, gently pull the arm out from the shoulder, shaking it slightly. Let the arm lie flat, extending it in a comfortable position out from the body.

Massage the upper left arm using both of your hands. Then hold the left wrist in your left hand and use your right thumb to massage down the Triple Burner Channel (see page 164). Then use your thumbs to work on the Large Intestine Channel (see page 163).

Bend the arm and locate Large Intestine 11 at the spot on the outside of the arm where the crease from bending the elbow ends (see page 206). Massage. Then work down the forearm with both of your hands.

Flex and extend the wrist. Work Large Intestine 4 (see page 206).

Turn the person's hand over, and using both thumbs, rub the palm of the hand from below the fingers to the wrist.

Pull and slightly twist the fingers.

Shake out the wrist and arm.

Move to right side of the person and repeat on the other arm.

LEGS AND FEET MASSAGE

Kneel at the person's left side. Make sure her or his toes are pointed slightly inward.

Put your left hand under the person's right knee and lift it up slightly. Place your right hand flat on the back of the knee and press gently, massaging the crease at the back of the knee.

Work the right calf with both hands, combining your thumbs and the flat of your hand.

Concentrate on Kidney 3 and Urinary Bladder 60 (see page 206).

Lift the leg and support the knee while turning the foot out. Place your right hand on the person's ankle. Use your left hand to rub the length of the Gallbladder Channel (see page 167) between the muscle and bone along the outside of the leg.

Then stretch the calf with one hand on the back of the knee and the other on the heel.

Switch to the other leg.

Sit cross-legged at the person's feet and place the feet in your lap.

On the right foot, press on Kidney 3 and Urinary Bladder 60 (see page 206). Then work the heel with both of your thumbs and move down to the center of the foot, through the arch. Stop at the big toe and massage the area and Stomach 41 (see page 206). Move to the top of the foot and work the spaces between the bones and tendons, Liver 3 (see page 206). Massage the toes and pull out gently from the foot.

Rotate the foot to stimulate the ankle. Then slap the bottom of the foot and stretch the foot one more time. Let the feet rest gently on the mat.

Massage the other foot.

## SHOULDER AND NECK LIFT

Have the person flip over onto his or her back. Place a small pillow under the person's knees to ease tension on the small of the back if necessary. Kneel or sit cross-legged at his or her head.

Place your hands under the person's shoulders along the shoulder blades. Draw the fingers of your left hand up along the person's spine to the head. Hold the head with your fingers resting on the bony ridge at the top of the neck and the base of the skull.

Use your right hand to massage the neck.

Rub Du 15, Du 16, and Gallbladder 20 with your left hand and thumb at the base of the skull (see page 206).

Cradle the person's head in both of your hands and turn it slowly from side to side and back and forth. Ask the person to inhale deeply. Then as he or she exhales, take the head and neck and ever so gently move it up and forward, stretching the back of the neck and moving the chin onto the chest. Release down slowly and carefully. Repeat.

## HEAD, EARS, AND FACE MASSAGE

With the person's head resting on the mat, move your hands to the ears and begin scratching lightly all around and behind. Then using your thumb and index finger, work the ear from the outer rim into the well. (For more extensive ear massage information, see page 202.)

Move to the scalp, rubbing vigorously. When you are finished, pull the hair gently.

Place one hand under the head, holding the lower part of the skull. Place your other hand so it is grabbing the person's chin. Gently pull the head out from the neck. Hold for a few seconds. Release gently. (For a detailed face massage, see page 200.)

## ABDOMEN MASSAGE

Rub the Ren Channel, starting at Ren 17 on the breastbone between the nipples (see page 40). Move to the ribs above the breastbone, using your thumbs to move from the center outward on both sides of the chest. Work Lung 1 and Lung 2 (see page 206).

Rub the stomach above the navel with both of your hands going clockwise. Use a rocking motion, alternating between the fingers and the heel of your hand. Move your hands down to the area below the navel. Focus on Ren 4 and Ren 6 (see page 40).

Hold your hands about 1 to 2 inches (2.5 to 5 cm) above the hara (or Dantien) area. Feel the flow of Qi.

## LEGS MASSAGE

Sit along the left side of the person. Starting at the top of the thigh, take the left leg in both of your hands and work your thumbs down the leg toward Stomach 36 (see page 206). Bend the person's left leg and draw his or her knee over toward your lap. Do not force it.

Use both of your hands and thumbs to work the Liver Channel that runs along the inside of the leg. Work Liver 8 and Kidney 10 along the calf (see page 206).

Straighten the leg out and squeeze along the top of the thigh to the knee. Massage the kneecap.

Move both of your hands alongside the shin bone, working the points on either side of it from the knee to the ankle.

Repeat on other leg.

## FINISH

Help the person sit up.

Stand behind him or her so your knees support the back.

Lean over and work your thumbs into the tops of the shoulders. Remember to brace your thumbs with your hands; don't jab. Then squeeze along the shoulders, working from either side of the neck out to the shoulders and down the arms, squeezing all of the time.

Pound the back and shoulders with your fist or open hand.

Breathe deeply, and shake out your hands.

Say thank you to the person.

# WESTERN MASSAGE TECHNIQUES

## Self and Partnered Hand Massage

Hand reflexology is a Western form of hand massage that correlates specific parts of the hand to internal organs and body parts as they are described in Western medicine. All hand massage can be done to yourself or by a partner.

To massage your hand using reflexology points, identify the location of your disharmony or disease in terms of Western anatomy and find the corresponding area for that body part on the chart. For example, if you hurt your knee jogging, use the hip and knee area on the chart. If you have irritable bowel syndrome, use all of the colon areas. If you have headaches, use the head area on the chart. If you have uterine cramps, use the womb area on the chart.

Use your thumb to rub the appropriate spot and use your fingers to hold the hand firmly but gently. Press with your thumb gently until you feel sensitivity, pain, or tenderness. Using the flat part of your thumb, draw it across the spot, rotating it gently in a clockwise motion. To use two thumbs, place them side by side on the appropriate area of the hand and draw them out and down in opposite directions, rubbing one in a clockwise and the other in a counterclockwise motion.

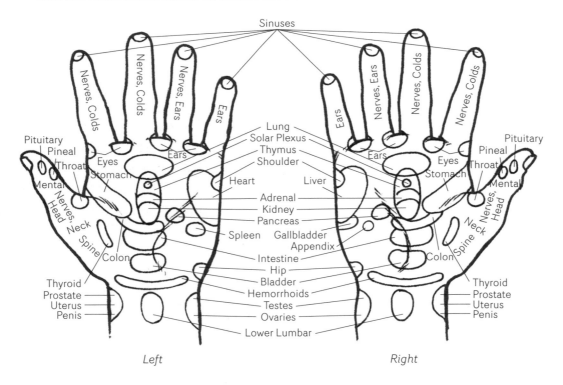

Left                                                    Right

## A REMINDER

For serious medical conditions, use these techniques in addition to medical treatment.

## Self and Partnered Foot Massage

Reflexology also has a system of foot massage that has identified specific points on the foot that correlate to specific internal organs and parts of the anatomy. To massage your foot using reflexology points, use the same technique as describe earlier for hand reflexology.

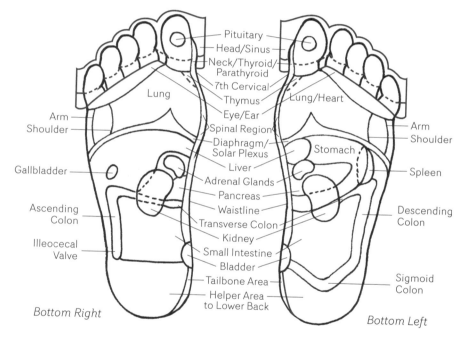

*Bottom Right*      *Bottom Left*

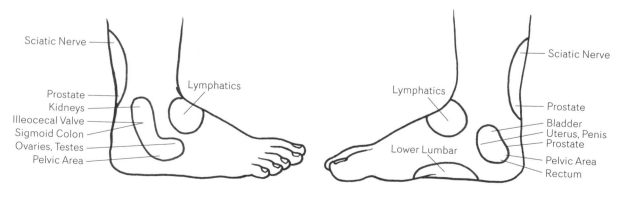

# HOT SOAKS, COMPRESSES, AND COOL SAUNAS

Hot soaks, compresses, and cool saunas can stimulate the flow of Qi and Xue and dispel Cold and Dampness. These immersion therapies should not be assaults on your body, making you turn beet red, sweat profusely, or become overheated. Instead, they should be gentle persuaders that soothe the Shen and calm the mind. They are often used to increase the effectiveness of acupuncture, massage, and herbal therapy.

## Hot Soaks

You may soak your whole body by slipping into a deep tub of water, or you can just dip your hands or feet into a basin. In general, to avoid dehydration, you should soak for no more than thirty minutes. Always drink lukewarm herb tea or room temperature water while soaking. When you get out of a soak, it is important to use a plant-based cream, oil, or moisturizer to seal the skin and prevent dehydration and flakiness. Avoid mineral oils and those that are full of dyes, preservatives, artificial colors, and aromas.

### GENERAL CALMING SOAKS

The following soaks are designed to calm the Shen and pacify the Heart.

### LATTE DELUXE

Because there are fats in milk that are moisturizing, this bath may be helpful for sunburns and to reduce itching and dryness caused by conditions such as eczema and psoriasis.

- 4 cinnamon sticks (omit if you have Heat-related problems or very sensitive skin)
- Bag made from unbleached cheesecloth
- 1 piece natural twine
- 1 tubful hot water
- 2 cups (470 ml) to 1 quart (1 L) whole milk (preferably organic)

Break the cinnamon stick into pieces, place them in the cheesecloth bag, and tie it closed with the twine.

Fill the basin or tub to the top with water from 100° to 106°F (38° to 41°C), depending on your comfort level. You will have to decide what feels good to you.

Stir in the milk. Drop in the bag of cinnamon sticks. Soak for 20 to 30 minutes.

## SLEEP EASE

If you are having trouble relaxing and going to sleep, this is the soak for you.

1 cup (16 g) loose chamomile, or ½ cup (8 g) loose chamomile and ½ cup (8 g) loose valerian

1 large square unbleached cheesecloth

1 piece natural twine

1 tubful warm to hot water

Place the chamomile or chamomile and valerian on the cheesecloth and tie it into a ball, securing it with the twine.

Fill a basin or tub with water. Select the temperature that feels relaxing to you.

Place the cheesecloth in the water and steep it for 10 minutes. Soak for 20 to 30 minutes.

# TO STIMULATE QI AND DISPEL COLD

## GINGER BATH

1 cup (125 g) grated or sliced fresh ginger

1 large square unbleached cheesecloth

1 piece natural twine

1 tubful warm to hot water

Place the ginger on the cheesecloth and tie it into a tea ball, securing it with the twine.

Fill a basin or tub with warm to hot water.

Place the cheesecloth in the water and steep it for 10 minutes. Soak for 20 to 30 minutes.

### THYME AND AGAIN

This bath is especially good if you are having sinus congestion.

1 tubful warm to hot water

2 to 5 drops thyme oil

Fill a basin or tub with warm to hot water. Place a few drops of thyme oil in the water. (Because the intensity of the oil varies, follow the instructions on the bottle.) Soak for 20 minutes. Rinse skin in cool water.

## TO DISPEL HEAT

### PEPPERMINT COOLER

For this soak, if you can buy or grow fresh peppermint, that is the best.

½ cup (48 g) fresh peppermint or other edible fresh mint

½ gallon (1.9 L) water

1 tubful cool water

Boil the mint in the ½ gallon (1.9 L) of water for 10 minutes to make peppermint tea. Using a strainer, strain the tea.

Draw a cool bath and add the peppermint tea to the tub. Slip in and soak until you begin to feel cool. Don't wait to get out until you are cold.

## TO FIGHT PERNICIOUS INFLUENCES

### BLEACH BATH

The following soak may trigger detoxification reactions, such as achy sensations and irritability. These are natural reactions and they are nothing to worry about. The National Eczema Association recommends bleach baths for eczema.[2] Other experts recommend bleach baths for various types of skin infections. However, if you have any negative reactions to bleach, do not use this soak and try others instead. Also, if you have any type of skin infection, ask your physician before using bleach baths. Only Clorox brand without any additives is recommended. If you are doing a cleansing diet, you may want to do this bath along with that.

1 tubful hot water

½ cup (120 ml) plain household bleach without additives, not concentrate (such as Clorox)

Add the Clorox to a hot bath and soak for 10 to 30 minutes.

Shower after bathing to make sure you don't leave a trail of bleach on your carpet or have bleach residue on your skin. Also, make sure that you apply moisturizer after the bath.

Do one soak per week. (Some sources, such as the Mayo Clinic, recommend two or three times per week for people with skin infections if cleared with your doctor.)

### SALTY DOG

Two of these baths a week are effective for muscle relaxation and detoxification.

1 tubful hot water

1 pound (455 g) sea salt

1 pound (455 g) baking soda

Fill a tub with hot water. Add the salt and baking soda to the water. Soak for 10 to 15 minutes. For a stronger cleansing, substitute Epsom salts for the sea salt in the same amount.

## HERBAL FOOT REST

½ cup (65 g) yarrow root

1 basin boiled water

Steep the yarrow in the water. After 5 to 10 minutes, it should be cool enough to slip your feet into the water. Soak your feet for 20 minutes.

### TO EASE DRYNESS

Prepared herbal oils, available at your local herb store or natural food store, can soothe or stimulate and keep your skin supple and smooth. They are a bonus for the senses when added to your soak. Choose those that appeal to you.

## Compresses

Compresses can be either warm or cool. Warming compresses have the advantage of being able to deliver concentrated heat or cool and herbal infusions directly to the spot on your body that needs the attention. Compresses are recommended for chronic and acute stomach problems, gynecologic discomfort, headaches, strains, and sprains. These are the ones we suggest you can do at home. Your practitioner may prescribe other compresses, depending on your constitution and the presence of any disharmonies.

### HOT SPOTS

These compresses are to dispel Stagnant Qi, Cold, and Dampness.

## GINGERLY

⅓ large ginger root, grated or finely chopped

1 square unbleached cheesecloth

1 piece natural twine

2 quarts (2 L) boiled water

Place the ginger on the cheesecloth, roll it into a tea ball, and tie it securely closed with the twine.

Place the ginger in a pan with the water. Boil for 10 minutes. Remove the cheesecloth from the water and set it aside.

Soak a washcloth in the ginger brew and apply it over the troubled area. Repeat until you feel warm and more comfortable.

## QUIET COUGH

½ cup (48 g) peppermint leaves, or ⅙ of a large ginger root, grated or finely chopped, and ¼ cup (24 g) peppermint leaves

1 square unbleached cheesecloth

1 piece natural twine

2 quarts (2 L) boiled water

Place the peppermint on the cheesecloth, roll it into a tea ball, and tie it securely closed with the twine.

Place the peppermint in a pan with the water. Boil for 10 minutes. Remove the cheesecloth from the water and set it aside.

Soak a washcloth in the tea. Apply the compress to the upper chest, breathing in the peppermint aroma.

## TO COOL A FEVER

3 or 4 drops eucalyptus oil

Cool water

Place 3 or 4 drops of eucalyptus oil on a washcloth saturated with cool water. Place on the chest. Breathe deeply. Repeat until the body temperature feels lower.

In addition to these homemade compresses, your practitioner may prescribe special herb compresses for problems such as eczema, psoriasis, acne, bruises, pain, and swelling.

You can also buy readymade compresses and herbal packs that become moist when warmed. You can buy these online or in your local cooperative or natural foods store.

## Cool Saunas

Saunas can hit a devastating 108° to 112°F (42° to 44°C). In Chinese medicine, these temperatures are understood to create disharmony and cause Deficient Qi. In Western terms, they are hard on the heart, skin, and immune system. Cool saunas, on the other hand, offer many benefits. They cleanse the skin (the largest organ in the body), ease nasal congestion, and help the body detoxify through the skin.

Set the sauna temperature for 102°F (39°C). When your skin becomes moist and you feel warmed throughout, gently scrub your skin with a loofah or a soft bristle brush. This gets rid of dead skin and excreted toxins.

# PART THREE

# WHERE THE PATHS MEET

## Comprehensive Healing Programs
## to Maintain and Restore Wellness

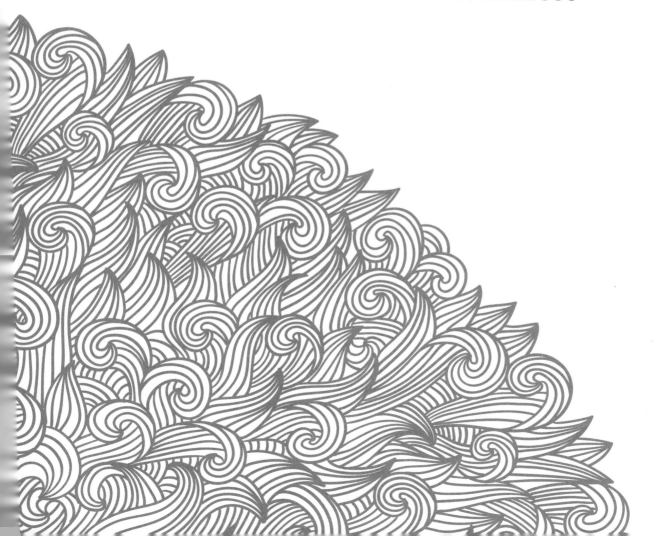

# INTRODUCTION TO NEW CHINESE MEDICINE'S COMPREHENSIVE PROGRAMS OF HEALING

The comprehensive programs in the following chapters are designed for you to use as a guide for your own self-directed healing. They bring together basic Chinese medicine therapies along with other healing arts so you can maintain harmony and treat disharmony in your mind/body/spirit. They are offered to you as plans that you can follow or adopt to suit your personal needs.

Maria is a client who aggressively followed her own comprehensive program and created an enormous difference in her life. When she came to the clinic in June 1994, she was complaining of chest pain, incredible fatigue, and low-level depression. She was so incapacitated that she had to take a leave of absence from her job as a registered nurse.

After examining her, I suspected she might have hepatitis and suggested she go immediately for blood chemistry tests that would reveal the function of her liver. If the levels were abnormal, I needed to know liver enzyme levels along with other lab levels, and she would need to have them retested throughout our treatment.

This way, along with diagnosing her using the traditional Chinese diagnostic procedures, I could follow the reduction in liver inflammation and shape acupuncture therapy to address the changing symptoms of the disease. This is an example of how important it is for Chinese and Western medicine to work together. Each therapy helps the client forge the most effective treatment possible.

Maria's blood work results showed she had elevated liver enzymes. We then tested her for hepatitis C, and the test came back positive for hepatitis C. Immediately she began searching the medical literature to find out about the disease and treatment options.

She said to me, "I'm in charge here. What I want are your suggestions."

My first recommendation was that she consult a liver specialist. Again, it's important that the client receive information about options from both Western and Eastern practitioners. The doctor said he could offer her only one possible remedy, interferon, which at that time had only a 10 to 20 percent success rate. It had many possible side effects, and often the virus returned after treatment.

Maria did not feel taking the medicine was worth the possible serious side effects. She refused Western treatment at that time. Her liver doctor agreed to monitor her while she pursued other therapies.

Maria started with a regular regime of herbs four times a day. She also had other herbs for use when certain symptoms would flare up. She received acupuncture twice a week and followed a strict self-care program of dietary therapy and moxibustion. In addition, she found she was beginning to examine her life from a spiritual side, seeking to eliminate high stress. She began practicing Qi Gong and meditating.

"I'll follow the whole regime for the rest of my life," Maria said. "It's improved my liver and my spirit and mind. I'm clearer and more centered."

When Maria had her initial blood work in June of 1994, two liver enzymes–ALT and AST—were high. After four months of herbal treatments and the full comprehensive program, she was retested.

"Those enzymes dropped forty-seven and fifty-nine units," she recalls. (Normal enzyme levels should be in the teens.) "[My liver] doctor was very impressed. In fact, he tested me three times to make sure of the results. I had also stopped drinking alcohol during that time, and that might account for a ten-point drop but not fifty-nine points. And it's only gotten better. The last time I had liver pain was March of 1995.

"If I met someone who was sick and couldn't find a solution, I'd tell them to try Chinese medicine and other forms of alternative healing," Maria added. "It doesn't hurt, it's not real expensive, and it's working."

As a follow-up, in 2014 Maria was still well. In the year 2000, she moved from San Francisco to rural Colorado. She continued to use all the modalities that she learned in 1994 and expanded her repertoire. She changed her career and has had a fabulous life.

However, with the advent in 2014 of new drug treatments for hepatitis C that do not include interferon and have much higher rates of success, Maria decided to add the Western drug treatment to her arsenal. By the end of 2014, she had cleared the virus from her body!

If you're ready to follow Maria's lead and try a comprehensive program, you may select from the following:

- A Comprehensive Program for Basic Good Health and a Strong Immune System (see page 223)

- A Comprehensive Program for Easing Stress, Anxiety, and Depression (see page 240)

- A Comprehensive Program for Gynecologic Health that includes special sections on PMS, menopausal symptoms, and fertility (see page 249)

- A Digestive Disorders Management Program (see page 288)

- A Comprehensive Program for Liver Support (see page 298)

- Cancer Support: A Comprehensive Approach from Diagnosis to Survivorship (see page 315)

Each comprehensive program contains a section on self-care therapies, including Chinese dietary therapy; Qi Gong exercise and meditation; acupressure, massage, and reflexology; and soaks and compresses. Each program also includes a section on assembling a healing team of health care providers, including Chinese medicine practitioners, standard Western doctors, and a variety of Eastern and Western healers.

# STRENGTHENING ORGAN QI AND PROTECTIVE QI

## A Comprehensive Program for Basic Good Health and a Strong Immune System

New Chinese Medicine offers each of us the opportunity to resist disease by strengthening the basic energy of the body. Combining Chinese medicine's ability to reinforce our Organ Qi and Protective Qi so the immune system can resist assaults + Western medicine's diagnostic technology and helpful medications + alternative therapies, such as Yoga, naturopathic medicine, Shiatsu, homeopathy, Ayurvedic medicine, Western herbs, and aromatherapy = New Chinese Medicine's program for becoming noticeably healthier and stronger.

## PART ONE: SELF-CARE: A SEVEN-STEP PROGRAM FOR STAYING HEALTHY

### Step One: Keeping a Daily Journal

At the core of every comprehensive program is the daily journal. This allows you to keep track of your physical and emotional actions and reactions. You should keep this journal for one to two weeks.

As a result, you will become conscious of the relationship between your daily habits and the way you feel in mind/body/spirit. That may indicate areas of your lifestyle that you want to change to support your Organ Systems, Protective Qi, and immune system.

These changes should be gradual. It's not necessary—in fact, it's not good for you—to make swift and extreme shifts in the way you live, your diet, or your activities. You want to allow your body and your consciousness to grow so that you are comfortable with the changes you make. This is central to the philosophy of balance and harmony in Chinese medicine.

To keep a journal, you may use any form of record-keeping that works for you. Track it in a notes app on your smartphone, iPad, or tablet or do the old-fashioned, tried-and-true approach and buy a small notebook that fits easily into your pocket or handbag. Whatever method you choose, give a copy of this record to your practitioner and Western physician and keep one for yourself. For one to two weeks, keep track of the following:

- Make note of everything you eat and when you eat it. Don't leave out that afternoon glass of juice or late-night snack.

- Write down how much physical activity you get, both formal exercise and in doing your daily chores or job.

- Keep track of your sleep pattern: when you go to sleep, if you awake during the night, and how long you sleep. Include information on snoring, night sweats, tingly limbs, nightmares, and dreams.

- List how much you drink, including water, sodas, coffee, tea, alcohol, and sugared drinks.

- Note the time of day you experience any changes in your blood sugar level, such as a sinking feeling, overwhelming fatigue without other causes, headache, a funny taste in your mouth, inability to concentrate, or a craving for sweets.

- Keep a record of your digestion, elimination, and urination. Note times you feel hungry, bloated, gassy, or constipated, or have loose stools, acid indigestion, or reflux, etc. Also note how often you urinate, the quantity, and what color it is.

- Record any prescription, over-the-counter, or recreational drugs that you take. Make note of the quantity and your reaction both during and after the initial sensation. If possible, note why you took that particular drug.

- Write down your emotions throughout the day, including grogginess or grumpiness in the morning (before you have coffee or tea), highs and lows, and feelings of depression, happiness, calmness, anger, frustration, etc. Try to pinpoint the times they occur and the triggers, if you know.

- Make note of your mental acuity—when you feel clear or unclear.

## Step Two: Implementing a Diet Program

**Review your journal.** After keeping your journal for one to two weeks, take some time to review it. Look for recurring symptoms of disharmony that might be associated with your diet. For example, ask yourself the following questions:

- Do you become bloated, gassy, tired, or grumpy after eating a particular food? Notice also if this happens several hours later or the next day.

- Notice foods that you eat frequently, foods that you have cravings for, and foods that you avoid. Can you associate those foods with physical symptoms of disharmony or mood changes?

- Do your symptoms of disharmony change depending on your meal schedule?

- Do your food-related symptoms change depending on what time of the month it is?

- Is there a correlation between your eating patterns, the amount of alcohol or caffeine you drink, and any symptoms of disharmony?

Once you've examined you daily journal for these and other associations between diet and well-being, you may target certain eating habits that you'd like to change—at least temporarily—to see if they eliminate troubling symptoms of disharmony in your mind/body/spirit.

**Start a cleansing routine.** Now that you've identified those elements of your diet that may be diminishing your ability to fight off disharmony and disease, you may want to give your body a little break. A cleansing diet removes irritants and toxins and soothes the system. The First-Step Diet Therapy (see page 113) can last from one day to one week. If you feel weak or unable to do a Phase, you may shorten it or skip it altogether.

**Use the power of food.** As you build a new approach to your diet, you want to harness the power of food. Chinese medicine considers diet to be the first line of defense against disease, and Western medicine is discovering new evidence almost daily of the relation between nutrition and disease prevention. This association between food and general health is the result of what the Chinese call "Food Energetics." This is the power within food that cools or warms the Organ Systems, dampens or dries the Organ Systems, and regulates the flow of Qi, Jing, and Xue. Keeping Food Energetics balanced is essential to maintaining harmony in Organ Qi and Protective Qi.

To protect the Food Energetics in the food you eat, choose organic foods and hormone- and antibiotic-free meats whenever possible and drink only filtered or spring water to eliminate sources of bacteria, protozoa, other organisms, and chemicals now commonly found in municipal water systems. It is important to use a water filter that eliminates all organisms. Keep fat intake between 20 and 30 percent of calories.

**Eat a balanced diet.** A Chinese medicine balanced diet delivers the right mix of Food Energetics. It includes warm foods, and it doesn't contain too many raw foods. It will include all five flavors. Eat food primarily in season from local sources. Food should be eaten with proper attitude and relaxation. For most healthy people, a three-meal-a-day plan offers the best sustenance. Breakfast should provide a moderate amount of whole grains, vegetables, fruit, and protein. Cooked, warming foods stimulate the Qi. Lunch should be the largest meal of the day, with a wide variety of vegetables, fruit, grains, and proteins in the form of legumes, fish, or meat if desired. For dinner, the smallest meal of the day, you want to avoid stimulating foods, such as a large amount of animal protein and spicy foods.

The traditional Chinese diet recommends 60 to 75 percent of your diet come from grains, vegetables, and legumes. (Of that, grains should account for two-thirds and vegetables and legumes/beans for the other third.) Fruits should be about 10 percent of your daily intake. Protein, including meats, dairy, and all other proteins, should add up to about 20 percent. Glycemic index (GI) and other modern concepts will help you modify these recommendations.

A practitioner will make final recommendations based on your constitution and Chinese diagnoses.

**Enjoy food tonics.** Therapeutic foods that combine Food Energetics with herbal actions tonify the Qi and Xue. Once a week, you may eat a congee made with American ginseng, codonopsis, or red dates or a serving of San Qi or Dang Gui Chicken. (For recipes, see page 121. For more information on how diet can support your immune system and maintain a well-balanced constitution, refer to chapters 6 and 7 on pages 91 and 112.)

## Step Three: Implementing an Exercise and Meditation Plan

Exercise/meditation is as important to a preventive health program as sound nutrition is. It keeps all of the Essential Substances in harmony, and it nourishes the Organ Systems. It also soothes the Shen and keeps the mind clear and alert. To help you figure out how you can use exercise/meditation in your preventive health care program, refer to your daily journal.

First, make note of those days you exercised—what form, for how long, and how you felt before and after. Reflect back and consider: Did some forms of exercise make you feel better than others? Or did you feel better exercising for a shorter length of time? A longer time?

Next, see if there is a correlation between anger, depression, or stress-related moods and maladies and your exercise schedule. Are you tenser when you don't exercise? Do you have more symptoms of disharmony after you don't exercise for a while? Does exercise exhaust you and make you feel blue?

Although each person should exercise to suit his or her Qi—so that Stagnant Qi is not encouraged nor is Qi depleted—a generally well-balanced weekly routine may incorporate a minimum of twenty minutes of exercise/meditation a day. Thirty to sixty minutes of moderate exercise and meditation, three to six days a week, is optimal. Your exercise should be a blend of aerobic movement—such as jogging, cycling, tennis, swimming, spinning, or step classes—as well as Qi Gong, weight-bearing exercises, stretching exercises including Qi Gong and Yoga, and breathing and meditation exercises.

## SUGGESTED WEEKLY EXERCISE/MEDITATION ROUTINE

| DAY 1 | DAY 2 | DAY 3 | DAY 4 | DAY 5 | DAY 6 | DAY 7 |
|---|---|---|---|---|---|---|
| 15 minutes Qi Gong warm-up (page 182) | 1 hour Qi Gong class (page 181) or Yoga | 30 minutes aerobics | 1 hour Qi Gong class (page 181) or Yoga | 30 minutes aerobics | 15 minutes Qi Gong warm-up (page 182) | Rest |
| 30 minutes aerobics | | 30 minutes weight-bearing exercises | | 30 minutes weight-bearing exercises | 30 minutes aerobics | |
| 15 minutes cool-down and meditation | | | | | 15 minutes cool-down and meditation | |

## Step Four: Using Soaks, Saunas, and Compresses

Soaks, saunas, and compresses are all effective ways to calm the Shen and keep the Qi and Xue flowing harmoniously. (See "Hot Soaks, Compresses, and Cool Saunas" on page 212 for details on how to use them for preserving your health.)

Once a week, take a twenty-minute sauna at 102°F (39°C) and/or a soak to help ease stress and eliminate Dampness or Excess. Soaks to stimulate Qi are recommended if you've had a sedentary week.

## Step Five: Using Massage and Moxibustion for Self-Healing

Moxa and many massage techniques can help maintain Organ System harmony and strengthen Protective Qi. (See "Acupuncture and Moxibusion" on page 89 for more information.) All of the various types of massage and bodywork will benefit your health and harmony. For attention to particular trouble spots, use your daily journal as a guide to the type of massage that will benefit you the most. Notice if you have a recurring complaint about neck, shoulder, or back pain and try the routines on pages 193 and 194. If you are bothered by pain with your monthly cycle, try the techniques on page 194. For a complete body massage and general Qi harmony, do the Ten Step Qi-Xue Self-Massage on page 191, and to ease discomfort try the partnered Shiatsu massage on page 204.

Acupressure can calm or invigorate and ease tension. For a listing of acupressure points you can self-massage and the symptoms they address, see page 197. Of particular benefit in a general program are Kidney 3, Ren 4, and Ren 6 (see page 40). Follow the acupressure techniques described for these points on pages 199 and 200. Repeat as often as desired. (*Note:* Unless you are a professional massage practitioner, do not use points below the navel such as Ren 6 during pregnancy.)

Moxibustion can be a regular part of your tonification routine. Use moxa on Stomach 36 one to seven times a week. Once a week, enjoy Spleen 6, Ren 6, and Ren 12. Ren 4 and Ren 6 are particularly good if you have a tendency toward Cold. Gallbladder 39 is especially good for Deficient Xue and often used for people with chronic immune weakness. For details on how to use moxibustion, see page 171. For the locations of the points, see the illustrations on pages 40 and 163 through 167. (*Note:* Unless directed by your practitioner, do not use points below the navel Spleen 6 during pregnancy.)

Ear massage can soothe the whole body. For general well-being, sit in a quiet room. Close your eyes and breathe evenly. Begin a general ear massage, using a gentle rubbing and pulling motion, start with the outer fold where it attaches on the top front of the ear and move slowly around the rim, into the inner cavities, and end with the ear lobe.

The process should take about two to three minutes. Repeat on your other ear. You may also target specific Organ Systems for re-harmonizing (see the ear massage chart and instructions on page 202). For overall rebalancing, massage the ear points called Shenmen, Lung, and Spleen.

## Step Six: Taking Nutritional Supplements

Follow the general supplement plan on page 135. Be sure to take *Lactobacillus acidophilus* because it maintains digestive flora, which are destroyed by antibiotics, hormones, and a poor diet. Don't take large doses of any supplement without the advice of a practitioner, doctor, or nutritionist.

### SEAN'S STORY

Sean came to the clinic for his allergies after he had given up on standard Western treatments.

"Taking a chance on a new kind of medicine seemed risky then, but I felt like it was riskier not to take the chance," Sean said. "And it turned me around."

Over time, Sean's exposure to another way of thinking about maintaining wholeness produced even greater changes. He began to meditate, improved his diet, and continued regular acupuncture and herbs, when needed.

After some soul-searching, Sean gave up his high-stress job, and he developed his own business. He also took up improvisational theater, which was a lifelong dream. Layers of stress and stress-related disharmonies fell away. Sean changed how he thought about his health care, and he also changed how he thought about himself as a whole person.

"When everything they were doing for me made me feel so much better, I got some confidence in myself," Sean said. "I started thinking I could probably take pretty good care of myself, or find people who could help me do it."

Four years later, Sean is healthier in mind/body/spirit.

"As it was happening, all of the changes seemed the most natural thing in the world. But looking back, I see I've come a long way," Sean said.

## Step Seven: Stocking Your Medicine Cabinet

To treat colds and flu, minor cuts, injuries, and stomach upset, you want to stock the most effective Chinese and other natural remedies. In this medicine cabinet, you will find, in addition to Chinese first aid, some homeopathic medicines for acute problems. For constitutional problems, I don't prescribe homeopathic medicine. If clients want to choose homeopathic treatment, I refer them to a homeopathic practitioner. But for acute problems, I often suggest that clients purchase the products listed below.

All of the suggested Chinese and Western remedies are generally safe, but they should not be used by children under twelve or by the elderly without the advice of a practitioner.

Many practitioners stock these formulas, or similar ones, and they can help you put together your Chinese and natural medicine cabinet. Just be careful to use products that have strict quality assurance and testing. (See "Choosing a Qualified Herbalist" on page 144 for more information.) Also, ask your practitioner for the correct dose for you.

### THE MEDICINE CABINET

| INDICATIONS | FORMULA | SUGGESTED USES | SUPPLIERS |
|---|---|---|---|
| Colds, flu | Cold Away | Early Heat type colds or fevers | Health Concerns |
| | Yin Chiao | Common cold, influenza | Many companies |
| | Loquat Cough Syrup | Cough (It's an expectorant.) | Plum Flower |
| Sinus congestion | Pe Min Kan Wan | Runny or stuffy nose, rhinitis, sinusitis, or sneezing | Plum Flower |
| | Allereze | Allergies, sneezing, or itching eyes, ears, and nose | Karuna |
| | Bi Yan Pian | Acute rhinitis and sinusitis | Many companies |
| | White Flower Oil | Use a few drops under nose or on chest for congestion | Pak Fah Yeow, distributed by many companies |
| Digestive problems | Quiet Digestion | Gastric distress, abdominal pain, nausea, abdominal distention, gastroenteritis, motion sickness, hangover, or jet lag (Do not use if appendicitis or intestinal obstruction is suspected.) | Health Concerns |

(continued)

| INDICATIONS | FORMULA | SUGGESTED USES | SUPPLIERS |
|---|---|---|---|
| Digestive problems (continued) | Ginger Tea | Nausea, morning sickness, or chemotherapy-related nausea | Can use fresh ginger root or 100 percent ginger tea bags from Triple Leaf |
| | Curing Pills | Nausea or diarrhea associated with stomach flu or food poisoning | Plum Flower |
| Trauma | Resinall K | Stagnant Xue or traumatic injury | Health Concerns |
| | *Zheng Gu Shui* | Traumatic injury, pain | Several companies |
| | Traumeel Cream | Muscular pain, joint pain, sports injuries, or bruising | Ask your practitioner |
| | Dr. Shir's Liniment | Injured joints, tendons, or ligaments where the skin is not broken | Spring Wind |
| | Medicated Plaster | Muscle and tendon pain, bruising, or traumatic injury | Wu Yang Brand distributed by many companies |
| | Moxa Stick | Traumatic injury, including bruise, sprains, and strains *(Do not use over open or bleeding wounds.)* | Ask your practitioner |
| Stress | Rescue Remedy | Stress due to traumatic events or emergencies and crises | Bach Flowers carried by many natural food stores |
| Skin irritation | Spring Wind Ointment | Dry skin, minor burns, sunburn, eczema, or psoriasis | Spring Wind |
| For massage | Warming Oil | For Cold conditions, increase circulation and warm an area such as the feet or abdomen | KW Botanicals |
| | Almond Oil | General massage on feet, face, or body | Any natural foods store, best if organic |

## THE HEALTHY TRAVELER

Traveling can cause all kinds of disharmonies, but you can protect yourself with a few easy-to-follow routines.

### FOR JET LAG

**Before you go:** Three days before you depart, begin the overcoming jet lag diet outlined in Dr. Charles Ehret's book, *Overcoming Jet Lag*. I've found it works to eliminate jet lag even after long flights.

Melatonin, the natural hormone that controls the body's clock, is available from your practitioner or over the counter. Taken at night for two days before you leave (and for two days upon arrival), it helps adjust your sleep cycle. Ask your practitioner for the dose that is best for you.

**On the plane:** To avoid dehydration and constipation, every hour you're in the air, drink a glass of water.

Limit alcohol or caffeine, which make dehydration worse.

Eat small, light meals when flying. Or follow Dr. Ehret's jet-lag diet.

Exercise on the plane by getting out of your seat and walking around at least once an hour.

Qi Gong exercise is also possible, particularly the exercises where you visualize your muscles tensing and relaxing. (See "Qi Gong" on page 175.) Some airlines offer in-the-seat aerobics on long flights.

**Upon arrival:** Take Curing Pills or Quiet Digestion (see "The Medicine Cabinet" on page 230) once a day for three days.

Take melatonin for at least two days after arrival.

Acupuncture treatments soon after arrival can reharmonize your system quickly.

### FOR DIGESTIVE PROBLEMS

Changes in water, stress, and time zones and bacterial infections can all contribute to digestive problems when you travel.

Before leaving home, take *Lactobacillus acidophilus* and continue to take it during your travels. At the first sign of cramping or diarrhea, take Curing Pills or Quiet Digestion. (See "The Medicine Cabinet" on page 230.)

# PART TWO: ASSEMBLING YOUR HEALING TEAM

When you're putting together a healing team for a preventive health care program, you want to blend the contributions of Eastern and Western practitioners. Although I practice Chinese medicine, I occasionally employ homeopathic remedies for acute conditions, such as sprained ankles, bruises, and the flu. I often refer clients for treatment to other practitioners, such as Western doctors, naturopathic physicians, chiropractors, physical therapists, and massage therapists.

Your Chinese medicine practitioner may provide regular checkups, offer advice on management of common colds and flu, and administer preventive acupuncture and herbal therapy. She may also help you develop a dietary and exercise/meditation routine that is tailored to your individual needs, help you maintain harmony of Shen, and work to rebalance your Essential Substances and Organ Systems before they develop full-blown disharmonies. The practitioner should become familiar with your constitution and medical history so diagnosis is as accurate as possible.

Your Western practitioner should provide regular diagnostic testing and a baseline evaluation. These exams may include Pap smears, mammograms, screening for sexually transmitted diseases, exams for colon and prostate cancers and breast cancers, skin cancer checkups, hepatitis C testing, diabetes screening, and cholesterol and cardiovascular monitoring.

Alternative or integrative practitioners who specialize in homeopathy, chiropractic, Ayurvedic medicine, Shiatsu, or other healing modalities are an important part of a preventive program. The key is to inform each member of your healing team about the various treatments you are receiving.

## Integrating Various Therapies

You may want to heed the following guidelines so that your eclectic approach doesn't create disharmonies either in your mind/body/spirit or among your various practitioners.

**Don't put off seeking a standard Western medicine baseline examination.** Western medicine provides many important healing tools, from surgical procedures to life-saving antibiotics and diagnostic tools. Using these modalities within the context of Chinese medicine is the best way to reap Western medicine's benefits and minimize its risks. For example, if you have a systemic infection from a wound, refusing antibiotics could lead to death. However, antibiotics also cause all kinds of systemic problems, and overdependence has led to bacterial mutations that antibiotics cannot kill. Chinese medicine and natural therapies, if used along with antibiotic therapy, can remove the negative systemic side effects such as yeast overgrowth and bowel disturbances and lessen the long-term need for antibiotics.

In short, Western medicine understands how to treat specific, narrowly defined health problems. Chinese medicine offers the opportunity to improve the strength and health of the whole body so that specific problems can be resolved. That's why New Chinese Medicine places such an emphasis on using other modalities in the context of Chinese medicine.

**Always inform all practitioners of the various healing arts that you are using.** Share the results of your Western examinations (and evaluations from other health care providers) with your Chinese medicine practitioner. The tests may help guide your treatment, and in the case of serious illness, they may allow your Chinese medicine practitioner, Western doctor, and other caregivers to work together to provide you the best care possible.

**Don't use yourself as a guinea pig.** If you have any questions, seek the guidance of a trained practitioner. Don't hesitate to get a second opinion on any health-related matter. Remember: You're the captain of your health care team.

**Don't mix drugs and/or herbal medications without the advice of a trained practitioner.** Seek a practitioner who is knowledgeable about drug/herb interactions. When looking for advice on herbal medications, ask a Chinese herbal practitioner, not someone without training in the contraindications, interactions, or possible side effects.

# PART THREE: BEGINNING THE COMPREHENSIVE PROGRAM

## Step One: Obtaining a Western Baseline

It's important to rule out cancer and other life-threatening problems and to identify an illness that can be treated quickly and effectively by Western medicine. The following are Western medicine guidelines for exams and diagnostic testing, adapted from the National Institutes of Health (NIH) guidelines of August 2014.

One test that is recommended by the Centers for Disease Control and Prevention starting in 2014 that is not in the NIH guidelines is one-time hepatitis C testing for all baby boomers (everyone born between 1945 and 1965) without ascertaining risk factors.

## WESTERN EXAMS AND DIAGNOSTIC TESTING

| TESTS | AGES 18 TO 39 | AGES 40 TO 64 | AGES 65+ |
|---|---|---|---|
| Health checkup | If healthy, two exams in 20s and 30s | Annually | Annually |
| Blood pressure | Every 2 years | Every 2 years | Annually |
| Cholesterol screening | Every 1 to 5 years | Every 1 to 5 years | Every 1 to 5 years |
| Breast self-exam (women) | Talk with provider | Talk with provider | Talk with provider |
| Breast exam by doctor (women) | During preventive exam | During preventive exam | During preventive exam |
| Mammogram (women) | Depends on family history | Every 1 to 2 years to age 50, then annually | Every 1 to 2 years, depending upon risk factors |
| Pap smear (women) | Age 21 to 29: every 3 years<br>Age 30 to 65: every 5 years, unless immunosuppressed | Every 5 years, unless immunosuppressed | Stop after three negative tests in 10 years, unless immunosuppressed |
| Diabetes screening | If BMI > 25, blood pressure 135/80 mm Hg | If BMI > 25, blood pressure 135/80 mm Hg; men every 3 years past age 45 | Every 3 years unless BMI > 25, blood pressure 135/80 mm Hg |
| Stool test for occult blood | At preventive exam if strong family history of colon cancer or polyps | At preventive exam if strong family history of colon cancer or polyps<br>After age 50: annually | Annually until age 75 |
| Sigmoidoscopy | As directed by physician | After age 50: every 5 to 10 years | Every 5 to 10 years until age 75 |
| Colonoscopy | As directed by physician | After age 50: every 10 years | Every 10 years until age 75 |
| Skin exam | Annually | Annually | Annually |
| Sexually transmitted infections | Screening according to lifestyle and risk | Screening according to lifestyle and risk | Screening according to lifestyle and risk |
| Eye exam | If problems, every 2 years | If problems, every 1 to 3 years | If problems, every 2 years |
| Dental exam | Annually | Annually | Annually |
| Dental cleaning | 2 to 3 times per year | 2 to 3 times per year | 2 to 3 times per year |

(continued)

| TESTS | AGES 18 TO 39 | AGES 40 TO 64 | AGES 65+ |
|---|---|---|---|
| Lung cancer screening | As required | After age 55, if history of 30 pack years or currently smoke or have in past 15 years | Until age 80 if history of 30 pack years or currently smoke or have in past 15 years |
| Hearing test | As required | As required | If symptoms of hearing loss: annually |
| Bone density test (DEXA scan) | As required | Men: after age 50 if risk factors, ask doctor Women: risk factors for osteoporosis; post-menopausal women with fractures | Women: have at least one DEXA scan after age 64 Men: risk factors, ask doctor |
| Prostate exam (men) | As required | Most men after age 50, African American men after age 45 | Most men after age 50, African American men after age 45 |

## Step Two: Obtaining Chinese Medicine Diagnosis and Treatment

When you go to a Chinese medicine practitioner, it's important to establish communication between the Chinese medicine and the Western medicine doctors. Both practitioners should be aware of what you are doing as director of your own healing process.

At the Chinese medicine practitioner, you can expect to be treated with acupuncture, moxibustion, and herbal medicine.

**Acupuncture and moxibustion:** For maintenance, when you are experiencing no troublesome disharmonies, you can receive an acupuncture treatment with the change of each season. The fluctuations in humidity, temperature, diet, amount of sunlight, and physical activity that happen from season to season make it helpful to get your Qi rebalanced seasonally. One set of points that would provide strengthening includes Large Intestine 4, Lung 7, Stomach 36, Kidney 3, Liver 3, and Spleen 6.

For most people, however, more frequent and more specific treatments may be recommended. Very few of us are so perfectly balanced that we don't have some complaint or could not improve upon our ability to fight off disease. The best acupuncture schedule can only be determined through individual diagnosis by your practitioner.

**Herbs:** The basic preventive health care routine is a blend of herb soups and congees and, if your practitioner suggests, a low dose of the supportive formulas Enhance, Cordyseng, Tremella American Ginseng (see "An Herbal Sampler" on page 145), or other formulas. When you are feeling susceptible to colds or flu or other viruses, you may use

Cold Away and *Yin Chiao* (see "The Medicine Cabinet" on page 230) to relieve the onset of symptoms. However, your practitioner will evaluate you according to traditional diagnosis and will most likely provide a formula for whatever specific diagnostic pattern and symptom-sign complex you have.

## IMMUNE SYSTEM FORMULAS

| FORMULA | CHINESE FUNCTION | INDICATIONS |
|---|---|---|
| Enhance | Tonify Qi, Xue, Yin, Yang, Jing; Clear Heat Clean Toxin; clear Phlegm; strengthen Spleen, Stomach, Kidney, and Wei Qi | Fatigue, immune dysfunction, frequent colds and flus, and chronic viral illness |
| Cordyceps PS | Tonify Kidney Yang, nourish Lung Yin, strengthen Wei Qi, stop Cough, and transform Phlegm | Fatigue, immune weakness, post-illness weakness, chronic cough, health maintenance, general tonic, supports athletic performance |
| Cordyseng | Tonify Qi and Yin through Fu Zheng action; strengthen Lung, Spleen, Stomach, and Kidney | Fatigue, recovery from serious illness or operation, supports immune function, supports lungs, improves athletic performance |
| Tremella American Ginseng | Tonify Yin, Qi, Xue, Jing; Clear Heat Clean Toxin; strengthen Wei Qi; strengthen Spleen, Stomach, Lung, and Kidney | Fatigue, immune dysfunction, frequent colds and flus, chronic viral illness, afternoon night sweats and fever, and chronic dry cough |

## Step Three: Bringing in Other Modalities

Many people will benefit from a monthly Shiatsu massage; visits to the chiropractor when muscle tension or soreness cause alignment problems; dietary or nutritional counseling from a Western nutritionist or registered dietician, macrobiotic, or Ayurvedic counselor; as well as exposure to other Eastern healing traditions such as Tibetan medicine or Yoga.

# WHAT TO DO WHEN THE IMMUNE SYSTEM IS WEAKENED

A comprehensive program of preventive health care is effective for people whose mind/body/spirit is in fairly good harmony. Unfortunately, people may be hit with unexpected assaults on their harmony, such as a car accident or serious illness. Or, if you undermine your naturally strong constitution by living with chronic stress or emotional upheaval, using drugs or alcohol, or engaging in excessive or unsafe sex, you become an easy target for viruses, bacteria, and other organisms.

However it happens, when the body is attacked and the immune system is weakened, people need extra-strong therapy to maximize their health.

If you have a disease that may be associated with a weakened immune system—such as herpes, chronic fatigue, chronic hepatitis, or diabetes or if you are HIV positive—a combination of aggressive Chinese and Western therapy can provide far-reaching benefits. With my colleagues, I have developed a therapeutic approach to managing such syndromes.

This approach relies upon modern herb formulas, traditional Chinese acupuncture and moxibustion treatments, and Western therapy. I have detailed comprehensive programs for hepatitis C in *The Hepatitis C Help Book*, Revised Edition[1] and for HIV in *The HIV Wellness Sourcebook*.[2]

## AT A GLANCE: THE COMPREHENSIVE PROGRAM FOR BASIC GOOD HEALTH AND A STRONG IMMUNE SYSTEM

| SELF-CARE PLAN | |
|---|---|
| Self-monitoring | Keep your daily journal; make note of your diet, physical activity, and body rhythms, including sleep, elimination, emotional changes, and mental acuity. |
| Implementing a dietary program | Step 1. Use information from your daily journal. Review your journal, look for symptoms of disharmony associated with your diet. Step 2. A cleansing routine. The First-Step Dietary Program removes irritants and toxins and soothes your system. Step 3. Use the power of food. As you build a new approach to your diet, you want to harness the Food Energetics. |

(continued)

| SELF-CARE PLAN *(continued)* | |
|---|---|
| Implementing a dietary program *(continued)* | **Step 4.** Establish a balanced diet. Eat warm and cooked foods, all flavors, in season. Other recommendations are made according to your constitution and Chinese diagnoses.<br>**Step 5.** Food tonics. Use therapeutic foods that combine Food Energetics with herbal action to tonify Qi and Xue. |
| Implementing an exercise/meditation plan | Use your daily journal to help you structure a plan that suits your constitution. The exercise should be a blend of aerobic movement—such as jogging, cycling, tennis, swimming, spinning and Qi Gong—weight-bearing exercises, stretching exercises including Qi Gong and Yoga, and breathing and meditation exercises. |
| Using massage and moxibustion for self-healing | Moxa and many massage techniques can help you maintain Organ System harmony and strengthen Wei Qi (Protective Qi). |
| Using soaks, saunas, and compresses | Soaks, saunas, and compresses are all effective ways to calm the Shen and keep the Qi and Xue flowing harmoniously. |
| Nutritional supplements | Follow the general nutritional supplement plan. Make sure you take a regular dose of *Lactobacillus acidophilus*. |
| ASSEMBLING THE HEALING TEAM | |
| Obtaining a Western baseline | It's important to rule out serious illnesses, cancer, and any life-threatening problems and to identify an illness that can be treated quickly and effectively by Western medicine. Regular diagnostic and screening tests are recommended. This information and information about any ongoing Western treatment should be shared with your Chinese medicine practitioner. |
| Obtaining Chinese medicine diagnosis and treatment | When you go to a Chinese medicine practitioner, it's important to establish communication between the Chinese and Western doctors. Follow the recommended preventive routine of acupuncture, moxibustion, and herbal medicine. |
| Bringing in other modalities | Most people will benefit from a monthly massage, occasional visits to the chiropractor, nutritional and dietary counseling, and exposure to other Eastern healing traditions. |

# 14

# CALMING THE SHEN
## A Comprehensive Program for Easing Stress, Anxiety, and Depression

In Chinese medicine, the mind/body/spirit is understood to be one entity. A peaceful mind and spirit are inseparable from the health of the body. A healthy body is part and parcel of a balanced mind and spirit. Depression, anxiety, and stress-related disorders are not singled out as symbols of an embarrassing failure of character, as they too often are in Western cultures. Instead, they are seen as a manifestation of a network of responses that are physical, spiritual, and psychological.

Relatively recently, Western doctors and scientists have begun to accept this expansive view of the origins of what the West calls mental illness. For example, depression is no longer seen as a linear result of bad thoughts or weakness. In a feedback loop reminiscent of Chinese medicine's concept of the role of Yin/Yang, depression is seen as a manifestation of outside stimuli, emotional reactions to those stimuli, brain chemistry, and genetic predisposition all working together to produce the disharmony that is identified as depression.

Blending the newest Western insights and the traditional Chinese therapies, New Chinese Medicine offers a four-pronged approach to managing anxiety disorders and depression.

## PART ONE: SELF-CARE TO CALM AND STRENGTHEN THE MIND/BODY/SPIRIT

Shen imbalances are usually caused by internal emotional disharmonies (traumas such as abuse and neglect) and by suppression of emotions (caused by denial and inability to contend with or express feelings). They are often associated with Qi Stagnation and disharmony in the Heart and Liver Systems.

There are two types of Shen imbalances: Disturbed Shen and Lack of Shen. Disturbed Shen causes forgetfulness, disorientation, memory lapses, insomnia, and lackluster eyes. Extreme disharmony is associated with madness, as described traditionally. Lack of Shen is associated with a flat affect and inability to communicate. Lack of Shen makes a person seem as though "the lights are on, but no one's home."

Alcoholism, depression, chronic headaches, digestive disturbances, panic attacks, anxiety, schizophrenia, and psychosis are all the manifestations of various degrees of Shen imbalance.

Any program to ease Shen imbalances focuses on restoring harmonious flow of Qi and Xue and balancing the Heart and Liver Systems.

## Step One: Implementing a Dietary Program

In addition to following the basic guidelines for sound nutrition set out in chapter 6, if you suffer from Shen imbalances, you can do the following:

- Eat foods that regulate or move Stagnant Qi and motivate stuck energy, such as basil, bay leaves, beets, black pepper, cabbage, chicken livers, coconut milk, garlic, ginger, kelp, leek, nori, peaches, scallions, and rosemary.

- Avoid alcohol, coffee, fatty foods, food additives, fried foods, excessively spicy foods, heavy red meat, unnecessary medicines, and overindulgence in sweets.

- Eat foods that sedate Excess Liver conditions, such as beef, chicken livers, celery, kelp, mussels, nori, and plums.

- Eat foods that help ease Xue Deficiency, such as oysters, sweet rice, liver, chicken soup, and Dang Gui Chicken (see page 121) if you do not have Stagnant Qi.

- Avoid raw fruit and vegetables, cold liquids, and ice.

Western nutrition offers evidence that foods and supplements high in omega-3 fatty acids may improve depression through several mechanisms.[1] These may include wild salmon, herring, tuna, sardines, coconut oil, flaxseed, and krill oil. Folic acid and folate supplements could help ease depression.[2] Folic acid in the form of folates are found in leafy greens, beans, lentils, avocado, okra, beets, seeds, and cruciferous vegetables, such as broccoli, brussels sprouts, and cauliflower.[3]

## Step Two: Implementing an Exercise and Meditation Plan

Qi Gong exercise and meditation are tremendously effective in soothing the Shen and balancing the flow of Qi and Xue. A daily routine that includes at least twenty minutes of Qi Gong exercises and twenty minutes of meditation can help ease anxiety, stress, and depression almost immediately. (See "The Basic Techniques" on page 178 for the basic Qi Gong routine.)

In addition, studies have shown that aerobic exercise has a positive effect on people suffering from chronic depression.[4] Although initial motivation may be difficult because of Stagnant Qi, the effort is vastly rewarding. Any aerobic activity—from walking to swimming or cycling—is suitable, depending on your level of fitness. One half hour every morning, in addition to the Qi Gong, is recommended for people with severe Shen disharmonies.

The following are some suggested routines:

**Gentle swaying:** This encourages flexibility both physically and psychologically. Practice this exercise from page 182 for five minutes.

**The bounce:** This gently massages the Organ Systems. For two to three minutes, practice this exercise from page 182.

**Refreshing meditation:** Spend ten minutes in visualization and stretching.

Lie, sit, or stand in a comfortable position.

Close your eyes halfway.

Breath slowly and evenly using the Buddha's Breath (see page 179).

Imagine yourself in an environment that is soothing to you—perhaps along the ocean, in the mountains, or in your own backyard.

Allow yourself to see the colors, feel the touch of the breeze on your face, smell the air, and feel the sun on your skin.

As you exhale, feel the stress leaving your body and drifting off, out of you, out of the scene.

Feel your chest rise and fall. Imagine your stress moving up, out of your left and right feet, up slowly through your legs, hips, and belly, moving out every time you exhale. Imagine it coming from your fingertips through your arms and shoulder, out with your breath. Imagine it moving up from your neck along the back of your head and out the top of your head with every breath.

Rest peacefully.

**Breathing cycle:** Use the Buddha's Breath technique (see page 179) to help disperse Stagnant Liver Qi, which is a common underlying pattern associated with Shen disturbance.

Sit on the floor with your legs crossed in lotus, half-lotus, or Indian style if you can. This is so the Qi does not become stagnant in the lower body, but follows the breathing path through the torso and the head.

Inhale to a count of four to eight, depending on what you are comfortable with. Extend your belly, filling it up from the bottom. As you inhale, turn your attention to your nose. Guide the Qi downward from your nose toward the Dantien, the area in your abdomen about 1 to 2 inches (2.5 to 5 cm) below the navel. (*Note:* Women should not concentrate on the Dantien during the menstrual period. Concentrate on the solar plexus instead.)

Exhale to a count of eight to sixteen and imagine the Qi moving down the torso, around the pelvic region, and up to the tailbone.

Inhale and visualize the Qi moving up the back to the top of the shoulders.

Exhale and feel the Qi move up the back of the head and back to the nose. One cycle may take about seventy seconds to complete. You want to set a pace that allows you to breathe comfortably and maintain concentration on the movement of Qi.

Repeat five times.

**Massage:** Self-massage is soothing to the Shen because it stimulates and regulates the flow of Xue and Qi and provides a period of pleasure and relaxation.

**Acupressure:** Every day you can massage Liver 3, Pericardium 6, the Si Shen Cong—the four points on the crown of the head—and the Yintang, between the eyebrows (see page 197).

Probe around the point until you feel tenderness and a slight emanation of energy. Applying a steady, even pressure, press down—don't stab—and then rock your finger gently around the point. Alternate holding the point steadily for about ten to thirty seconds with periods of active massage.

**General head massage:** This can help ease headaches, anxiety, or depression. (Follow the instructions on page 192.)

**Ear massage:** Focus on the Shenmen and the Brain, Heart, Sympathetic, and Liver points. (See pages 202 to 203 for the locations of the points.)

**Reflexology:** Use the head, brain, and adrenal points on your foot and hand. (See pages 210 to 211 for the locations of the points.)

**Professional massage:** In addition, receiving a professional massage once a week to once a month can provide the kind of thorough Shen relaxation and Qi stimulation that is difficult to do for yourself. Chinese foot massage, available in many cities, is often very affordable. Other types of massage and bodywork are excellent as well. You should choose the style of massage that is most soothing to you.

**Soaks and compresses:** Soaks and compresses are effective in calming the Shen because they can help move the Qi and offer spirit-lifting time of self-indulgent pleasure.

Sleep Ease, a chamomile-valerian soak, is especially recommended (see page 213).

**Nutritional supplements:** Several supplements, when combined with the other elements of this comprehensive program, can offer support for the Shen. SAM-e has extensive literature on relief of depression.[5] Magnesium has been shown to help people recover from depression.[6] Vitamin D, often found to be low in people who are depressed, is also prescribed for mood disorders and depression.[7] Melatonin may be used to overcome insomnia, which is often associated with depression and anxiety. Ask your naturopathic physician, psychiatrist, or other qualified professional for additional supplement recommendations.

# PART TWO: USING A CHINESE MEDICINE PRACTITIONER

When practical, you may want to try therapies, such as acupuncture and herbs, before taking Western medications for anxiety and depression, because the medications all have potentially troubling side effects. But if you decide the benefits of Western medications are worth the risk (and they often are), then Western medicine can be used to complement the Shen-calming powers of acupuncture and herbs.

## Acupuncture

Regular acupuncture sessions targeted to address your specific diagnosis can provide relief from anxiety, panic attacks, and depression. However, because depression may indicate the presence of a serious undiagnosed illness or can be life-threatening itself, you should always see a Western doctor for evaluation.

Shen disturbances, including depression, anxiety, and other issues, can be associated with Stagnant Liver Qi, the Heart and Kidney failing to communicate, and the Spleen not feeding the Heart Xue. Anxiety and depression may be associated with Liver Fire, Heart Fire, Heart and Liver Yin Deficiency, and Xue Deficiency. Treatment with specific points can be determined only after an individualized diagnosis.

## JEFFREY'S STORY

Six months after Jeffrey first came to the clinic, curious to find out what Chinese medicine could do for his anxiety and depression, he was able to go off Prozac.

"My anxiety is finished, gone," Jeffrey said. "I am much more centered, more balanced."

Jeffrey's initial program included a blend of Eastern and Western therapy. He was seeing a psychiatrist who prescribed the Prozac, and he was receiving acupuncture—twice a week for the first month, then once a week, and now once every two weeks. He also takes herbs daily.

"I never believed it would really work," Jeffrey said. "But it did. And although Misha talks to me each time I come for a treatment to see how I am, the therapy is physical as much or more than it's verbal."

## Herbal Therapy

Herbal therapy is generally gentler on the system than Western medications, with fewer and less serious side effects and no danger of addiction. However, if you have panic attacks, deep depression, or have not been able to sleep, you may want to take a Western sleeping medication for two or three days to break the cycle of agitation and get some rest. Then you can go on herbs that address the underlying problems associated with Shen disturbances.

Because Shen disturbances are usually deeply rooted, it is particularly important to take herbs and Western medications only under the ongoing supervision of a medical doctor and/or a qualified practitioner.

## EXAMPLES OF CHINESE HERBAL FORMULAS FOR SHEN DISTURBANCES

| FORMULA | CHINESE FUNCTION | INDICATIONS |
|---|---|---|
| Calm Spirit | Calm Shen, nourish Heart Yin and Xue, moisten Intestines | Depression, anxiety, insomnia, constipation, stress-associated emotions, poor memory |
| Chai Hu Su Gan San (Bupleurum Powder to Spread the Liver) | Regulate Liver Qi, vitalize Liver Xue, ease pain | Abdominal distension, hypochondriac and chest pain, indigestion, depression, constipation, belching |
| Ease Plus | Invigorate Liver Qi, sedate Liver Yang, tonify Spleen Qi, calm Shen | Insomnia, stress disorders, migraines, drug and alcohol withdrawal symptoms |
| Gui Pi Tang | Tonify Qi and Xue, strengthen Heart and Spleen (Do not use with Heat patterns.) | Insomnia, palpitations, forgetfulness, tiredness, poor appetite due to stress, pale face |
| Schizandra Dreams | Nourish Heart, calm Shen | Insomnia, anxiety attacks, daytime agitation |
| Shen Gem | Vitalize Heart Xue; calm Shen; tonify Spleen, Heart, Qi, and Xue | Insomnia, memory loss, palpitations, nervousness, anxiety, pallor |
| Xiao Yao San (Rambling Powder) | Spread Liver Qi, relieve Stagnation, tonify Spleen, nourish Xue | Irritability, depression, moodiness, fatigue, headache, dizziness, breast distention, irregular menstruation, menstrual pain |

# PART THREE: GOING TO A WESTERN DOCTOR

Depression, panic attacks, anxiety, and stress-related disorders can benefit enormously from Western intervention, particularly if used in conjunction with Chinese medicine. Chinese therapy can often ease the negative impact of the Western medication without interfering with positive therapy.

The reason to use Western drugs to treat what the West identifies as psychological disorders is twofold. First, in the past three decades, there has been a revolutionary change in Western medicine's understanding of the role of body chemistry in neuropsychological problems, such as depression, anxiety, and obsessive-compulsive disorder. This has led to the development of medications that help compensate for deficiencies and produce changes in the underlying chemistry of the body. That in turn eases the symptoms of the disharmony. (Western medicine is actually getting closer to the Chinese viewpoint in these areas.)

Second, some Western syndromes that are related to Shen disturbance, such as depression, may be life-threatening if not ameliorated immediately. Often, Western intervention can remove the short-term threat.

Your Western baseline should include a physical work-up to eliminate the presence of a serious underlying disease, evaluation to determine possible physical origins of the disorder, and discussion of your options, including talk therapy and medications and their benefits and side effects.

## PART FOUR: CONSULT WITH OTHER HEALERS

Psychotherapy, bodywork practitioners, self-help and support groups, spiritual healers, and twelve-step programs are tremendously important in any program to restore harmony to the Shen. Chinese medicine recognizes the positive influence of functioning as a member of a group. The balance of Yin/Yang that joins the mind/body/spirit also connects each person to the world at large and to each individual in it. When that connection is reinforced and strengthened by positive interdependence, the internal harmony of the mind/body/spirit is also strengthened.

If you decide to see a therapist, psychologist, psychiatrist, or healer, try to arrange for her or him to talk with your Chinese medicine practitioner so they can work in concert. The therapist's diagnosis can help guide the Chinese practitioner toward targeted therapies. Chinese medicine treatments may resolve some Shen problems, allowing the therapist to focus on others.

## AT A GLANCE: THE COMPREHENSIVE PROGRAM FOR CALMING THE SHEN

| SELF-CARE PLAN | |
|---|---|
| Dietary guidelines | Start with the First-Step Dietary Therapy Program (see page 113) that removes irritants and toxins and soothes the system. Then, according to your Chinese diagnosis, eat foods that regulate or move Stagnant Qi and motivate stuck energy, sedate Excess Liver conditions, and/or help ease Xue Deficiency and Xue Stagnation. Avoid excess caffeine, reduce or eliminate alcohol, reduce fatty foods, decrease raw foods and excess sweets, and eliminate icy drinks or foods. |
| Exercise/meditation | Daily practice at least twenty minutes of Qi Gong exercises and twenty minutes of meditation. If you have severe Shen disharmonies, a half hour of aerobic exercises such as walking or cycling is recommended in addition to Qi Gong. |
| Massage | Acupressure: Stimulate Liver 3, Pericardium 6, Si Shen Cong, and Yintang. You may also use the General Head Massage (see page 192) and Amazing Ear Massage (see page 202). Reflexology: Focus on the head, brain, and other related points on the foot and hand (see pages 210 and 211). Professional massage once a week can provide Shen relaxation and Qi stimulation. |
| Soaks and saunas | Sleep Ease (see page 213), a chamomile-valerian soak, is especially recommended. |
| Nutritional supplements | Follow the nutritional supplement plan with the modifications made in this chapter. Ask your naturopathic physician or psychiatrist for additional recommendations. |
| USING A CHINESE MEDICINE PRACTITIONER | |
| Acupuncture | Treatment of specific points are determined after an individualized diagnosis. |
| Herbal therapy | A number of Chinese herbal formulas may be used for Shen disharmonies, such as Calm Spirit, *Gui Pi Tang*, *Shen Gem*, *Xiao Yao Wan*, and Schizandra Dreams. Your practitioner will give you formulas based upon your diagnosis. |
| GOING TO A WESTERN DOCTOR | |
| Obtaining a Western baseline | Your Western baseline should include a physical work-up to eliminate the presence of a serious underlying disease, evaluation to determine possible physical origins of the disorder, and a complete discussion of your options, including talk therapy and medications and their benefits and side effects. |
| Other healers | Psychotherapy, bodywork practitioners, self-help and support groups, spiritual healers, and twelve-step programs are tremendously important in any program to restore harmony to the Shen. |

# HARMONIOUS CYCLES
## A Comprehensive Program for Gynecologic Health

At one time or another, most women contend with some unpleasant physical symptoms, such as bloating, irritability, or pain, before or during their menstrual periods. These are not signs of illness but rather indicate that there is a degree of disharmony in the reproductive system. By following this comprehensive program, you can lessen or eliminate those unpleasant symptoms and restore harmony without resorting to over-the-counter medications or prescription drugs.

Before beginning this program, let's review the Chinese and Western concepts of women's reproductive system and the origins of disharmonies and disorders.

## WOMEN'S HEALTH IN CHINESE MEDICINE

The monthly cycle depends on the harmonious functioning of the Stomach, Spleen, Liver, and Kidney systems and a balanced flow of Qi and Xue. Irregular periods, pain, bloating, mood swings, and cramps are signs that one or more of the governing Organ Systems and Qi and Xue are not in balance. It's also possible that gynecological problems have a more complex origin in your emotional history that has caused damage along the Chong Mai (Penetrating Channel). (For more detail on the Chong Mai, see "The Chong Mai" on page 41.)

Such emotional and physical disharmonies can produce a combination of symptoms. The Kidney System controls the formation and release of the egg from the ovaries. If Kidney Qi, Yin, or Yang is weak, infertility may result. Kidney Deficiency can accompany a kind of chronic fearfulness that causes tension, irritability, or depression associated with the monthly cycle. The Liver Qi promotes the free flow of Qi in all areas of the body and triggers the release of Xue and the onset of the period. Therefore, menstrual problems, such as cramps before or during onset of the monthly period and mild premenstrual headache, are usually due to Stagnant Qi. If Liver Qi is not flowing smoothly, depression and anxiety may occur in the days before the period. Liver Excess can accompany generalized anger. Conversely, anger and emotional suppression can damage Liver Qi. Stagnant Liver Qi is associated with menstrual cramps and mild headaches that subside with onset of the period. Stagnant Liver Qi with Heat is associated with irritability, flashes of anger, a feeling of a hot sensation in the upper part of the body, and breast pain. When combined with Stomach Heat, you may experience acne, increased appetite, and breast pain.

When Stagnant Liver Qi leads to Stagnant Xue, there may be blood clots with severe headaches during the menstrual period. When Stagnant Xue is accompanied by Cold, you may experience a cold sensation in the abdomen, darker flow with dark clots, and cramps that are eased by the application of warmth.

Disharmony in the Spleen develops as either Deficient Spleen Qi or Spleen Deficient Qi with Dampness. These syndromes are associated with digestive disturbances, sugar cravings, and fluid retention. When Deficient Spleen leads to Deficient Xue, it is associated with lengthening of the cycle or missed periods and difficulty falling asleep.

## THE MENSTRUAL CYCLE IN CHINESE MEDICINE

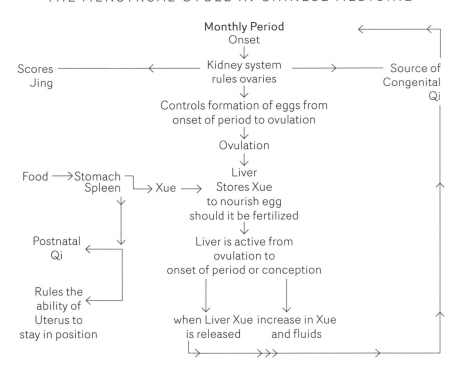

# WOMEN'S HEALTH IN WESTERN MEDICINE

Women show considerable variation in the lengths of their menstrual cycles. Normal cycle length may vary between twenty-one and thirty-six days, but most sources use twenty-eight days as the average number for the total menstrual cycle.

Convention uses the onset of menstrual bleeding to mark the beginning of the cycle, so the first day of bleeding is called "Cycle Day One (CD1)." The menstrual cycle can be divided into several phases. Although the length of each phase varies widely from woman to woman and cycle to cycle, most references use the following average numbers.

## MENSTRUAL CYCLE PHASES

| NAME OF PHASE | CYCLE DAYS |
| --- | --- |
| Menstrual phase | 1 to 4 |
| Follicular phase (also known as proliferative phase) | 4 to 14 |
| Ovulation (not a phase, but an event dividing the phases) | 14 |
| Luteal phase (also known as secretory phase) | 15 to 26 |
| Ischemic phase (some sources group this with the secretory phase) | 27 to 28 |

The phases of the menstrual cycle are controlled by the interaction of three hormone-secreting organs: the hypothalamus, pituitary, and ovaries. They secrete gonadotropin-releasing hormone (GNRH), gonadotropin, luteinizing hormone (LH), follicle-stimulating hormone (FSH), and steroidal hormones (estrogen and progesterone).

For fertility to be robust, the luteal phase needs to be from twelve to fourteen days long. Menstruation itself runs one to seven days. Longer than seven days is considered abnormal. Disorders such as premenstrual syndrome (PMS) and endometriosis (an often painful disorder in which tissue that normally lines the inside of your uterus grows outside your uterus) are not entirely understood by current science. No one is sure of what triggers either condition.

## THE CHINESE CYCLE AND THE WESTERN CYCLE

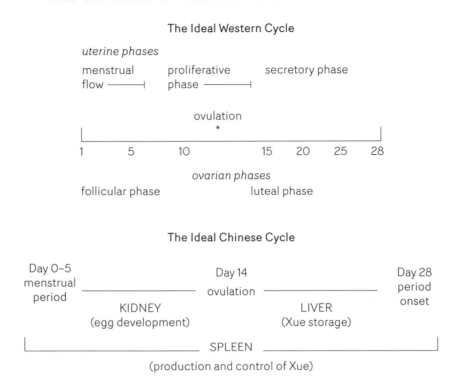

### The Ideal Western Cycle

*uterine phases*

menstrual flow ⟶ | proliferative phase ⟶ | secretory phase

ovulation
*

1    5    10    15    20    25    28

*ovarian phases*

follicular phase          luteal phase

### The Ideal Chinese Cycle

Day 0–5 menstrual period ⟶ Day 14 ovulation ⟶ Day 28 period onset

KIDNEY (egg development)          LIVER (Xue storage)

SPLEEN

(production and control of Xue)

*Although this is the "ideal" cycle, Chinese medicine considers any regular cycle to be a healthy cycle. One woman may have a period every twenty-one days, another every thirty-five. If they are both regular, no disharmony is indicated.*

When PMS is diagnosed in Western medicine, recommendations typically include hormonal therapy, anti-prostaglandins and analgesics (pain medications such as NSAIDS), dietary changes such as avoiding caffeine, exercise, and psychotherapy. For endometriosis, the alternatives usually prescribed are surgery and potent but often difficult drug therapy with many side effects and mixed results.

Until recently, emotional components of gynecological disorders were dismissed or trivialized by Western physicians. A relatively new field in Western medicine is called psychoneuroimmunology (coined in 1975), the study of the interaction between psychological processes and the nervous and immune systems of the human body. Psychoneuroimmunology recognizes that emotional stressors can be related to disease development. In general, however, Western therapies offer few targeted treatments to ameliorate emotional disturbances and associated physical complaints.

## BASIC FACTS

- The average age of menarche in North America is 12.47 years old.[1]

- The perimenopausal stage can last from two to ten years. In the beginning, there are usually shorter cycles—probably caused by the luteal phase becoming irregular. As menopause nears, menstrual periods generally come farther apart due to cessation of ovulation. The beginning and end of the fertility cycle are marked by long anovulatory cycles with progesterone deficiency.

- The average age for menopause is fifty-one.[2] In the United States, smokers reach menopause earlier.[3] (A recent study shows this may be a genetic variation in white women, but it's not known for others.)

# PART ONE: SELF-CARE FOR PREVENTION AND THERAPEUTIC TREATMENT

Except in severe life-threatening situations, I believe that self-care is 80 percent of all care. Your ability to take care of yourself often determines how well you will be and how much you can enjoy yourself—in the short term and also for your whole life. In this section, you will learn how to take care of yourself in a step-by-step method to create wellness and wholeness.

## Step One: Adopt the Comprehensive Program for Strengthening Organ Qi and Protective Qi

A general, preventive health care routine that includes a balanced diet, regular exercise and meditation, self-massage, and other stress-reduction techniques is essential for reproductive health. That's why the Comprehensive Program for Gynecologic Health integrates the Comprehensive Program for Basic Good Health and a Strong Immune System (see page 223), including preventive techniques tailored to suit the unique needs of women's bodies.

If you suffer from specific complaints, such as PMS or menopausal symptoms, or who need fertility support, you will find targeted therapies at the end of this chapter to consider.

## Step Two: Expand Your Daily Journal

When starting a Comprehensive Program for Gynecologic Health, the first step is to expand your daily journal to a monthly log. It should include information on your cycle and associated physical and emotional responses. You should develop a habit of making these notations every day for at least six months—even if you stop keeping your general journal after two weeks. In fact, this would be a good practice for a lifetime. If you have a well-balanced cycle, it will help alert you to the development of any disharmonies. If you are currently working to remedy an imbalance, it will alert you to triggers and help you track improvements.

The monthly log should include information on the following:

- Food cravings or times when you lose your appetite for specific foods or food in general

- Alcohol and caffeine consumption

- Energy levels and ability to exercise

- Times when sore breasts, overall heaviness, bloating, depression, or fatigue makes it difficult to exercise

- Emotional ups and downs—especially times when you are irritable, cry or feel like crying, get angry, or become depressed as well as when your emotions are positive

- Physical symptoms you suspect are associated with your cycle, such as headaches, blood sugar problems, insomnia, swollen ankles, tender breasts, swollen abdomen, cramps, acne, or lower back pain

- Information about the quality of your period itself: date of ovulation and feelings surrounding it, date of onset, and description of quality of flow, color, texture, intensity, and duration

A review of this information over the course of several months should reveal correlations between your monthly cycle, diet, exercise, emotions, and physical symptoms. This information indicates how you can control or eliminate some of the troubling symptoms associated with your cycle. You'll see which times of the month you should be particularly vigilant about exercising, curtailing stress, and avoiding foods that exacerbate symptoms.

## Step Three: Implementing a Dietary Program

In addition to the diet guidelines outlined in the Comprehensive Program for Basic Good Health and a Strong Immune System (see page 223), you may tailor your diet to remove Dampness and promote a balanced flow of Qi and Xue with the following recommendations:

- Eat a diet of warm, cooked foods. Be particularly careful not to eat cold, raw foods during your period, because it may increase cramping and discomfort.

- Avoid excess dairy products to decrease Dampness and strengthen the Spleen.

- Eliminate caffeine and drink a minimum of alcohol, which increases PMS symptoms and is linked to increased breast cancer risk. Artificial stimulants of all kinds amplify gynecological disharmonies, causing Stagnant Liver Qi along with Liver and Heart Fire.

- Eat an optimal fat diet. Too little or too much body fat affects estrogen production and can lead to various gynecological problems. Too fatty a diet, especially poor-quality fats, can also increase Stagnant Qi and Dampness, which is associated with depression and lack of energy. Too little fat can lead to Deficient Yin and Dryness.

- Increase fiber and include whole grains in your diet to avoid premenstrual constipation.

- Eliminate excess salt from your diet to ease water retention. Pure foods contribute enough salt to the diet to maintain health. Eating processed and packaged foods and adding salt to home-cooked meals is unnecessary, and it can be detrimental to your health. According to Five Phases diagnoses, excess salt injures the Kidney Water, counteracts Earth, and injures the Spleen.

- Once a week, you may enjoy a bowl of San Qi Chicken (see the recipe on page 121) to promote proper Xue movement.

- Eliminate any foods that your daily journal indicates are associated with PMS, cramps, irregularity, or any of the emotional and physical symptoms surrounding the progress of your cycle. You may try reintroducing them after a one-month break by using the First-Step Dietary Therapy Program (see page 113).

## Step Four: Implementing an Exercise Plan

To regulate and move Qi and Xue so they flow smoothly, avoid excessive aerobic activities. If you're trying to reestablish a regular, symptom-free cycle, the first step is to use Yoga, Qi Gong warm-up exercises (see page 182), and walking to stimulate balanced flow. Once a routine is established (daily for thirty minutes), you can expand your exercises to include aerobics such as jogging, cycling, and swimming. Walking 10,000 steps per day can meet the exercise goal. For example, if you walk a lot at work or to and from work, you may want to wear a pedometer (such as a Fitbit) to monitor your walking.

Guidelines from the Centers for Disease Control and Prevention (CDC) recommend that adults ages eighteen to sixty-four engage in at least two hours and thirty minutes (150 minutes) of moderate-intensity aerobic activity weekly (or an hour and fifteen minutes of vigorous activity), and also do muscle-strengthening activities that work all major muscle groups (legs, hips, back, abdomen, chest, shoulders, and arms) such as push-ups or weight lifting, at least two days a week.[4]

Exercising five times a week, forty-five minutes a day will strengthen Qi, but you should avoid exercising to the point of exhaustion or you will deplete your Qi. Your optimal exercise time in a week should be about five to seven hours, including Yoga and/or Qi Gong, walking, and aerobics.

If you have any gynecological disharmony, do weight-lifting exercises only three days a week. The process of tearing down and building up muscle tissue may cause Spleen Deficiency in susceptible women, which could lead to Deficient Xue and increased menstrual problems.

## Step Five: Implementing Meditation

Stress is both a trigger and a result of gynecological problems. Meditation can alleviate the stress and diminish associated symptoms, such as premenstrual depression and anxiety. Use the Lotus Blossom Meditation (see page 189) for a quick time-out from cycle-related discomfort and stress. Use the Buddha's Breath exercise (see page 179) to help ease Stagnation. Regular practice of the longer Qi Meditation (see page 186) can produce constitutional improvements that will do much to restore harmony.

## Step Six: Using Self-Massage and Moxibustion for Preventive Care

Massage and acupressure are extremely helpful in relieving gynecological problems. For example, Qi Gong abdominal massage (see page 194) is effective while you are having cramps. When used regularly throughout the month, it can dispel Stagnation and Dampness, relieving PMS and dysmenorrhea.

You may also use reflexology on the hands and feet, particularly on the abdomen, womb, uterus, lower back, and brain points. (See the hand illustration on page 210.)

For reducing symptoms associated with Stagnant Liver Qi, you may perform acupressure on Liver 3. (See the acupressure illustration on page 206.)

In addition, perform a monthly breast self-exam, using the following procedure:

- All women over age twenty are encouraged to examine their breasts regularly for changes in texture, shape, and color of the skin and for evidence of discharge from the nipples.

- If you notice a change, such as the development of a lump or swelling, skin irritation or dimpling, nipple pain or retraction, redness, or scaliness of the nipple or breast skin, or a discharge other than breast milk (such as staining of your sheets or bra), you should see your health care provider as soon as possible.[5]

- In addition to the traditional Western self-exam, Western herbalist Susun Weed advocates an herbal massage, which is done in the bath.[6] This is a less intimidating process, and it also combines the monthly checkup with stress reduction. To enjoy this therapeutic soak, follow these steps:

  - Buy or make your own herbal oil by infusing olive or almond oil with fresh thyme, rosemary, basil, peppermint, or rose petals.

  - Draw a warm bath.

  - Pour herbal oil into the palm of your hand.

  - Place both of your hands around one breast, with your thumbs pointing to the ceiling and your fingers cradling the breast from underneath.

  - Touch the tips of your thumbs at the top of your breast and draw them down toward the nipple.

  - Repeat this motion slowly, pressing down as hard as is comfortable, but spreading the thumbs apart ½ inch (1.3 cm).

  - Repeat this motion until your thumbs are halfway down your breast on opposite sides.

  - Add more oil at any time.

  - Now use your fingers under you breast to draw up toward the nipple. Spread them farther and farther apart until you have massaged the whole breast.

As with the more traditional massage, if you repeat this at the same time in your cycle every month, you will become acquainted with the texture of your breasts and become alert to any variations that may require diagnostic testing by a Western doctor.

Perform self-moxa on Spleen 6 and Ren 6 once a week for three weeks, with a week off during your period.

## Step Seven: Using Soaks, Saunas, and Compresses for Self-Healing

In general, warming compresses and brief soaks can ease some of the discomfort associated with cramps and lower back pain during the onset of your period. You have to tune into what temperature is best for you. If you are already feeling too hot or dizzy, keep water and sauna temperatures below 101°F (38°C). If you have Cold Dampness, hotter compress, soaks, and saunas can be beneficial.

Use Sleep Ease, a chamomile-based soak, to which you may also add valerian (see "Sleep Ease" on page 213). Enjoy this soak for up to a half hour. You can also prepare and use ginger soaks and Gingerly compresses (see "Gingerly" on page 217).

## Step Eight: Taking Nutritional Supplements

All women should adopt a daily supplement program. Ask your practitioner for specific dosing recommendations, because individual needs are different for different women. Your regimen should include essential fatty acids, such as krill oil and flaxseed oil that are sources of omega-3 fatty acids. Vitamin D is prescribed from 2000 IU to 10,000 IU. It is best to dose this according to lab results, although 4000 to 6000 IU is the average dose I give to women. Antioxidants such as lycopenes are important. Also, if you can tolerate it without diarrhea, include 1 to 3 grams of vitamin C a day. Calcium is recommended daily; use from 500 to 1500 milligrams of calcium hydroxyapatite (prion free) or calcium citrate, which contains all of the substances needed to help absorb and build bone mass, including vitamin C, vitamin K, vitamin E, magnesium, and boron. A combination of vitamin $B_{12}$/folic acid/vitamin $B_6$ is another daily recommendation. The sublingual form is great for absorption. Daily *Lactobacillus acidophilus* can also be taken to protect against yeast infections and keep the digestive tract healthy. The Mayo Clinic recommends that "1 x 109 living *L. acidophilus* cells by mouth in divided doses daily is an adequate dose for most people."[7]

# PART TWO: ASSEMBLING THE TEAM

When it comes to gynecological health, you need to include both Western-trained and Eastern-trained practitioners to optimize your preventive health care plan. When you use practitioners of both types of medicine in concert, it will give you the opportunity to create an individualized comprehensive treatment plan, share diagnoses, reduce side effects, make better choices for treatments and self-care, and attain the best outcomes.

## Western Medicine

The American Cancer Society recommends that every woman have a Pap smear every three years from age twenty-one to twenty-nine, then every five years along with HPV testing until age sixty-five.[87] The American Cancer Society recommends mammograms yearly starting at age forty as long as a woman is in good health. Yearly screening for sexually transmitted disease, including HIV, is essential for sexually active women.

## Eastern Medicine

Chinese medicine is particularly effective for treating the powerful confluences of emotional and physical forces that influence the harmony of a woman's cycle. For information on Chinese medicine therapies for PMS, menopausal symptoms, and fertility support, see the specific treatment plans that follow the general gynecologic health plan.

## Step One: Obtaining a Western Baseline

It's important to use Western screening techniques to rule out sexually transmitted diseases and cancer as the cause of any gynecological irregularities or discomfort. Western doctors may also be able to offer quick therapies for some other problems. If you opt for Western treatments, take your baseline diagnosis and information on the treatment to a Chinese medicine practitioner. Always tell your Western doctor that you are seeking Chinese medicine therapy as there may be interactions with Western treatment. Also, if you are not using the medicine the Western physician prescribed and you have gotten better, any caring doctor will want to know this information.

Telling doctors what is actually working for you is a major way that Western physicians and practitioners learn that Chinese medicine can help their patients and make recommendations. By seeing a Chinese medicine doctor, you can receive treatment that will ease any negative side effects of Western treatment, and you can benefit from the balancing powers of acupuncture, herbs, and other Chinese medicine therapies.

## IRENE'S STORY

"At forty-six, I was diagnosed with fibroid tumors, which caused prolonged bleeding, sometimes for a month at a time," Irene said. "My gynecologist recommended that I take Provera [a drug that stops abnormal uterine bleeding]. My blood pressure was up to 140/90, and I was feeling pretty bad." Irene had a hard time taking Provera, which made her vision blurry, moods manic, and body bloated. She decided to try acupuncture for the bleeding.

"After a few treatments, the bleeding stopped. I went back to my gynecologist and he told me that my blood pressure was also down—to 130/88. I didn't immediately see the connection. But after a few months, I could tell that it was the acupuncture treatments. The treatments had taken care of the bleeding and my high blood pressure. Today at fifty-three, my blood pressure is 110/70, and I have acupuncture treatments twice a month for a half hour. The treatments also kept my condition under control for five years.

"One more thing: After observing my success with acupuncture, my seventy-seven-year-old mother tried it for arthritis and neck pain and has continued treatment for three years now," Irene said. "She drives an hour each way to receive treatments she considers life prolonging."

## Step Two: Obtaining a Chinese Medicine Diagnosis and Treatment

To ascertain your gynecological health, a Chinese medicine practitioner does not do a direct examination of your reproductive organs. This is not part of the scope of practice of acupuncturists and Chinese medicine doctors in the United States. A Chinese medicine doctor will read the reports from the Western physician for this information. Rather, using the Four Examinations (see page 76), the practitioner conducts an interview to determine what disharmonies are present and to find out what symptoms are troubling you. Using this set of traditional diagnostic techniques, the practitioner is able to design a course of treatment that will restore harmony to your Organ Systems and Essential Substances and, as a consequence, alleviate your gynecological problems.

### ACUPUNCTURE AND MOXIBUSTION

The inclusion of Qi and Xue harmonizing treatments once a month will promote gynecological harmony. They are effective in influencing the Spleen, Liver, and Kidney at appropriate stages of the cycle to preserve or restore regularity and harmony. Acupuncture can also be used to impact the Channels that are particularly important in maintaining a harmonious reproductive cycle. The four Extraordinary Channels that govern the cycle are the Chong Mai (Penetrating Channel), Dai Mai (Belt Channel), Ren Mai (Conception Channel), and Du Mai (Governing Channel).

The Chong Mai is known as the Sea of Qi and Xue. It is the root of the other Extraordinary Channels.

The Ren Mai is related to all of the Yin Organs and Channels and is in charge of transporting the Jing, Xue, and Jin-Ye. As conduit of the Xue—which is a Yin Substance, the Ren Mai plays a large part in the woman's cycle. It also supports Qi, Xue, and Jin-Ye for supply to the fetus. If Ren Mai is weak, women may miss periods, become infertile, or have difficulty with pregnancy or labor.

The Du Mai is the master of all Yang energy, and with the Ren Mai it regulates the balance of Yin/Yang, which in turn regulates Qi and Xue and keeps the functions of the uterus normal. The lack of Yang due to a Du Mai disturbance might lead to spotting accompanied by vaginal discharge.

Another Channel that is important is the Dai Mai, which is closely associated with the Liver and Gallbladder. If the Liver is not moving Qi correctly, it cannot absorb female hormones as it should. Headaches associated with the menstrual period may occur.

## MOXIBUSTION

For general gynecological health, maintenance centers on Ren 4, Ren 6 (see page 40), Spleen 6 (see page 163), and Zi Gong (Uterus) (see page 206), plus back points along the Urinary Bladder—Urinary Bladder 20 and 23 (see page 166)—and the sacrum or lower back.

## HERBAL TREATMENTS

Most herbal formulas are designed to treat specific disharmonies and are not appropriate for preventive care. However, some herbal soups can help regulate the flow of Qi and Xue and as such offer general herbal support for gynecological health. (For herbal treatments for specific gynecologic complaints, see the sections that follow on PMS, menopausal and premenopausal symptoms, and fertility support.)

### HERBS FOR GENERAL GYNECOLOGICAL HARMONY

| HERB SOUP | HERBAL CONTENT | CHINESE THERAPEUTIC INDICATIONS |
| --- | --- | --- |
| Dang Gui Chicken Soup (page 121) | Dang Gui (*Angelica sinensis*) | Eat once to four times per month to strengthen Spleen and tonify Xue. |
| San Qi Chicken Soup (page 121) | San Qi (pseudoginseng) | Eat once to four times per month to strengthen Spleen and circulate Xue. |

## PART THREE: BRING IN OTHER MODALITIES

Your treatment plan can be expanded in several ways. To increase Shen harmony and to reduce irritability, mood swings, stress, and/or depression, you may want to include other forms of Eastern meditations, biofeedback, hypnosis, or psychotherapy. To alleviate digestive problems associated with the cycle, some women adopt an Ayurvedic diet or other diets such as Paleo to dispel the imbalances. Japanese abdominal massage can also ease digestive problems and alleviate pain associated with the period.

## FREEING THE QI: THE COMPREHENSIVE PROGRAM FOR PMS MANAGEMENT

To ease PMS symptoms, you will expand the Comprehensive Program for Gynecologic Health to include targeted therapies.

PMS is a loose collection of symptoms triggered by hormonal shifts that afflict an estimated 80 percent of all women during the last week or two of their menstrual cycles. The symptoms include increased appetite and sugar cravings, fatigue, headaches, dizziness, palpitations, depression, weight gain, breast tenderness, emotional volatility, vaginal infections, constipation, worsening of allergies, and acne or skin eruptions. For 10 to 20 percent of women, the syndrome is incapacitating.

In Chinese medicine, these symptoms are associated with various disharmonies: Stagnant Liver Qi, Depressive Liver Fire, Heart Fire, Deficient Heart and Liver Xue, Stomach Heat, and Deficient Spleen Qi with Dampness.

To eliminate debilitating symptoms and restore harmony to the Organ Systems, Essential Substances, and Channels, follow the Comprehensive Program for Gynecologic Health (see page 249), plus the following steps.

### Step One: Additional Dietary Guidelines

In addition to the general gynecologic guidelines given earlier, women with PMS should eliminate all refined sugars from the diet; eliminate decaffeinated coffee, chocolate, and dark sodas; reduce the fat content of their diet to 25 percent of daily calories; avoid over-the-counter diuretics and instead adjust diet to eliminate excess salt; increase grains and fiber; and drink 48 ounces (1.4 L) of filtered or spring water a day.

## Step Two: Additional Nutritional Supplements

Do not take nutritional supplements before talking to your Western doctor and/or Chinese practitioner because there may be contraindications you don't know about.

Vitamin $B_6$ may provide some relief in doses between 250 and 500 milligrams a day. The proof that it works is anecdotal at this point.[9]

*The American Journal of Epidemiology* reports that women with PMS may benefit from taking zinc[10] as well as non-heme iron (plant-based iron not the iron found in red meat). However, only take supplements under the direction of your practitioner. The highest limit of zinc that should be consumed without a physician recommendation is 40 milligrams per day. Higher doses may interfere with copper and iron metabolism, leading to a negative impact on serum lipids (fat in the blood) and immune function. Non-heme iron should only be consumed up to a maximum 45 milligrams per day in menstruating women unless a physician prescribes it.[11] High potassium levels may increase PMS symptoms because it can increase fluid retention, causing symptoms of PMS like extremity swelling and bloating.

Calcium (best as hydroxyapatite or citrate) and magnesium should be considered. Chocolate cravings associated with PMS may in fact result from magnesium deficiency because chocolate is relatively high in magnesium. So, if you eat chocolate (best in small amounts), you are getting some extra magnesium. Magnesium deficiency can lead to symptoms such as leg muscle cramps, especially at night. Daily consumption of 200 milligrams of magnesium (best is citrate or hydroxyapatite) can alleviate mild symptoms of PMS-related fluid retention.[12] And calcium is important for general gynecologic health plus as a preventive measure against osteoporosis, the brittle bone syndrome that afflicts so many women after menopause.

## Step Three: Additional Herbal Treatments

Several Chinese herbal formulas are designed to treat disharmonies associated with symptoms of PMS. It is advised that you do not take herbs without a practitioner's direction and prescription because you may take the wrong formula, which at the least may not work and at the most may be harmful. A licensed practitioner should do a thorough diagnostic examination and then prescribe appropriate herbal therapy. Many formulas are associated with PMS symptoms. Your practitioner may recommend some of the formulas in the following table or other herbal formulas, depending on your diagnosis.

EXAMPLES OF CHINESE HERBAL FORMULAS FOR PMS

| FORMULA | CHINESE FUNCTION | INDICATIONS |
| --- | --- | --- |
| *Xiao Yao San* (Rambling Powder) | Spread Liver Qi, relieve Stagnation, tonify Spleen, nourish Xue | Irritability, depression, moodiness, fatigue, headache, dizziness, breast distention, irregular menstruation, menstrual pain |
| Woman's Balance | Regulate Qi, nourish Liver Xue and Yin, strengthen Spleen Qi, harmonize Liver and Spleen | Menstrual disorders, PMS, swollen breasts, depression, menstrual pain, irregular periods, abdominal bloating |

## Step Four: Bringing in Additional Modalities

Some practitioners—especially naturopathic physicians (N.D.s) and some natural medicine M.D.s—use natural progesterone topical creams to combat PMS.

A common theory about PMS is that is stems from elevated levels of estrogen. But another view holds that it is the relative lack of progesterone in relation to the amount of estrogen that causes PMS. Western science and many physicians prescribe synthetic progestin to counter menopausal symptoms, but this chemical is not a satisfactory replica of natural progesterone. In fact, progestin has been posited by some researchers to actually inhibit the body's natural synthesis of progesterone, and it may worsen symptoms.

WARNING

Never use natural progesterone cream without a practitioner's supervision and never in conjunction with other hormones or medicines without consulting both your Chinese and your Western doctors.

# SUPPORTING THE YIN: THE COMPREHENSIVE PROGRAM FOR MENOPAUSAL SYMPTOMS

To ease menopausal symptoms, you will expand the Comprehensive Program for Gynecologic Health to include targeted therapies.

In Chinese medicine, the symptoms of menopause—hot flashes, palpitations, emotionality, depression, vaginal dryness, change in libido, urinary problems, and changes in skin texture—are associated with Deficient Kidney Yin, Deficient Liver Xue, Deficient Kidney Yang, and Deficient Yin and Yang of Kidney. It is important to emphasize that menopause is not a disease or a disorder. Menopause is part of the natural progress of a woman's life. Any physical or emotional discomfort associated with menopause can be eased or eliminated.

To relieve your symptoms, implement the guidelines in the general gynecologic program plus the suggestions that follow here.

## Step One: Expanding the Daily Journal

Along with your daily journal of your cycle, symptoms, diet, sleep patterns, exercise, stress, and emotions, record the following information:

- Changes in length of cycle (shortening or lengthening) and how long your period lasts

- The quality of menstrual blood, including color, heaviness of flow (light or heavy), and clotting (small, large, color)

- How you feel during mid-cycle: Is there mid-cycle bleeding or spotting? Is there mittelschmerz (pain at mid-cycle)? What about emotional changes?

- How you feel during the week prior to the onset of your period: Is there increased depression, bloating, or breast tenderness?

- Any increase in skin dryness and vaginal dryness and changes in secretions

- Fluctuations in your body temperature: Are you hotter or colder, less tolerant to changes in external temperature? Do you have hot flashes or sweating? How often? What time of day or night?

## Step Two: Additional Dietary Guidelines

Some foods contain isoflavones that are biochemically similar to estrogens. These are sometimes called phytoestrogens because they are plant foods that contain estrogen-mimicking substances.

Eating foods that contain isoflavones may help ease the symptoms of menopause that are associated with lowered estrogen. In some societies, up to half the dietary intake contains foods that have isoflavones, but in the United States less than 10 percent of the diet comes from such sources.

Isoflavone-containing foods include soy and foods made from soy—such as tofu, tempeh, edamame, and miso—as well as flaxseed, red clover, oats, barley, and beans.

Two of the primary isoflavones, genistein and diadzen, can act similarly to estrogen in the body. However, they have a very small fraction of the potency of the estrogen produced and circulating in women's bodies.

While isoflavones may act like estrogens, because they have much lower potency, they also are considered to have anti-estrogenic properties. This means that isoflavones potentially could block natural estrogens from binding to the estrogen receptors in tissues in the breasts and uterus, which could potentially lower the risk for these types of cancers.

Isoflavones are also thought to stop the formation of estrogens in fat tissue and stimulate production of a protein that binds estrogen in the blood (to make it less able to bind to the receptor). In addition, isoflavone-containing foods have antioxidants and are anti-inflammatory.

Studies conducted in Asian women have found a lower risk of breast cancer with eating more soy products. However, studies in the United States have tended to not find any association between how much soy a woman consumes and her risk of breast cancer. However, in general, women in the United States have a much lower soy intake overall than women in other countries do.[13]

Foods high in calcium and magnesium are recommended as well, although dairy products, especially those that are not organic, are generally discouraged in high quantities. Nondairy, high-calcium–containing foods include tahini, sesame seeds, curly kale, sardines, kidney beans, figs, and many types of nuts.[14]

Dietary fat (especially animal fats) should be kept relatively low, especially during perimenopause, when estrogen levels are unopposed by progesterone.

## Step Three: Additional Exercise Guidelines

Weight-bearing exercise is an important part of any perimenopausal or menopausal program. It is associated with increased calcium uptake and increased bone density. It's important to work both the lower and the upper body. Doing weight-bearing exercises on only one part of the skeleton will not spread the benefit throughout the body. You should only do weight-lifting exercises three times a week to avoid damaging the Spleen Qi and thus cause Deficient Xue.

Aerobic exercise is recommended for women who find they gain weight through menopause or who are at higher risk for heart disease. Remember, heart disease is the major killer of women older than age fifty.

## Step Four: Additional Soaks

For hot flashes, cooling soaks such as Peppermint Cooler are recommended (see page 214).

## Step Five: Additional Self-Massage

**Ear massage:** For general menopausal symptoms, try additional ear massage every day using the following points: Uterus, Endocrine, Ovaries, Sympathetic point, Shenmen, and Kidney. (See page 203 for the locations of the points.)

**Acupressure:** Rub the following points once a day for about ten minutes: Spleen 6, Kidney 3, and Stomach 36. For hot flashes, massage Heart 6, Kidney 7, Liver 2, and Kidney 6. (See pages 163 through 167 for the locations of the points.)

**Moxibustion:** If you are having hot flashes, only use moxa after consulting a practitioner. However, moxa can be soothing for fatigue and vaginal dryness. Moxa Stomach 36, Spleen 6, and Ren 6.

## Step Six: Assembling the Team

When it comes time to bring in a Western doctor, Chinese practitioner, and others who offer health care and healing, you want to remember the following:

- Menopause is not a disease. Avoid practitioners who treat you as though it were.

- Perimenopausal and menopausal women should be vigilant about having regular mammograms, Pap smears (even after the period has stopped), and cardiovascular checkups. For women in high-risk groups (white women, fair-haired women, those who are very thin, smokers, and those with a family history), a bone density scan may be recommended.

- The smartest approach to menopause is to try the least harsh, most natural treatments first. That means first changing your diet, increasing supplements, reducing stress levels, increasing aerobic exercise, avoiding caffeine, using acupuncture and herbs, trying massage and meditation, and stopping smoking—which is the single worst trigger of symptoms.

A growing number of physicians use hormone replacement therapy (HRT) only as a last resort for menopausal symptoms. Several recent studies have shown that women using HRT have increased risk of breast cancer, stroke, heart disease, and blood clots. The Women's Health Initiative (WHI), a study conducted over fifteen years that tracked more than 161,800 healthy, postmenopausal women, found that women who took HRT had an increased risk of heart disease. This study showed that the overall risk of long-term HRT use outweighed its benefits. However, newer data show that very low dose estrogen, either given systemically or vaginally, may be beneficial for menopausal symptoms, such as hot flashes, vaginal dryness, and osteopenia.[15]

## Step Seven: Additional Herbal Therapy

In addition to the herbal soups outlined in the general gynecologic program, your Chinese medicine practitioner may suggest that you take the following herbal formulas or others, according to your individual Chinese patterns.

### EXAMPLES OF CHINESE HERBAL FORMULAS FOR MENOPAUSE

| FORMULA | CHINESE FUNCTION | INDICATIONS |
| --- | --- | --- |
| Da Bu Yin Wan | Nourish Kidney Yin, remove Deficiency Heat | Night sweats, chest and face flushing, hot sensation in the palms and soles, difficulty staying asleep, irritability, fidgeting/restlessness, ear ringing, steaming bones (which feels like hot bones from inside) |
| Great Yin | Nourish Kidney Yin, clear Heat, subdue Deficiency Fire, stop Sweating | Night sweats, afternoon fevers, hot flashes, hot sensations, steaming bones |
| Zhi Bai Di Huang Wan | Enrich Yin, nourish Liver and Kidney Jing, reduce Deficiency Fire | Night sweats, dry mouth and tongue, urinary difficulty, weakness and pain in the lower back, knees, and extremities, steaming bones |

## Step Eight: Acupuncture and Moxibustion

Treatment is individualized to suit changing symptoms over the course of the pre-menopausal and menopausal interval. Whenever you receive treatment, you need to make a commitment of at least three months. If you go once a week and your practitioner is adept, you should see a dramatic change by your fourth cycle—for women who are still having menstrual periods.

A recent meta-analysis of 104 randomized controlled trials showed acupuncture's effectiveness in relieving menopause-related symptoms. It was published in the peer-reviewed journal *Menopause* in July 2014. This meta-analysis confirmed that acupuncture improves hot flash frequency and severity, menopause-related symptoms, and quality of life in women who are undergoing natural menopause.[16]

## Step Nine: Additional Supplements

For information on the use of natural progesterone to ease the symptoms of menopause, see the PMS section on page 262.

# CONSCIOUS CONCEPTION: THE COMPREHENSIVE PROGRAM FOR NATURAL FERTILITY SUPPORT

According to the Centers for Disease Control and Prevention (CDC), about 11 percent of women ages fifteen to forty-four in the United States have difficulty getting pregnant or carrying a pregnancy to term, regardless of marital status (impaired fecundity). Infertility is not just a problem for women, but also for men.

A CDC study analyzed data from the 2002 National Survey of Family Growth and found that 7.5 percent of all sexually experienced men younger than age forty-five reported seeing a fertility doctor during their lifetime. This equals 3.3 to 4.7 million men. Of the men who sought help, 18 percent were diagnosed with a male-related infertility problem.[17]

Women need functioning ovaries and fallopian tubes and a uterus to get pregnant. Conditions affecting any one of these organs can contribute to female infertility. We'll talk about a few of them here: ovarian function, fallopian tube patency, and uterine contour.

BETH'S STORY

"When you want to have a child, but your body betrays you, it is the most helpless, frustrating, world-shaking experience," Beth said. "Since I was a teenager, when I thought of who I was, I saw myself as a mother. To not be able to become pregnant brought my whole world crashing down on me. I'm sorry it took me so long to try acupuncture and herbs. I could have saved myself and my husband a whole lot of heartache."

Beth, age thirty-four, tried for five years to conceive. Her daughter, Faith, is a thriving toddler.

## Ovarian Function

Having regular, predictable periods generally means you are ovulating. Your ovulation can be predicted by using an ovulation predictor kit, and it can be confirmed by a blood test to check your progesterone level.

On the other hand, a woman who is having irregular periods is likely not ovulating, at least some of the time. This may be because of several conditions, and she should be evaluated by a Western doctor. The most common hormone imbalance that causes lack of ovulation is polycystic ovarian syndrome (PCOS), which is lack of periods due to physical or emotional stress and diminished ovarian reserve. Several tests exist to evaluate a woman's ovarian function.

As far as tests for fertility, several tests are currently used to predict fertility: follicle-stimulating hormone (FSH) on day 3 to 5 of the menstrual cycle, anti-mullerian hormone (AMH), and ultrasound for the antral follicle count (AFC). However, there is no infallible predictor of fertility.

## Fallopian Tube Patency

This term refers to whether the fallopian tubes are open, blocked, or swollen. Blocked fallopian tubes may be a result of pelvic infection, a ruptured appendix, gonorrhea or chlamydia, endometriosis, or abdominal surgery. The tubes may be checked through a type of X-ray called a hysterosalpingogram (HSG) or by chromopertubation (CP) during a laparosopic surgical procedure.

## Uterine Contour

This term refers to the physical characteristics of the uterus. Uterine function can be evaluated by ultrasound to look for fibroids or other abnormalities. If suspicion exists that the fibroids are blocking pregnancy, a sonohysterogram (SHG) or hysteroscopy (HSC) may be performed.

Because many fertility symptoms are not obvious as overt health conditions, sometimes underlying issues are only discovered once a woman starts trying to conceive. Some symptoms that may indicate the need for closer examination include painful periods, missed or irregular periods, no periods, mid-cycle bleeding or pain, and abdominal masses. Also, if a woman has gone through treatment for cancer, it would be good to have a Western evaluation before trying to conceive.

### CENTERS FOR DISEASE CONTROL AND PREVENTION (CDC) SUMMARY OF INFERTILITY RISK IN WOMEN[18]

Female fertility is known to decline with:

Age: Many women are waiting until their thirties and forties to have children. In fact, about 20 percent of women in the United States now have their first child after age thirty-five, and this leads to age becoming a growing cause of fertility problems. About one-third of couples in which the woman is older than thirty-five years have fertility problems. Aging decreases a woman's chances of having a baby, and it also increases her chances of miscarriage and of having a child with a genetic abnormality. Aging decreases a woman's chances of having a baby in the following ways:

- Her ovaries become less able to release eggs.

- She has a smaller number of eggs left.

- Her eggs are not as healthy.

- She is more likely to have health conditions that can cause fertility problems.

- She is more likely to have a miscarriage.

Other factors that affect fertility include:

- Smoking

- Excessive alcohol use

- Extreme weight gain or loss

- Excessive physical or emotional stress that results in amenorrhea (absent periods)

## Fertility Support in Chinese Medicine

Evidence that acupuncture and herbal medicine have been used to aid fertility can be found in early medical literature dating back to 3 CE. The condition of infertility was first recorded by Zhang Zhong-Jing, a famous physician from the Han Dynasty, in his discussion of diseases in women in the *Jin Gui Yao Lue* (*Essentials of the Golden Cabinet*).

The benefits of using Chinese medicine treatments—acupuncture, Qi Gong, herbs, and nutritional therapy—to support healthy fertility and to remedy infertility have been used since before that time.

Modern researchers have confirmed that these therapies benefit in the following areas:

- Regulating the menstrual cycle
- Helping to overcome hormonal imbalances
- Eliminating immune system incompatibilities
- Easing tubal obstructions
- Enhancing general health
- Reducing stress, controlling anxiety, enhancing sleep, and increasing energy
- Balancing the endocrine system
- Improving blood flow in the pelvic cavity
- Invigorating sperm, enhancing a man's sperm count and motility
- Reversing ejaculatory defects and erectile dysfunction
- Increasing the chance of pregnancy for women undergoing in-vitro fertilization (IVF)

By following the Comprehensive Program for Natural Fertility Support, you can identify methods for optimizing your reproductive health and potentially avoiding more invasive procedures. And when necessary, you can support your body for potentially incorporating appropriate Western medical treatments for family building.

Before beginning this program, let's expand on the Chinese and Western concepts of a woman's reproductive system that we outlined in the general gynecology section and delve into more specific origins of disharmonies and disorders as they relate specifically to the pursuit of fertility.

The primary Organ Systems involved in Chinese reproductive medicine are the Spleen, Liver, Kidney, and Heart Systems. By enriching the blood in the uterus, the Spleen System governs the nutrition in the uterus, such as to the uterine lining (endometrium). The Liver System dictates the timing of menstruation and ovulation. The Kidney System is associated with the entire endocrine and reproductive system, including all of the important hormone-producing glands, such as the pituitary, thyroid, and adrenal glands.

In Chinese medicine, the mind is stored in the Heart, and the Heart Xue descends to nourish the uterine Xue. This can be thought of as an ancient description of the hypothalamus-pituitary-ovarian axis, which in Western medicine we know is a pivotal piece of assessing and treating fertility.

Chinese medicine diagnoses for fertility-related problems include Deficient Jing, Deficient Qi and Xue, Heat Injury of the Channels, Stagnant Qi and Xue, Deficient Yin of Kidney and Liver, Cold Uterus, and Deficient Yang, along with Extraordinary Channel disturbances.

## Fertility in Western Medicine

While Chinese medicine looks at the Organ Systems to determine a woman's fertility potential, Western medicine uses markers such as hormone panels, age and assessment of the fallopian tubes, and uterine environment to arrive at a diagnosis or prognosis for fertility.

### CHARTING BASAL BODY TEMPERATURE AND CERVICAL MUCUS

Experts say the best way to detect ovulation is to combine a daily reading of your basal body temperature with monitoring the texture of your cervical mucus. Chart your cycle for a few months so you can recognize your pattern and have a better chance of predicting your most fertile days.

**Charting basal body temperature:** Basal body temperature (BBT) is your temperature when you first wake up in the morning. Before you ever get out of bed to brush your teeth or start your day, pop a basal thermometer (available at drugstores) into your mouth. This particular type of thermometer shows the minute incremental degree changes that a regular thermometer does not show. It is important to try to wake up and take this reading about the same time each morning.

Your BBT probably ranges from 97.2°F (36.2°C) to about 97.7°F (36.5°C) before ovulation. During the two or three days after you ovulate, hormonal changes cause a rise in your BBT of between 0.5°F and 1.6°F, which lasts at least until your next period. You'll probably notice your temperatures spiking on other days, but unless it stays that way, you probably haven't yet ovulated. If you become pregnant, your temperature will stay elevated throughout your pregnancy.

It's helpful to chart your temperature for a few months so you can see whether there is a pattern to your cycle. If you're sick or fail to take your temperature immediately upon awakening, any pattern you find may be inaccurate.

**Charting cervical mucus:** There are many different types of vaginal discharge, one of which is cervical mucus. The type of mucus your body produces provides clues to your fertility. You can check your cervical mucus using either your fingers or toilet paper. On days when you're not fertile, the mucus from the cervix is either light or sticky (about the same texture as sticky rice).

During the few days leading up to ovulation, when you are most fertile, you'll have more discharge that is clear and slippery with the consistency of raw egg white. You are most fertile on the last day you notice egg white–type cervical mucus. It usually happens either the day before, or the day of, ovulation.[19]

**Putting them together:** Start keeping track of your temperature on the first day of your period using a basal body thermometer. Take your basal body temperature, and plot it on a chart. Then check the consistency of your cervical mucus and plot it on the same chart.

Most women will see a spike in temperature, signaling that you've ovulated, and notice that their mucus looks and feels like raw egg white around the same time. When the two coincide, you are more fertile.

## Basic Fertility Work-Up for Women

Have the following tests ordered at any time by your practitioner or physician to get a clear picture of the current state of your body:

- Comprehensive metabolic panel (glucose, kidneys, fluids and electrolytes, calcium, and liver)
- Lipid profile (total, HDL, LDL, risk ratio, and triglycerides)
- Complete blood count (CBC) with differential
- Luteinizing hormone (LH)
- Thyroid panel (TSH, T3, T4, etc.)
- Testosterone

On day three of your menstrual cycle (the third day of your period), have the following tests:

- Cycle day 3 FSH (Follicle Stimulating Hormone)
- Cycle day 3 E2 (Estradiol)
- Cycle day 3 LH (Luteinizing Hormone)
- Prolactin

Seven days (ideally) before your next period, have the following test:

- Mid-luteal progesterone

For example, if you have a twenty-eight day cycle, you would have this test done on cycle day 21.

The following optional tests can be done at any time:

- Anti-mullerian hormone (AMH) is a substance produced by granulosa cells in ovarian follicles. Because AMH is produced only in small ovarian follicles, blood levels of this substance have been used to attempt to measure the size of the pool of growing follicles in women. Research shows that the size of the pool of growing follicles is heavily influenced by the size of the pool of remaining primordial follicles (microscopic follicles in "deep sleep"). Therefore, AMH blood levels are thought to reflect the size of the remaining egg supply or "ovarian reserve." An AMH test can be done on any day of a woman's cycle.

- Ultrasound: It is important that you have an ultrasound done to check your ovarian follicle development, providing information about the number and size of developing follicles and the reaction of the uterine lining (endometrium) to follicle growth. Ask your fertility physician to guide you as to time in the cycle.

## RECURRENT PREGNANCY LOSS

While one in three women experience a pregnancy loss in the context of a normal reproductive history, miscarriage does not mean you cannot have a healthy successful pregnancy and birth.

Recurrent pregnancy loss (RPL) is the occurrence of three or more consecutive pregnancies that end in miscarriage of the fetus during the first trimester or one or more second-trimester miscarriages.

With RPL, it is important to be evaluated by a reproductive endocrinologist for clotting factors, genetic abnormalities, and autoimmune problems (including sperm allergy).

## Assisted Reproduction Technologies

If you are unable to become pregnant naturally and have exhausted everything else, your body may need some additional Western medicine treatments. The Centers for Disease Control and Prevention (CDC) defines assisted reproduction technologies (ART) to include all fertility treatments in which both eggs and sperm are handled. These include procedures that involve surgically removing eggs from a woman's ovaries, combining them with sperm in the lab, and returning them to the woman's body or donating them to another woman. The CDC does not include treatments in which only sperm are handled or procedures in which a woman takes medicine only to stimulate egg production without the intention of having eggs retrieved. However, for our purposes I am including all conventional treatments that are in addition to natural fertility support.

In addition to ART, you will still use all the natural fertility support modalities previously discussed. The less invasive, the better. Here is a brief list of the ART treatments. Discuss these with your physician. It is best to see a reproductive endocrinologist (RE) for evaluation and treatment if you can.

**Fertility drugs:** These are often the first line of treatment if you are not becoming pregnant naturally. These may include drugs to stimulate ovulation, such as clomiphene and gonadotropins. There is a small risk of ovarian hyperstimulation syndrome in which the ovaries are overstimulated and too many follicles are produced and get very large.

**Intrauterine insemination (IUI):** IUI is when sperm are "washed" and placed in sterile fluid, concentrated, and injected directly into the uterus. Drug treatment is commonly used to increase the success of IUI.

**In vitro fertilization (IVF):** IVF is the most common ART. Currently, 99 percent of all ART in the United States is IVF. In IVF, the woman injects fertility drugs to develop several eggs, may take other drugs to prevent premature release of the eggs, and egg development is monitored by ultrasound along with hormone testing. When the follicles are the correct size, human chorionic gonadotropin (HCG) is injected to complete the maturation of the egg. Thirty-six to forty-eight hours later, eggs are removed from the ovary under anesthesia. During the same time, sperm is collected from the partner or donor. Then the eggs and sperm are combined and monitored for fertilization. For the next two to five days, the fertilized eggs develop, and then the embryos are ready to be transferred into the uterus. Unused embryos may be frozen and saved for future use.

In my opinion, IVF as a first line treatment should be limited to women who have difficulty conceiving due to severely scarred and blocked fallopian tubes, poor sperm quality in the partner or donor, or fertility unexplained after every possible evaluation.

IVF is very expensive, comes with risk of multiple pregnancies, includes risks of high doses of drugs to support the IVF procedures, and possibly increases the risks of birth defects and low birth weight. Acupuncture is often used to improve the outcomes of IVF treatments.

**Intracytoplasmic sperm injection (ICSI):** ICSI is a type of IVF in which one sperm is injected directly into an individual egg. Generally, the best times to use ICSI are for low sperm count, poor sperm motility, poor morphology (structural problems), or for a male partner or donor who had a vasectomy.

**Other transfer options:** These options are generally out of date; however, they are part of ART. These include gamete intrafallopian transfer (GIFT) and zygote intrafallopian transfer (ZIFT).

**Donor eggs:** Donor eggs are generally used for women over the age of forty-three whose eggs are damaged or insufficient in some way, or not enough are produced when using fertility drugs. Eggs are donated by another woman, and they are fertilized by sperm from either a male partner or donor. This is a similar process to IVF; however, it is the woman donating the eggs who is given the fertility medications and her eggs are collected. The woman receiving the eggs also takes drugs to synchronize her estrogen levels with the donor's levels and is also given progesterone to build the uterine (endometrial) lining to accept the donor embryo during the IVF procedure.

## Step One: Expanding the Daily Journal

As you begin this program, to support natural fertility, you will expand the Comprehensive Program for Gynecologic Health to include targeted therapies. Follow the guidelines in the general gynecologic program plus the suggestions that follow here.

Along with your daily journal of your cycle, symptoms, diet, sleep patterns, exercise, stress, and emotions, record the following information:

- Chart your cycle for a few months.
- Track your basal body temperature (BBT).
- Monitor the texture of your cervical mucus.
- Monitor the quality of menstrual blood, including color, heaviness of flow (light or heavy), and clotting (small, large, color).
- Jot down how you feel during ovulation: Is there ovulation-related bleeding or spotting?

## Step Two: Additional Dietary Guidelines

In addition to the general gynecological guidelines, you should make extra sure that you are getting plenty of high-quality protein. During menstruation, make sure that you are eating foods rich in iron.

To support the Kidney and Spleen Systems and maintain enough Yang Qi for development of the egg, make sure that 90 percent of your diet is cooked and that the foods you eat eliminate Dampness.

During the time between your period and ovulation, protein consumption is very important. It is best to eat foods that support the Kidney System to nourish the follicles as they mature. Foods that support the Spleen System are important for maintaining uterine function. Vitamin-E-rich foods such as cold-pressed organic oils, nuts, seeds, and avocados support the developing egg as well. During this time, it is important to completely avoid alcohol.

During ovulation, eat foods that support the Liver System and Spleen System. Make sure you are taking a sublingual vitamin B that includes folic acid, $B_{12}$, and $B_6$ during this time to support egg release and implantation. Eat foods high in zinc, such as eggs, whole grains, and fish to support progesterone production.

After ovulation, consider eating organic ripe pineapple. Bromelain, contained in pineapple, has been shown to help with egg implantation. After confirmed ovulation or embryo transfer during IVF, begin consuming one to two slices of pineapple each day. Stop when implantation has occurred.

## Step Three: Additional Exercise Guidelines

Moderate exercise is best for women trying to conceive. Also, proper weight is associated with improved chances of becoming pregnant. Research shows that being underweight or overweight can reduce the chances of becoming pregnant. Ovulation can be compromised in women who don't consume enough calories and good fats every day. Being overweight or obese can also create difficulty in conception because obesity can interfere with normal hormone function and therefore fertility.

However, just being skinny by itself is only part of the issue. We know that estrogen is stored in fat tissue, and it is an important part of conceiving and holding a pregnancy. Even if you are thin, if you are eating enough good fats and exercising moderately, you are fine.

While you are trying to get pregnant, don't stop exercising if you are doing moderate exercise. Exercise increases the flow of Qi and Xue, helps endorphin production, decreases pain, decreases stress, and improves your mood. If you exercise throughout your time of trying to conceive, it becomes natural for you to continue throughout pregnancy. During pregnancy, exercise is important for many reasons.

## Step Four: Additional Soaks and Compresses

You may use the Gingerly compress during the time before conception to warm the uterus and ovaries and to improve blood flow in these areas (see page 217).

You can buy readymade compresses and herbal packs in your local herb or natural foods stores for supporting fertility.

## Step Five: Additional Self-Massage

**Ear massage:** For supporting fertility, you can perform ear massage every day using the Uterus point, the Endocrine point, the Ovaries point, the Sympathetic point, the Shenmen point, and the Kidney point. (See page 203 for the locations of the points.)

**Uterine massage:** To increase blood flow to the uterus, or if you have a history of endometriosis, fibroids, or scar tissue, you can perform uterine massage. Find your uterus just above the pubic bone on the midline of your lower abdomen. Massage using lifting and pressing motions over the uterus area. Then use all of your fingers or the heel of your hand to make a pumping movement to increase blood flow in the area. To be on the safe side, do not do this massage during your period or after you have ovulated.

**Ovary massage:** To increase blood flow to the ovaries, or if you have a history of ovarian cysts, scarring, or adhesions, you can perform ovary massage. The ovaries are approximately four fingers from the midline, about two fingers above the pubic bone. The acupressure point Zigong (uterus) is located here. Massage over each ovary with your fingers or thumbs in circles. You can go deeper as you find areas of tenderness; however, don't go so deep as to bruise yourself and cause pain. Make a pumping movement over the whole area to increase blood flow. To be on the safe side, do not do this massage during your period or after you have ovulated.

**Reflexology:** You may massage the areas of the ovary, uterus (womb), and pelvic area on both the hands and feet (see pages 210 and 211).

Ask your practitioner to show you other types of massage for additional issues.

## Step Six: Additional Self-Moxibustion

You may perform moxibustion over the whole lower abdomen from the navel to the pubic bone out to ovary areas. The points Ren 3, Ren 4, Ren 6 (page 40), and Zi Gong (page 206) are especially important. Ask your practitioner what points you may use if you become pregnant.

## Step Seven: Assembling the Team

When it comes time to bring in a Western doctor, Chinese practitioner, and others who offer health care and healing, you want to remember the following:

- If you are trying to get pregnant naturally, although you may not be seeking Western treatment for infertility, make sure you have had your yearly gynecological checkup and all of your other regular medical exams. Men involved as partners or sperm donors should also have regular checkups to make sure they are healthy.
- The first approach to natural fertility support is to try the least harsh, most natural treatments first. That means changing your diet, increasing supplements, reducing stress levels, increasing your exercise routine, avoiding caffeine, stopping smoking, and using acupuncture, Chinese herbs, massage, and meditation.
- After a certain amount of time trying to conceive without success, most Western experts recommend that you see a fertility specialist. If you are younger than thirty-five, most experts suggest you try to become pregnant every month for at least one year. However, if you are thirty-five years or older, you should see a fertility specialist after six months of trying unsuccessfully.

Conventional wisdom is that the chance of having a successful pregnancy and birth rapidly decreases each year after the age of thirty. Because some health problems also increase the risk of infertility, you should talk to a health care provider if you have any of the following:

- Irregular menstrual periods
- No menstrual periods
- Very painful menstrual periods
- Diagnosed endometriosis
- History of pelvic inflammatory disease (PID)
- More than one miscarriage

Ideally, it is appropriate for any woman, and her male partner or donor, to talk to a fertility-knowledgeable Western medical provider prior to trying to get pregnant. The provider can help you get your body ready for a healthy baby, and she or he can also answer questions on fertility and give tips on proper conception.

Seeking a fertility support consultation from a Chinese medicine practitioner is important as well. You can learn your Chinese medicine diagnosis, decide if you would like to use acupuncture to support becoming pregnant, and learn which herbs, supplements, and foods are appropriate for your particular Chinese medicine patterns.

## Step Eight: Additional Herbal Therapy

In addition to the herbal soups outlined in the general gynecologic program, your Chinese medicine practitioner may suggest that you take the following herbal formulas or others according to your diagnosis.

### EXAMPLES OF CHINESE HERBAL FORMULAS FOR FERTILITY

| FORMULA | CHINESE FUNCTION | INDICATIONS |
|---|---|---|
| Channel Flow | Regulate Qi and Xue, warm the Channels | Menstrual pain and cramps, menstrual clotting, abdominal pain, infertility |
| Women's Precious Pills | Tonify Qi and Xue | Irregular menstruation, painful menses, light or no menstrual flow, pale complexion, irritability, poor memory |
| Maternal Herbal | Tonify Liver Yin and Kidney Yang, relax Shen, invigorate Qi and Xue, nourish Xue, tonify Qi | Promote fertility, reduce coldness |

## Step Nine: Acupuncture and Moxibustion

Acupuncture and moxa treatments are individualized to suit your specific Chinese diagnoses and your specific menstrual issues, timing, and age. With acupuncture and herbal fertility support, it is often a long-term treatment, anywhere from one month to one or two years. If you have normal menstrual cycles, are eager to become pregnant immediately, or are older than age thirty, you may want to start fertility support treatment right away.

If your cycle is irregular or absent, or if you have endometriosis, PCOS, or other conditions associated with higher rates of infertility, it is best to address these issues for some period of time prior to focusing on direct fertility support. Some of the treatments for those issues are inappropriate while trying to actively become pregnant. After several months or even a couple of years, you then would be ready to support treatment for becoming pregnant.

You should plan to make a commitment of at least three months minimum, especially if cycle regulation is the first part of your treatment. Because it can take a year for normal conception to occur, plan on at least twelve months of treatment. When you become pregnant, plan to get acupuncture treatments throughout pregnancy.

In general, the best candidates for acupuncture and Chinese herbal medicine for natural fertility support are women (and men) who have a functional, rather than structural, reason for infertility. Infertility due to hormonal problems, immune disorders, amenorrhea, irregular menstruation, stress, and age-related factors all fall into the category of functional infertility.

Acupuncture is also used for support during in vitro fertilization (IVF).

A very important study, published in 2002 in *Fertility and Sterility,* found that acupuncture significantly increases the chances of a woman becoming pregnant. In this study, eighty patients received two 25-minute acupuncture treatments—one prior to having fertilized embryos transferred into their uterus, and one directly afterward. A second group of eighty patients, who also underwent embryo transfer, received no acupuncture treatments.[20]

Some evidence suggests that needle stimulation may improve blood flow to the uterus. Researchers are looking at whether acupuncture might make the uterine wall more receptive to the embryo. Also, egg production may be improved with the use of acupuncture.

## Step Ten: Additional Supplements

Follow the supplement recommendations in the Comprehensive Program for Gynecologic Health (see page 241). Your practitioner should guide you as to doses, depending on your specific conditions and where you are in your fertility process.

Prenatal nutritional supplements are recommended while you are trying to conceive and throughout pregnancy.

Coenzyme Q10 ($CoQ_{10}$) improves pelvic blood flow and reduces miscarriages. Studies in IVF and ICSI show that women who take $CoQ_{10}$ have higher pregnancy rates.[21] L-arginine also increases blood flow to the pelvis; however, it should not be taken if you have herpes. Women with higher rates of miscarriage have low glutathione; glutathione is made in the body from N-acetyl cysteine (NAC). Therefore, supplemental NAC or whey protein is often recommended. Royal jelly is another Chinese food substance that may help fertility.

Your naturopathic physician, Chinese medicine doctor, or integrative physician will give you additional recommendations according to your specific situation.

## SUPPLEMENTS FOR ENHANCING MALE FERTILITY

- L-Carnitine 3 grams per day increases motility[22]
- L-Arginine 4 grams per day increases motility (Do not take if you have herpes.)
- Zinc Sulfate 24 milligrams per day increases testosterone and sperm count
- Vitamin E 600 milligrams per day increases motility (Take with food.)
- Selenium 1000 milligrams per day increases sperm count
- Folic acid 800 micrograms per day improves sperm quality
- Vitamin $B_{12}$ 1000 milligrams per day increases motility
- Vitamin C 1000 milligrams per day increases motility
- $CoQ_{10}$ 100 milligrams per day increases sperm count and motility[23]
- Chinese herbal formulas from your practitioner

## AT A GLANCE: COMPREHENSIVE PROGRAM FOR GYNECOLOGIC HEALTH

| SELF-CARE PLAN | |
|---|---|
| Self-monitoring | In addition to the general guidelines, your daily journal will include the following in relation to your monthly cycle: food cravings, changes in appetite, alcohol and caffeine consumption, energy levels, symptoms that make it difficult to exercise, emotional ups and downs, when you ovulate, when your period starts, description of the flow, color, texture, intensity, and duration. |
| Dietary guidelines | Eat a diet of warm, cooked foods. Avoid excess dairy products, eliminate caffeine, and drink a minimum of alcohol. Increase fiber and use whole grains to avoid premenstrual constipation. Eliminate excess salt from your diet to ease water retention. Eliminate any foods that your daily log indicates are associated with premenstrual syndrome (PMS), cramps, irregularity, or any of the emotional and physical symptoms surrounding the progress of your cycle. |

*(continued)*

| SELF-CARE PLAN *(continued)* | |
|---|---|
| Exercise | Use Yoga, Qi Gong warm-up exercises, and walking to stimulate balanced flow. Once a routine is established daily for thirty minutes, you can expand your exercises to include aerobics, such as jogging, cycling, and swimming. Try to walk 10,000 steps per day. |
| Meditation | Use the Lotus Blossom Meditation for a quick time-out from cycle-related discomfort and stress. Use the Buddha's Breath exercise to help ease Stagnation. Regular practice of the longer Qi Meditation does much to restore harmony. |
| Moxibustion | Perform self-moxa on Spleen 6 and Ren 6 once a week for three weeks, with a week off during the period. |
| Massage | Practice Qi Gong abdominal massage for cramps and to dispel Stagnation and Dampness. Use reflexology as well as acupressure on Liver 3. A monthly breast self-exam and massage are important for all women. |
| Soaks and Compresses | Use ginger compresses and soaks to ease cramps and lower back pain. A Sleep Ease soak can help you relax. |
| Nutritional supplements | Follow the general nutritional supplement guidelines with the modifications made in this chapter. Include omega-3 fatty acids, vitamin D, antioxidants, calcium with other substances, and sublingual $B_{12}$/folic acid/$B_6$. Make sure you take a regular dose of *Lactobacillus acidophilus*. |
| PMS SELF-CARE (GENERAL GUIDELINES ABOVE PLUS . . .) | |
| Dietary guidelines | In addition to the general guidelines, women with PMS should eliminate all refined sugars from the diet; eliminate decaffeinated coffee, chocolate, and dark sodas; reduce fat content of diet to 25 percent of daily calories; avoid over-the-counter diuretics. Adjust diet to eliminate excess salt and increase grains. Drink 48 ounces (1.4 L) of filtered or spring water a day. |
| Nutritional supplements | Considering taking zinc and non-heme plant iron for PMS symptoms only with your practitioner's advice. Increase magnesium for leg cramps and fluid retention, if necessary. See the chapter for additional recommendations. |
| MENOPAUSE SELF-CARE (GENERAL GUIDELINES ABOVE PLUS . . .) | |
| Self-monitoring | In addition to the daily journal of your cycle, note changes in the length of your cycle and how long your period lasts and the quality of your menstrual blood. See if there is mid-cycle bleeding or spotting or pain. Is there increased depression, bloating, or breast tenderness? Note skin dryness, vaginal dryness, and changes in secretions. Are you having temperature changes, hot flashes, or sweating? |
| Dietary guidelines | In addition to the general guidelines for gynecology, isoflavone-containing foods may help ease the symptoms of menopause associated with lowered estrogen. Foods high in calcium and magnesium are recommended. Dietary fat (especially animal fats) should be consumed moderately, especially during perimenopause, when estrogen levels are unopposed by progesterone. |

*(continued)*

| MENOPAUSE SELF-CARE *(continued)* | |
| --- | --- |
| Additional exercise recommendations | Weight-bearing exercise three times a week. Aerobic exercise is important for women who gain weight or are at higher risk of heart disease. |
| Soaks | For hot flashes, cooling soaks such as Peppermint Cooler are useful. |
| Additional self-massage | Ear massage daily plus ten minutes of acupressure on varying points. |
| Moxibustion | If you are having hot flashes, moxa should not be used without consulting a practitioner. However, it can be soothing for problems of fatigue and vaginal dryness. Moxa Stomach 36, Spleen 6, and Ren 6. |
| FERTILITY SUPPORT SELF-CARE (GENERAL GUIDELINES ABOVE PLUS . . .) | |
| Self-monitoring | In addition to the daily journal of your cycle, chart your cycle for several months, check your basal body temperature, monitor your cervical mucus, and observe your menstrual blood and how you feel during ovulation and whether there is bleeding or spotting. |
| Dietary guidelines | In addition to the general guidelines for gynecology, make sure you are eating enough high-quality protein, eat 90 percent of your diet cooked and follow the guidelines in the chapter for the correct foods during the different parts of your menstrual cycle. |
| Additional exercise recommendations | Proper weight is associated with improved chances of becoming pregnant. Exercise moderately and don't stop while trying to conceive. Exercise throughout your time of trying to conceive and then it becomes natural for you to continue throughout pregnancy. |
| Soaks | Use ginger compresses during the time before conception to warm the uterus and ovaries and improve blood flow in these areas. |
| Additional self-massage | Ear massage daily plus regular uterine massage and ovary massage. Reflexology on the ovary, uterus, and pelvic areas can be done. |
| Moxibustion | You may perform moxibustion over the whole lower abdomen from the navel to the pubic bone out to ovary areas. The points Ren 3, Ren 4, Ren 6, and Zi Gong are especially important. Ask your practitioner which points you may use if you become pregnant. |
| GENERAL PROGRAM: ADDING PRACTITIONERS TO THE HEALING TEAM | |
| Obtaining a Western baseline | For screening for cancer, HIV, and sexually transmitted diseases, see your gynecologist yearly. Other tests according to the general program. |
| CHINESE MEDICINE | |
| Evaluation and diagnosis | Using the Four Examinations, the practitioner is able to design a treatment course that will restore harmony to your Organ Systems and Essential Substances and, as a consequence, alleviate your gynecological problems. |
| Acupuncture | The inclusion of Qi and Xue harmonizing acupuncture treatments at least once a month will promote gynecological harmony. |

*(continued)*

| CHINESE MEDICINE (continued) | |
|---|---|
| Moxibustion | In addition to the points you can do at home, the practitioner may use those points plus ones on your back such as Urinary Bladder 20 and Urinary Bladder 23. |
| Herbs | For prevention of disharmonies, you can eat Dang Gui Chicken Soup and San Qi Chicken Soup. |
| Other therapies | To increase Shen harmony and to reduce irritability, mood swings, stress, and/or depression, include other forms of Eastern meditation, biofeedback, hypnosis, or psychotherapy. To dispel digestive imbalances, some women adopt an Ayurvedic diet or Paleo diet. Abdominal massage can also ease digestive problems and alleviate period pain. |
| PMS PROGRAM: ADDING PRACTITIONERS TO THE HEALING TEAM | |
| Herbs | Formulas such as Woman's Balance, *Xiao Yao Wan*, and Heavenly Water alleviate PMS symptoms. A trained practitioner should prescribe any herbal formulas. |
| Additional modalities | Some practitioners—especially naturopathic physicians (N.D.s) and some natural medicine M.D.s—use natural progesterone topical creams to combat PMS. |
| MENOPAUSE PROGRAM: ADDING PRACTITIONERS TO THE HEALING TEAM | |
| Herbs | Formulas such as *Da Bu Yin Wan*, Great Yin, and *Zhi Bai Di Huang Wan* alleviate menopausal symptoms, such as hot flashes, mood swings, and urinary problems. A trained practitioner should prescribe any herbal formulas. |
| Acupuncture and moxibustion | Treatment is individualized to suit changing symptoms over the course of the premenopausal and menopausal interval. Make a commitment of at least three months to see the changes in your cycles and symptoms. |
| Additional modalities | Your doctor may prescribe use of natural progesterone to ease the symptoms of menopause. |
| FERTILITY SUPPORT PROGRAM: ADDING PRACTITIONERS TO THE HEALING TEAM | |
| Obtaining a Western baseline | If you are trying to get pregnant naturally, make sure you have had your yearly gynecological checkup and all your other regular medical exams. Men involved as partners or sperm donors should also have regular checkups. If you are thinking about becoming pregnant, see a fertility specialist if you are having irregular periods or no periods, have a history of endometriosis or PID, have a history of more than one miscarriage, are older than thirty-five, have been a smoker, have used excessive alcohol, have had extreme weight gain or loss, have excess physical or emotional stress, or have a history of treatment for cancer. Also, if you are not becoming pregnant after a year of trying monthly if age thirty-five or younger, or after six months if over age thirty-five, you should seek evaluation with a Western fertility specialist. You may need to consider ART. |

*(continued)*

| CHINESE MEDICINE | |
| --- | --- |
| Evaluation and diagnosis | Seek a fertility support consultation from a Chinese medicine practitioner. Learn your Chinese medicine diagnosis, decide if you would like to use acupuncture to support becoming pregnant, and learn which herbs and supplements are appropriate for your particular Chinese medicine patterns. |
| Herbs | Some herbal formulas used in fertility treatment are Channel Flow, Women's Precious Pills, and Maternal Herbal. Your practitioner will prescribe formulas based on your individual diagnosis. |
| Acupuncture and moxibustion | Treatment is individualized to your Chinese diagnoses and menstrual issues, timing, and age. Acupuncture is often a long-term treatment, anywhere from one month to one or two years. Acupuncture can also support IVF cycles. |
| Additional supplements | Prenatal vitamin supplements, $CoQ_{10}$, NAC, or whey protein to support glutathione production and royal jelly might be used. Your naturopathic physician, Chinese medicine doctor, or integrative physician will give you additional recommendations according to your specific situation. |

# 16

# SUPPORTING THE CENTER
## A Digestive Disorders Management Program

For thousands of years, Chinese medicine doctors have had a profound understanding of how important a nutritious diet and good digestion are in preventing disharmony in the mind/body/spirit. Recently, Western science has made breakthroughs in research confirming exactly how powerful diet is in preventing and/or causing a whole range of illnesses—from colon and breast cancer to fatty liver to allergies and irritable bowel syndrome. Yet millions of us suffer daily digestive upset and chronic digestive illnesses. Antacids, laxatives, proton pump inhibitors—we down millions of over-the-counter stomach remedies in a futile attempt to make our bellies feel better. Millions of dollars' worth of prescription drugs, from steroids to Tagamet, are taken to ease problems that stubbornly resist Western treatments.

## PART ONE: A SIX-STEP SELF-CARE PLAN FOR PREVENTION AND THERAPEUTIC TREATMENT

Whether you have a chronic digestive disorder or an acute attack, the following comprehensive program offers a way for you to use self-care and assemble a team of practitioners to support your healing efforts.

### Step One: Keeping a Daily Journal

When starting a comprehensive digestive program, the first step is to keep a one- to two-week journal, paying special attention to your diet in relationship to daily activities, your sleep patterns, and your physical and emotional responses throughout the day. Over time, possible correlations among diet, emotion, and symptoms of digestive problems should emerge. These will then give you clues as to wise self-care and will help your practitioner(s) prescribe effective treatment. (For information on how to establish and interpret your journal see page 223.) In your journal, note the following:

- Your diet: When considering your diet in relation to digestive disorders, note foods that obviously make you feel sleepy, tired, or gassy; foods that increase nervousness, change stools, or trigger sneezing or congestion within an hour of eating or the next day; and foods that cause stomach or intestinal pain.

- Your emotions: When considering diet in relation to emotions, compare your journal of times when you eat certain foods with your journal of times when you notice an increase in worry, agitation, or tension. Also, write down if becoming emotional causes pain or tension in the area beneath your breastbone. Note if you become more gassy when you eat while you are upset or if your appetite increases or decreases with a particular emotion.

- Overall energy levels: Track the daily ebb and flow of your energy: Do you have morning grogginess or an afternoon slump? Do you get tired after eating certain foods or eating in general? What time of day is your energy at the lowest? Compare your findings with your journal for diet and emotions. Can you see a pattern between low energy, eating certain foods and experiencing certain emotions?

- Physical symptoms: Make a note of your general aches and pains; stiff joints; headaches; stuffy or runny nose; itchy eyes; grumbly, gassy, or upset stomach; and cravings for sugar, chocolate, or caffeine. Again, you want to see if there is a relationship between emotions, diet, and physical symptoms.

## Step Two: Implementing a Diet Program

For preventive self-care, it's a good idea to increase your intake of high-quality protein, legumes, grains, and vegetables. At the same time, decrease sugars, cut down on red meats and trans-fats, and follow a varied diet that includes many foods. (See the dietary guidelines in chapter 6, page 91.)

For self-care treatment of digestive disorders, it is vital that you eat a diet of cooked, warm foods and limit raw and uncooked foods. That will help strengthen your Spleen/Stomach Organ Systems, which are generally weak when digestive disharmony occurs.

In addition, eat as simply as possible to give your body time to heal. Do not overeat or skip any meals. Too much or too little food can create additional digestive problems.

Generally, you should have your largest meal at midday. Eating large meals in the evening or eating before going to bed puts a strain on the Spleen and Stomach Systems. If you already have a weakened Spleen, however, you may find that you feel best if you eat small meals frequently throughout the day.

Follow the First-Step Dietary Therapy Program to break the cycle of digestive upset (see page 113).

Identify the foods that you suspect may aggravate the condition by evaluating your self-monitoring journal. Eliminate those foods from your diet. After four days, introduce one back into your diet. Observe the results. If all goes well, you may continue eating that food, but no more than once every four days. You may introduce each eliminated food back into your diet on a four-day rotation. If one produces a symptomatic reaction, it should be taken out of your diet, at least for the next several months.

Take *Lactobacillus acidophilus* for both prevention and treatment of digestive upset and parasites. Yogurt doesn't pack enough live cultures into one serving to provide as much help as the pill or powder form.

## Step Three: Implementing an Exercise and Meditation Plan

The methods of exercise you'll choose to help digestive disharmony depend on your Chinese diagnosis. If the Qi is weak and you experience fatigue, lack of appetite, and a feeling of fullness after eating very little, try mild Qi Gong exercises, such as exercise one and two on page 182 and breathing exercises on page 185. Done three to four times a week, they will help strengthen the Qi and ease your symptoms.

If Stagnant Qi is your diagnosis with symptoms such as gas, irritability, and bloating, the digestive disorder will respond to more vigorous exercise five to seven days a week. Recommended exercises such as jogging, cycling, fast walking, and other aerobics should not be done to the point of exhaustion because that can deplete Qi, instead of building it. Too much exercise can also deplete Xue. Women who overdo aerobic exercise may have light or no periods because of Xue Deficiency related to Qi Deficiency.

Weight-lifting on machines or using free weights should only be done every other day, because the process of tearing down the muscles to build them up can cause a Deficient Spleen, which would worsen any digestive problems.

You can, however, engage in Yoga, Qi Gong exercises, and Tai Chi without worry about detrimental effects.

## Step Four: Using Compresses and Soaks for Digestive Problems

In general, warming compresses and brief soaks ease some of the discomfort of digestive disorders. However, don't use them directly after eating. And if you are feeling weak, use warm, not hot, water.

Use ginger compresses to warm and strengthen the abdominal area. To make a ginger compress, grate one-third of a large ginger root. Place the grated ginger in an unbleached square of cheesecloth and tie it securely. Place in 1 to 2 quarts (1 to 2 L) of boiling water for ten minutes. Remove the bag of ginger from the water and set aside. Take 1 cup (235 ml) of tea from the pot. Add ½ to 1 teaspoon dried ginger before drinking. Soak a washcloth in the remaining ginger brew in the pot. Wring it out. Apply it to your abdomen. Repeat applications until you feel very warm and comfortable. Drink the ginger tea.

Other compress alternatives include hydrocollator packs that you heat in a boiling pot of water and microwaveable herbal heat packs that become damp when heated.

For a soak, draw a chamomile bath using the recipe for Sleep Ease on page 213.

## Step Five: Using Massage for Self-Healing

Many massage techniques can ease discomfort and restore balance in digestive disorders.

Self-acupressure can ease the discomfort of digestive disorders. Concentrate on Stomach 36, Spleen 6, and Stomach 34 (for stomach pain) (see pages 163 through 167). Follow the acupressure techniques described for these points on page 197. Repeat at least once a day.

Moxibustion is a powerful self-care tool. Focus your moxa treatment on these points for Deficiency and Cold conditions: Stomach 36, Spleen 6, Ren 6, Ren 12, and Stomach 25. Du 20 strengthens the Xue and brings up Qi. It is particularly effective for Qi Deficient diarrhea and organ prolapse. Almost anyone can moxa Stomach 36 to tonify Qi unless you have a high fever. Don't moxa when there is a sign of heat problems—such as fever, bloody stools, or burning diarrhea—without a practitioner's prescription. (See pages 40 and 206 for the locations of these points.)

Try ear massage. See the illustration of the ear on page 203 with the points for massage: Ear-Shen Men, Ear-Stomach, Ear-Spleen, and Ear-Large Intestine. Follow the massage techniques for these points explained on page 202.

Use reflexology. See the illustration of the foot with points highlighted on page 211.

Hara massage, a Japanese abdominal massage, is especially soothing to people with digestive disorders.

Qi-Xue abdominal self-massage instructions are on page 194.

## Step Six: Additional Nutritional Supplements

Nutritional supplements may be difficult for a person with severe digestive disorders to absorb. That's why the program begins with dietary changes, acupuncture, mild herbal formulas, and exercise. Once digestive stability has been established, you can add supplements, although several of them require the supervision of a doctor or practitioner. General recommendations include the following:

- *Lactobacillus acidophilus*: Take ½ teaspoon of this probiotic as a refrigerated powder once or twice a day in unchilled water thirty to sixty minutes before a meal.

- Sublingual vitamin $B_{12}$/folic acid/$B_6$: Trader Joe's carries one we use in the clinic. The sublingual version avoids the digestive tract and is easily absorbed.

- Vitamin $D_3$: There is evidence that taking vitamin $D_3$ helps chronic inflammatory bowel problems, improves irritable bowel syndrome (IBS) symptoms, and may reduce the incidence of intestinal cancer in persons with intestinal problems. Dosage can range from 2000 IU to 8000 IU per day, depending on the level of deficiency.

- Ground flaxseed: For both constipation and loose stools, sprinkle ground organic flaxseed over your food. Buy it in vacuum-sealed packages, not in bulk, to avoid rancidity. Some people prefer psyllium seed and husk. However, flaxseed has the advantage of having omega-3 fatty acids.

- Lactase pills or milk digestant pills, for lactose intolerance, can help when it's difficult to avoid all dairy products. Better yet, avoid dairy altogether because dairy products tend to promote Dampness. People with chronic digestive problems tend to be Spleen Deficient and Damp, and eating dairy can be a stress on the digestive system.

- Additional forms of probiotics may be prescribed, depending on the Western diagnosis of your digestive problem. For example, if you are having trouble in your upper small intestine, then *Bifidus* may be recommended.

- Digestive enzymes are generally good for people who have trouble digesting specific types of food, who are diagnosed as having decreased hydrochloric acid, or who can't digest any meat. (This is especially a problem for people who have been vegetarians for many years and begin to eat meat again.) Some people with wheat or gluten sensitivity may also use special enzymes to counteract the effects if those products are eaten inadvertently. Many Chinese herbal formulas are enzymatic, and the need for enzymes decreases or is eliminated when receiving Chinese herbal medicines from your practitioner. To determine if you need digestive enzymes, consult a naturopathic physician or Western nutritionist for recommended therapy.

· Additional supplements should be prescribed by a qualified practitioner. For example, a naturopathic doctor might recommend additional supplements such as d-limonene or deglycyrrhizinated licorice (DGL) for chronic indigestion, heartburn, and gastroesophageal reflux disease (GERD).

Always ask your practitioner to review your self-care plan as well.

# PART TWO: ASSEMBLING THE TEAM

Often when people turn to Chinese medicine, they have been suffering with chronic problems that Western medicine has not been able to relieve. If you are suffering from severe gastrointestinal disorders, such as Crohn's disease, ulcerative colitis, or irritable bowel syndrome, or if you have bloody diarrhea, expanding the treatment to include a combination of acupuncture, moxibustion, dietary changes, herbal medicine, and exercise may create the breakthrough that's needed. However, improvement doesn't usually happen overnight. Because the disharmonies that trigger these disorders are deep-rooted, it can take a full year before the problem is completely resolved. However, people with digestive disorders frequently are able to cut back on interventions such as acupuncture and herbal medicine before the year is up. They slowly return to a more normal diet. Because they have been involved in all aspects of their healing, the person knows when to return to a stricter, more therapeutic diet before the problem recurs.

## Step One: Obtaining a Western Baseline

It's important to rule out cancer and other life-threatening problems, a genetic disorder such as celiac disease, or to identify an illness that can be treated quickly and effectively by Western medicine. Follow the general guidelines in the basic comprehensive program for working with a Western practitioner. Find an expert in digestive disorders who can outline your treatment options. This information and information about ongoing Western treatment should be presented to your Chinese medicine practitioner.

### RENE'S STORY

Rene came into the clinic suffering from ulcerative colitis. She was afraid to go anywhere for fear that she couldn't get to a bathroom. She was about to get fired, and she was running out of hope.

"At the clinic, I was diagnosed with Deficient Spleen, and told I needed to bolster my immune system, change my diet, and eliminate some stress from my life," Rene said. "My Western doctors mentioned none of those things. They just said they had no idea how I got the disease or how to get rid of it.

"I was taking steroid enemas that made me gain sixteen pounds, then I had a bad reaction to the drug they gave me to compensate for the bloating. And I was taking oral medication that gave me severe headaches.

"I came for acupuncture and herbal therapy when it was clear that Western medications weren't going to help—at least not enough and not by themselves. Misha gave me Source Qi, an herbal formula that she developed.

"I'm still on some Western medication, but now after ten months of Chinese medicine treatments, I'm feeling much better and taking far fewer drugs," Rene said. "I still get acupuncture and moxibustion on my navel and legs once a week. I also get lots of other positive effects from it. If I have any other issues in my health—stress or allergies or painful periods—the acupuncture helps them, too."

## Step Two: Obtaining a Chinese Medicine Diagnosis and Treatment

When you go to a Chinese medicine practitioner, it's important to establish communication between the Chinese medicine and the Western doctor. Both practitioners should be aware of what you are doing as director of your own healing process.

At the Chinese medicine practitioner, you can expect to be treated with herbs, acupuncture, and moxibustion.

### HERBS

The following chart outlines some examples of Chinese herbal formulas that I've found are most effective and indicate the Chinese function and Western diagnosis they address. Under no circumstances should you self-administer these medicines unless they are also listed in the Medicine Cabinet (see page 230).

## EXAMPLES OF CHINESE HERBAL FORMULAS FOR DIGESTIVE PROBLEMS

| FORMULA | CHINESE FUNCTION | INDICATIONS |
|---|---|---|
| Artestatin | Expel parasites, clear Summer Heat, circulate Stagnant Qi, tonify Spleen and Stomach, anti-malarial | Nausea, vomiting, diarrhea caused by contaminated food and amebic dysentery, protozoal infestations |
| Chai Hu Su Gan San (Bupleurum Powder to Spread the Liver) | Regulate Liver Qi, vitalize Liver Xue, ease pain | Abdominal distension, hypochondriac and chest pain, indigestion, depression, constipation, belching |
| Curing Pills | Regulate the Middle Burner, improve digestion, expel Wind-Cold during the summer, disperse Dampness | Stomach upset, nausea, bloating, gas, diarrhea, food poisoning, motion sickness, gastroenteritis, jet lag (Do not use if appendicitis is suspected.) |
| Gui Pi Wan | Tonify Qi and Xue, strengthen Heart and Spleen (Do not use with Heat patterns.) | Poor appetite, mild abdominal pain and distention, fatigue, insomnia, palpitations, forgetfulness, pale face |
| Quiet Digestion | Disperse Wind-Damp, resolve Spleen Dampness, regulate Stomach, resolve Phlegm | Nausea, vomiting, diarrhea, poor appetite, gas, abdominal pain and cramping, motion sickness, gastroenteritis, hangover, jet lag (Do not use if appendicitis is suspected.) |
| Shen Ling Bai Zhu Wan | Strengthen Spleen, tonify Qi, harmonize Stomach functions, eliminate Dampness | Chronic gastroenteritis, chronic fatigue, loose stools, diarrhea, burping |
| Source Qi | Strengthen Spleen and Stomach, tonify Qi, astringe Fluid, increase digestive functions | Intestinal parasites, diarrhea, chronic shigella, Crohn's disease, intestinal bacterial infections |

## ACUPUNCTURE AND MOXIBUSTION

For severe bowel disorders such as Crohn's disease and acute irritable bowel syndrome symptoms, the recommended therapy is acupuncture and moxibustion two or three times a week to begin with and once a week for an extended period—from twelve to fifty-two weeks.

Moxibustion may include additional points on the Stomach and Urinary Bladder Channels (Stomach 37, Stomach 25, and Urinary Bladder 20). (See pages 163 through 166 for the locations of the points.)

## Step Three: Bringing in Other Modalities

The comprehensive program includes diverse therapeutic approaches, including nutritional supplements, massage, Western lab tests and medicines, psychotherapy, and Ayurvedic nutritional counseling.

Digestive disorders often demand comprehensive treatment plans. For example, Maggie came to the clinic with severe digestive complaints after having traveled through India. I sent her for Western lab tests for bacterial infections and parasites. The labs found bacterial infections, systemic candidiasis, and parasites.

Chinese medicine can treat yeast infections and many parasites, but I knew that unless Maggie took antibiotics for the bacterial infection, she could not benefit from the other therapies. Even though the antibiotics were going to aggravate her yeast infection, she needed to knock out the bacterial infection first. While she took the antibiotics, our clinic provided *Lactobacillus acidophilus* and treatments to tonify the Spleen and Stomach, remove Dampness, and combat the yeast overgrowth. Once Maggie was done with the course of antibiotics, we could treat the increased yeast infection and parasites. Over six months, Maggie's digestive system regained harmony.

If Maggie's treatment had not included both Western and Chinese modalities, her therapy would not have been as effective or her recovery as rapid.

## AT A GLANCE: COMPREHENSIVE PROGRAM FOR DIGESTIVE DISORDERS

| SELF-CARE PLAN | |
|---|---|
| Evaluation | Even if your focus is self-care, if you suffer with a digestive disorder, you should first get a Western baseline evaluation and a Chinese medicine evaluation. You should rule out life-threatening disorders before proceeding. |
| Self-monitoring | If your diet journal reveals you have a negative reaction to particular foods, eliminate those foods for four days and reintroduce them one at a time. |
| Dietary guidelines | Follow the recommended diet plan in this chapter. Make sure you limit raw foods, cold foods, and dairy if you have a diagnosis of Dampness. Reduce caffeine and alcohol intake. |
| Moxibustion | Highly recommended unless there are Excess Heat problems, such as a fever, acute bloody stools, or burning diarrhea. Then use only if prescribed by a practitioner. |
| Exercise/ meditation | If you have Deficient Qi, do mild Yoga and Qi Gong exercises. With Stagnant Qi, do more vigorous exercise five to seven days per week. |

*(continued)*

| SELF-CARE PLAN *(continued)* | |
|---|---|
| Massage | Qi Gong massage, reflexology, and ear massage are recommended. |
| Soaks and saunas | Ginger compresses or hot packs can be used on the abdomen for Cold and Deficiency. Use Sleep Ease, a chamomile-valerian soak, for stress. |
| Nutritional supplements | Follow the nutritional supplement plan with the modifications made in this chapter. Ask your naturopathic physician or gastroenterologist for additional recommendations such as d-limonene or deglycyrrhizinated licorice (DGL) for chronic indigestion, heartburn, and GERD. |
| Medicine cabinet | Always have Quiet Digestion or Curing Pills on hand for acute problems. |
| **USING A CHINESE MEDICINE PRACTITIONER** | |
| Evaluation and diagnosis | Bring your daily journal, Western diagnosis, and lab tests. Together, the practitioner(s) and client will create a healing plan. |
| Diet | Using the daily journal as a guide, the practitioner can help you create a diet that restores digestive harmony. |
| Herbal therapy | A number of Chinese herbal formulas may be used for digestive disorders. Your practitioner will prescribe formulas based upon your specific Chinese diagnosis. |
| Acupuncture | Treatment of specific points is determined after an individualized diagnosis. These points are often on the Spleen and Stomach Channels plus additional points for other patterns. |
| Moxibustion | The practitioner might recommend moxibustion for home self-treatment along with using moxa during your clinic treatment session. |
| Qi Gong exercise/ meditation | The practitioner may recommend you see a Qi Gong instructor. You should ask your instructor for specific exercises/meditations for your diagnoses. |
| **OTHER PRACTITIONERS** | |
| Obtaining a Western baseline | Your Western baseline should include a physical work-up to eliminate the presence of a serious underlying disease. Western doctors may prescribe medications, such as antibiotics for bacterial infections and antiparasite drugs. Supplements may also be recommended. |
| Other healers | Naturopathic physicians, homeopaths, psychotherapists, and others may contribute to the healing process. Professional massage focused on the abdomen, such as Qi-Xue abdominal massage, Hara massage, Ayurvedic hot oil massage, and Chi Nei Tsang, can be very helpful. |

# 17

# FATTY LIVER
## A Comprehensive Program for Liver Support

The liver is the second largest organ in your body, and it is located under your rib cage on the right side. It weighs about 3 pounds (1.4 kg), and it is shaped like a football that is flat on one side.

The liver performs many jobs in your body. It processes what you eat and drink into energy, and it stores nutrients your body can use. The liver also detoxifies harmful substances and drugs from your blood. It is responsible for correct blood clotting, sex hormones, many metabolic processes, making bile for proper digestion, as well as other functions.

If the liver is not working correctly, it can affect your overall health, energy levels, sexual functioning, mood, digestion, and many other area of your mind/body/spirit.

## WHAT IS FATTY LIVER?

Fatty liver, also known as steatosis, has become an important medical problem in the United States and around the world. Fatty liver is the buildup of fat in liver cells. While alcohol consumption is the main reason for the development of fatty liver disease, the type of fatty liver disease we are addressing in this chapter is found in people who drink little or no alcohol.

Fatty liver affects up to one out of four adults, one of whom might be you. In fact, fatty liver is the leading cause of chronic liver disease. After hepatitis C and long-term alcoholism, complications of fatty liver is the third most common reason for liver transplants in the United States. There are different medical terms for fatty liver, depending on whether or not inflammation is present.

If no inflammation is present, fat stored in the liver cells is called steatosis. In people who drink little or no alcohol, this steatosis is called nonalcoholic fatty liver disease

(NAFLD). The word *hepatitis* means "inflammation of the liver." The presence of fat in liver cells along with inflammation is called steatohepatitis. In people who drink little or no alcohol, this hepatitis is called nonalcoholic steatohepatitis (NASH).

According to a review in *Clinical Science*, it is estimated that 20 to 30 percent of adult populations in developed countries have NAFLD. NAFLD is also increasing in children. Approximately 2 to 3 percent of people with NAFLD will progress to NASH. NAFLD is also associated with an increased risk of developing insulin resistance and type 2 diabetes.[1]

NASH is a common and often "silent" liver disease, and it affects up to 5 percent of people in the United States. Most people with NASH feel well and do not know they have liver disease. However, like other forms of hepatitis, NASH can lead to severe liver scarring (cirrhosis) and poor liver function, liver cancer, and/or liver failure.

Both NAFLD and NASH have become more common as people get fatter. Obesity is highly associated with fatty liver. In the United States alone, from 2004 to 2014, the rate of obesity doubled in adults and tripled in children according to the National Institutes of Health (NIH).[2] Half of obese people have fatty livers, meaning it is likely that more that 25 percent of the U.S. population has steatosis.

Obesity is defined medically as having a body mass index (BMI) of greater than 30, and it affects up to 50 percent of the U.S. population. BMI is a measure of body fat based on dividing height by weight and applies to adult men and women. Compare this to a normal BMI that runs between 20 and 25.

TIP

The National Institutes of Health (NIH) provides a free body mass index (BMI) calculator at www.nhlbi.nih.gov/health/educational/lose_wt/BMI/bmicalc.htm.

# FATTY LIVER RISK, DIAGNOSIS, AND METABOLIC SYNDROME

NAFLD tends to develop in people who are overweight or obese or who have type 2 diabetes, high cholesterol, or high triglycerides. Rapid weight loss and poor eating habits also may lead to NAFLD. However, some people develop NAFLD even if they do not have any risk factors.

Most people with NASH are between the ages of forty and sixty. NASH is more common in women than in men. NASH often has no symptoms, and people can have NASH for years before symptoms occur. NASH is one of the leading causes of cirrhosis in adults in the United States. Up to 25 percent of adults with NASH may have cirrhosis.

Also, people with hepatitis C—the leading cause of liver transplants in the United States—who have NAFLD have an increased risk of cirrhosis of up to 15 percent. As discussed previously, if you are suspected of having NAFLD or NASH, having a liver biopsy can help you and your doctor know if you have fat in the liver as well as the level of liver damage. Fibroscan and Fibrosure are noninvasive tests that are often used instead of biopsy. However, liver biopsy is still the gold standard for determining the amount of liver damage.

Usually, the first suspicion of NASH is when you have elevated liver enzyme levels found in routine blood tests, such as increased levels of alanine aminotransferase (ALT) or aspartate aminotransferase (AST).

If liver enzyme elevation is found upon routine blood testing, you should be evaluated to determine why there are abnormal elevations. Elevated liver enzymes can come from ingesting certain medications and sometimes herbs, viral hepatitis B or C, weight reduction surgery, or excessive alcohol consumption. If there is no other reason determined for these high liver enzymes, further testing is done with X-rays, ultrasounds, or other imaging studies that may show fat in the liver.

The gold standard for determining a final diagnosis of NASH, rather than just NAFLD, is a liver biopsy. A liver biopsy can determine if there is fat in the liver, if there is hepatitis, and if you have a damaged liver and early stages of liver disease, fibrosis, or cirrhosis.

When symptoms occur, they are not necessarily specific or severe. Fatigue, aching or pain over the area of the liver, and general weakness are examples of the symptoms associated with NAFLD and NASH.

The good news is that NAFLD is a reversible condition. Having NAFLD alone, before any disease progression, is a good sign. NAFLD can be reversed with weight loss, dietary changes, exercise, and eliminating medications and substances that might have caused the fat to accumulate.

The treatment of NAFLD and NASH depends on the possible causes. If you are overweight, losing weight can usually normalize elevated liver enzymes, decrease inflammation, and decrease liver fat. If weight loss is undertaken when there is just NAFLD, you can generally prevent cirrhosis. It is best that you do not attempt a severe weight

## METABOLIC SYNDROME

Fatty liver can be part of a complex of symptoms called "metabolic syndrome." Metabolic syndrome is a group of conditions that puts a person at risk for cardiovascular disease and type 2 diabetes.

A consensus between the International Diabetes Foundation and the American Heart Association/National Heart, Lung, and Blood Institute defines metabolic syndrome as the presence of at least three of the following symptoms:

- Increased waist circumference of ≥40 inches (102 cm) in men and ≥34 inches (88 cm) in women

- Elevated blood pressure of ≥130/85 mmHg

- Elevated blood sugar of fasting glucose ≥100 mg/dL

- High triglycerides of ≥150 mg/dL

- Low high-density lipoprotein of 40 mg/dL or less in men and 50 mg/dL or less in women

You may also suffer from this in addition to having liver disease. This syndrome is more prevalent in people with advanced liver disease.

The questions to ask yourself are:

- Are you gaining belly fat around the middle?

- Are you fatigued after you eat?

- Do you have a family history of diabetes or elevated glucose levels?

- Do you have "borderline" high blood pressure?

- Are your cholesterol levels elevated?

- Do you have liver disease?

If you recognize some of these issues as your own, you are most likely suffering from metabolic syndrome.

Metabolic syndrome affects one in three people in the United States, and it occurs more frequently with age. Metabolic syndrome is also known as metabolic syndrome X, syndrome X, and insulin resistance syndrome.

loss diet, but rather lose weight gradually using a controlled plan of diet and exercise. Very fast weight loss can cause an advancement of liver disease. Also, weight loss must be maintained, or the disease may return.

Discontinuing any medications or substances that can cause fat to accumulate in the liver can reduce progression of disease. If done early enough, it can prevent liver damage altogether. In type 2 diabetes, reducing glucose levels is not enough. Weight loss is key for overweight people to reverse liver damage.

Unfortunately, for people who are not overweight and for whom NAFLD or NASH is not associated with intake of substances, there is currently no recommended Western treatment.

# PART ONE: SELF-CARE PLAN FOR PREVENTION AND THERAPEUTIC TREATMENT

The following comprehensive program offers a way for you to use self-care and assemble a team of practitioners to support your healing efforts.

### Step One: Adopt the Comprehensive Program for Strengthening Organ Qi and Protective Qi

A general, preventive health care routine that includes a balanced diet, regular exercise and meditation, self-massage, and other stress-reduction techniques is essential for a healthy liver. The liver health comprehensive program integrates the Comprehensive Program for Basic Good Health and a Strong Immune System (see page 223) with additional liver support.

If you have NASH, you should consider the following additional targeted therapies.

### Step Two: Expanding Your Daily Journal

When starting a Comprehensive Program for Liver Support, the first step is to expand your daily journal. The journal will help alert you to the development of any disharmonies. If you are currently working to remedy an imbalance, it will alert you to triggers and help you track your improvements.

## THE HIGH FRUCTOSE CORN SYRUP CONNECTION

In July 2006, Raphael Merriman, M.D., a hepatologist specializing in fatty liver disease at the University of California, published an article for the American Liver Foundation called "High Fructose Corn Syrup (HFCS) and Its Potential Role in Fatty Liver Disease." Here is an excerpt:

> *Nonalcoholic steatohepatitis (NASH) is characterized by fat in the liver, causing variable amounts of inflammation and scarring in people who drink little or no alcohol. Obesity is a major risk factor for NASH, which is becoming increasingly common in adults and children. Obesity is also the major risk factor for insulin resistance. Insulin, a hormone secreted by the pancreas, helps the body use glucose (blood sugar), allowing it to enter muscle and liver cells for use as energy or storage. Insulin resistance occurs when those cells are less sensitive to normal amounts of insulin, causing the pancreas to increase secretion. This can lead to diabetes and elevated cholesterol, both of which are also strongly associated with NASH. Therefore it is not surprising that insulin resistance has recently emerged as the main underlying metabolic abnormality in NASH.*
>
> *As obesity has escalated to epidemic levels, there has been an increase in both total caloric consumption and the consumption of certain substances in the typical American diet. The nutrition labels of most processed foods will show the near ever-presence of high fructose corn syrup (HFCS), which is made by converting inexpensive cornstarch into a high fructose mix. Fructose is nearly twice as sweet as 'regular' sugar (sucrose), and it now accounts for over 40 percent of caloric sweeteners added to food products. HFCS has largely replaced sucrose in sodas, fruit juices, dairy products, most baked goods, and numerous processed products. For example, 60 percent of the calories in apple juice come from fructose.*
>
> *But why has concern been expressed about HFCS? Is it simply that we are consuming more calories (and added sweeteners) in larger portion sizes? Though that also appears true, recent research indicates a more troubling side of HFCS. The metabolism of fructose is substantially different from that of the main human sugar, glucose. Unlike glucose, fructose does not stimulate insulin release from the pancreas or leptin release, another hormone important in regulating appetite. As a result, the brain does not sense the need to limit food intake. This leads to further caloric intake, weight gain, and obesity. Of even greater concern, when large quantities of fructose are consumed, it bypasses the usual control mechanisms and is preferentially converted to fat, leading to liver fat accumulation and high cholesterol. Additionally, the long-term consumption of HFCS-laden diets has recently been implicated in the development of insulin resistance. Therefore many aspects of HFCS use point to its potential role in the development of NASH.*

Recent research has supported this hypothesis.[3]

The journal should include additional information on the following:

- Food cravings or times when you lose your appetite for specific foods or food in general

- Alcohol and caffeine consumption

- Energy levels and ability to exercise

- Times when fatigue, abdominal pain, digestive problems, depression, or weakness make it difficult to exercise or to work

- Physical symptoms you suspect are associated with your liver, such as fatigue, headaches, blood sugar problems, changes in sleep patterns, swollen legs, swollen abdomen, and pain over the liver area

- Cognitive problems, such as "brain fog," feeling sleepy during the day and wakeful at night, excessive forgetfulness, changes in moods, irritability, or anger

Paying close attention to this information over time can reveal very important information about your liver health as well as overall health. This information indicates how you can control or eliminate some of the troubling symptoms as well as whether there is disease progression or regression. This will help you report to your Chinese medicine practitioner as well as your Western providers about improvement or worsening of symptoms.

## Step Three: Implementing a Dietary Program

In addition to the diet guidelines outlined in the Comprehensive Program for Basic Good Health and a Strong Immune System (see page 223), you may tailor your diet to remove Dampness, promote a balanced flow of Qi and Xue, improve insulin sensitivity, and lose weight. Consider the following:

- Eat a diet of warm, cooked foods. Reduce cold and raw foods to a minimum unless you have Excess Heat.

- Eliminate or drastically reduce dairy products to decrease Dampness and strengthen the Spleen. Eliminating dairy products can help increase weight and fat loss.

- Eliminate alcohol completely.

- Reduce caffeine if it increases your symptoms.

- Eat less fatty foods. A fatty diet can also increase Qi Stagnation and Dampness and increase weight.

- Eat a diet high in protein, especially fish and vegetable protein. People with liver disease should eat 90 to 100 grams of high-quality protein every day. If it is difficult to eat the full amount in a normal diet, you can add protein powders (with no sugar added), such as organic grass-fed whey protein (contains dairy) or hemp protein, to your diet by combining with other foods or creating shakes that are not cold and do not have added sugar.

- Adopt a diet focused on balancing high-glycemic foods with lower-glycemic foods and proteins. Visit www.glycemicindex.com and www.nutritiondata.com/topics/glycemic-index for glycemic index information on all foods; use this as a guide for keeping your meals on the low end of the glycemic index. In general, adopt a diet focused on balancing high-glycemic foods with lower-glycemic foods to reduce issues with metabolic syndrome.

- Try to eliminate any foods that contain high fructose corn syrup.

- Eliminate excess salt from your diet to reduce fluid retention. Pure foods contribute enough salt to the diet to maintain health. Eating processed and packaged foods and adding salt to home-cooked meals is unnecessary, and it can be detrimental to your health. According to Five Phases diagnoses, excess salt injures the Kidney Water, counteracts Earth, and injures the Spleen.

## Step Four: Implementing an Exercise Plan

Excessive exercise can trigger a flare-up of symptoms for anyone who has liver disease. If you are already suffering from fatigue, it is particularly important that you don't overtax yourself. On the other hand, it is vital to oxygenate your system and maintain muscle tone if you are to stay as healthy as possible. Exercise should really be according to your level of disease and energy. To regulate and move Qi and Xue so they flow smoothly, avoid excessive aerobic activities. Use the Qi Gong warm-up exercises (see page 182) and walking to stimulate balanced flow.

If you need to lose weight, you can walk 10,000 steps per day to meet the exercise goal. For example if you walk a lot at work or to and from work, you may want to wear a pedometer (such as a Fitbit) to monitor your walking. This will help in your weight loss goals.

To support your Spleen and prevent further Deficient Spleen Qi and Dampness, weight lifting should be done a maximum of three times a week.

You may practice Tai Chi, Qi Gong, or moderate Yoga exercises every day to increase muscle strength, improve balance, and support all of your Organ Qi.

## THE GLYCEMIC INDEX

The University of Sydney Human Nutrition Unit has been the world leader in the development of the concept known as glycemic index. In their own words from their website:

*The glycemic index (GI) is a ranking of carbohydrates on a scale from 0 to 100 according to the extent to which they raise blood sugar levels after eating. Foods with a high GI are those which are rapidly digested and absorbed and result in marked fluctuations in blood sugar levels. Low-GI foods, by virtue of their slow digestion and absorption, produce gradual rises in blood sugar and insulin levels, and have proven benefits for health. Low GI diets have been shown to improve both glucose and lipid levels in people with diabetes (type 1 and type 2). They have benefits for weight control because they help control appetite and delay hunger. Low-GI diets also reduce insulin levels and insulin resistance.*

*Recent studies from Harvard School of Public Health indicate that the risks of diseases such as type 2 diabetes and coronary heart disease are strongly related to the GI of the overall diet. In 1999, the World Health Organization (WHO) and Food and Agriculture Organization (FAO) recommended that people in industrialized countries base their diets on low-GI foods in order to prevent the most common diseases of affluence, such as coronary heart disease, diabetes and obesity.*

## Step Five: Implementing a Meditation Plan

Meditation can alleviate the stress and diminish associated symptoms. First, just start with taking a deep breath. Then use the Buddha's Breath exercise (see page 179) to help ease Stagnation. Regular practice of the longer Qi Meditation (see page 186) can produce constitutional improvements that will do much to restore harmony. Even if you have severe fatigue, Qi Gong breathing and Qi-stimulating movements can be done with minimal effort and still produce great results. (You can even lie down to do them!)

As your strength returns, you can increase your routine. Add Zen walking and more aerobic activities for ten minutes a day. Always include the breathing exercises. To decide if you are strong enough to add more vigorous exercise, ask yourself, "Could I walk comfortably at a steady pace for ten minutes? How about for twenty minutes?" If the answer is yes, a daily ten- or twenty-minute Qi Gong workout can provide the Qi nurturing and stimulation you need.

## Step Six: Using Self-Massage and Moxibustion for Preventive Care

Massage and acupressure are extremely helpful for liver support. For example, Qi Gong abdominal massage (see page 194) is effective in dispelling Stagnation and Dampness.

You may also use reflexology on the hands and feet, particularly on the liver points (see pages 210 and 211).

For reducing symptoms associated with Stagnant Liver Qi, you may perform acupressure on Liver 3 (see page 206). For support of the Stomach and Spleen Qi and to reduce fatigue and digestive problems, perform acupressure on Stomach 36 and Spleen 6 (see page 163).

For swelling in the extremities and abdomen, you may perform acupressure on Spleen 9, Ren 9, and Kidney 3 (see pages 36, 40, and 206).

Ear massage is also very helpful for supporting digestion as well as decreasing fatigue and hunger. Follow these suggestions for a total of ten minutes once a day. For fatigue relieved by activity and for Stagnant Liver Qi, use Ear Liver, Ear Sympathetic, and Ear Lung. For fatigue with digestion problems, use Ear Stomach and Ear Spleen. For fatigue related to negative side effects of medications, use Ear Liver (see the ear chart on page 203).

## Step Seven: Using Soaks, Saunas, and Compresses for Self-Healing

In general, warming compresses and brief soaks can ease some of the discomfort associated with abdominal pain and swelling. Don't make the water too cold or too hot, especially if you have later stage liver disease.

Use Sleep Ease for relaxation (see page 213). Enjoy this soak for up to half an hour. You can also prepare and use ginger soaks and compresses. (For instructions, see "Comprehensive Program for Digestive Disorders" on page 96.)

## Step Eight: Taking Nutritional Supplements

To support liver health, you should adopt a daily supplement program. Ask your practitioner for specific dosing recommendations because individual needs are different for different people. Also, different stages of liver disease require different types of supplementation. Your regimen should include omega-3 fatty acids, as well as eating healthy sustainable seafood. Visit www.seafoodwatch.org for accurate health and ecological information on seafood. You may take krill oil for your omega-3 fatty acids. Evidence suggests that vitamin D deficiency may be associated with progression of steatosis into

NASH.[4] Vitamin D is generally prescribed from 2000 IU to 10,000 IU. It is best to dose this according to lab results, although 4000 to 6000 IU is the average.

NASH guidelines from the American Association for the Study of Liver Disease include the following recommendations for vitamin E:

- Vitamin E (alpha-tocopherol) administered at a daily dose of 800 IU per day improves liver histology in non-diabetic adults with biopsy-proven NASH, and therefore it should be considered as a first-line pharmacotherapy for this patient population.

- Until further data supporting its effectiveness become available, vitamin E is not recommended to treat NASH in diabetic patients, NAFLD without liver biopsy, NASH cirrhosis, or cryptogenic cirrhosis.[5]

People with compromised livers should never take iron supplements or vitamin A unless prescribed by a doctor after being tested for deficiencies.

Daily *Lactobacillus acidophilus* can also be taken to keep your digestive tract healthy. Probiotics are also used in liver disease to reduce brain swelling (encephalopathy) through reducing toxins.[6] The Mayo Clinic recommends that "1 x 109 living *L. acidophilus* cells by mouth in divided doses daily is an adequate dose for most people."[7]

## PART TWO: ASSEMBLING THE TEAM

When it comes to liver health, you need to include both Western-trained and Eastern-trained practitioners to optimize your preventive and therapeutic health care plan. When you use practitioners of both types in concert, it will give you the opportunity to create an individualized comprehensive treatment plan, share diagnoses, reduce side effects, make better choices for treatments and self-care, and attain the best outcomes.

### Western Medicine

Everyone in the United States should be tested regularly for liver enzymes. Remember, the vast majority of people found to have NAFLD and NASH have elevated liver enzymes upon routine lab testing. Also, checking your blood pressure, cholesterol, triglycerides, and blood glucose levels along with calculating your BMI will help determine if you have metabolic syndrome.

### GRACE'S STORY

Grace told me this is how she felt when she came to see me for the first time: "Everything was a problem because I was so sick and tired. Physically, my 20+ years of symptoms went up and down in severity and were generally flulike symptoms, exhaustion, muddy thinking, chemical and food sensitivity, nausea and poor digestion, chronic gynecological problems, irritability, fevers, sores, insomnia, headache, and depression. After several years, I realized I was on a gradual slide toward full-on chronic symptoms. I found myself unable to push through it physically, emotionally, or mentally, and the biggest problem became my attitude of complete and utter demoralization.

"When I left after my first acupuncture treatment, I felt like a huge weight of anxiety and indecision had been lifted for me. I knew that I had found the right treatment for myself."

## Eastern Medicine

Chinese medicine is particularly effective for treating the symptoms associated with liver disease as well as helping to maintain metabolic balance. Fatigue, weakness, brain fog, swelling, and other issues are often improved or resolved with Chinese medicine treatment and self-care along with Western therapies for metabolic issues.

## Step One: Obtaining a Western Baseline

Everyone in the United States should be tested regularly for liver enzymes during regular medical visits (see page 308). If there is elevation in the enzymes, your doctor needs to rule out whether you are taking a medicine or substance that can cause high enzyme levels, if you have viral hepatitis or another form of hepatitis or liver disease, or if it could be caused by overconsumption of alcohol. If these are all ruled out, you should have imaging tests such as an ultrasound or magnetic resonance imaging (MRI) to see if you have fat in the liver. If the imaging reveals any indication of fat, you should see a hepatologist and have a liver biopsy to determine if you have NAFLD or NASH, and if there is liver disease, what the stage of disease might be. Also, if you already have cirrhosis, you should have regular scans for liver cancer.

If you are overweight, creating a weight loss and weight management program is the best step toward reducing fat in the liver. You can normalize your liver enzymes and reduce symptoms by losing weight alone. To be able to lose weight effectively, you may need a medical program, a program such as Weight Watchers or Overeater's

Anonymous, therapy groups, individualized therapy, a structured exercise program, or any combination of these. You may add Chinese medicine to these therapies to support you.

Always tell your Western doctor that you are seeking Chinese medicine therapy or other treatments that may affect your overall treatment plan. By seeing a Chinese medicine doctor, you can benefit from the balancing powers of acupuncture, herbs, and other Chinese medicine therapies.

## Step Two: Obtaining a Chinese Medicine Diagnosis and Treatment

To ascertain your liver health, a Chinese medicine practitioner may or may not directly examine your liver. However, palpating your abdomen is a normal part of the Chinese medicine examination. The Chinese medicine practitioner will conduct an interview and use the Four Examinations (see page 76) to determine which disharmonies are present and to find out what symptoms are troubling you. Using this set of traditional diagnostic techniques, the practitioner will design a course that will restore harmony to your Organ Systems and Essential Substances and, as a consequence, alleviate your symptoms, support your liver health, help you lose weight, and improve your metabolic health. In addition, it is best if your Chinese medicine doctor can also read the lab tests, imaging reports, and biopsy reports from the hepatologist or other Western physician for information on your liver health from a Western medicine perspective.

Treatment for severe fatigue and other symptoms associated with liver disease must be tailored to an individual diagnosis, but in each case an intensive routine for several months is recommended. Your practitioner will help you determine the frequency of treatment to maintain strength and vigor as well as support your liver. Moxibustion will follow the individualized diagnosis that guides acupuncture.

### ACUPUNCTURE

Treatment to strengthen the Spleen and Stomach Qi are very important for liver support, especially when there is Dampness involved. This is often the case with metabolic syndrome. Treatment of the Liver and Gallbladder is essential as well. NAFLD and NASH are often found in conjunction with other problems, such as high blood pressure and obesity. Your practitioner must be able to understand all the complexities to diagnose and treat correctly.

If you have liver disease, it would be a good idea for you to ask your practitioner how much experience he or she has in treating people with liver disease; how much Western knowledge he or she has of lab reports, imaging, and other testing; and if he or she will communicate with your Western practitioners.

## MOXIBUSTION

To support the Liver, you can moxa over the liver at Liver 14 and Gallbladder 24. For Deficient Spleen and Stomach Qi with Dampness, you can apply moxa to Stomach 36 and Ren 12. If there is abdominal swelling, you may use Ren 9. For leg or ankle swelling, use Spleen 9 and Spleen 6. Your practitioner might teach your partner, family member, or friend special acupuncture points on your back that he or she can treat for you at home. See *The Hepatitis C Help Book,* revised edition, for more specific information on hepatitis.[8]

## HERBAL TREATMENTS

Most herbal formulas are generally designed to treat specific disharmonies that are diagnosed by your Chinese medicine practitioner. Your practitioner should be able to determine any drug-herb interactions as well as know if there are any herbs that are contraindicated during your stage of liver disease.

### EXAMPLES OF CHINESE HERBAL FORMULAS FOR LIVER SUPPORT

| FORMULA | CHINESE FUNCTION | INDICATIONS |
| --- | --- | --- |
| *Chai Hu Su Gan San* (Bupleurum Powder to Spread the Liver) | Regulate Liver Qi, vitalize Liver Xue, ease pain | Abdominal distension, hypochondriac and chest pain, indigestion, depression, constipation, belching |
| Ecliptex | Vitalize Qi and Xue, tonify Kidney and Liver Yin, tonify Xue | Protects liver from damage from environmental chemicals, drugs, and alcohol |
| HepatoPlex One | Regulate Qi, invigorate Xue, tonify Qi, Kidney, and Spleen, clear Damp Heat | Hepatitis symptoms, particularly viral hepatitis |
| Cordyceps PS | Tonify Kidney Yang, nourish Lung Yin, strengthen Wei Qi, stop cough and transform Phlegm | Fatigue, immune weakness, post-illness weakness, chronic cough, health maintenance, general tonic, supports athletic performance |

*(continued)*

| FORMULA | CHINESE FUNCTION | INDICATIONS |
|---|---|---|
| Cordyseng | Tonify Qi and Yin through Fu Zheng action; strengthen Lung, Spleen, Stomach, and Kidney | Fatigue, recovery from serious illness or operation, support immune function, support lungs, improve athletic performance |
| Tremella American Ginseng | Tonify Yin, Qi, Xue, and Jing; Clear Heat Clean Toxin; strengthen Wei Qi; strengthen Spleen, Stomach, Lung, Kidney | Fatigue, immune dysfunction, frequent colds and flus, chronic viral illness, afternoon night sweats and fever, chronic dry cough |
| *Xiao Yao San* (Rambling Powder) | Spread Liver Qi, relieve Stagnation, tonify Spleen, nourish Xue | Irritability, depression, moodiness, fatigue, headache, dizziness, breast distention, irregular menstruation, menstrual pain |
| *Xiao Chai Hu Tang* (Minor Bupleurum Decoction) | Harmonize Shao Yang Stage Disorders, harmonize and tonify Middle Jiao | Alternating chills and fever, dry mouth and throat, bitter taste, irritability, dizziness, fullness and discomfort in the hypochondria and chest, loss of appetite, nausea, vomiting, heartburn |

# STEP THREE: BRING IN OTHER MODALITIES

Your treatment plan can be expanded in several ways. You may want to include other forms of Eastern meditations, biofeedback, hypnosis, or psychotherapy. To alleviate digestive problems, some people adopt an Ayurvedic diet or other diets such as Paleo to dispel the imbalances. Japanese abdominal massage can also ease digestive problems and alleviate pain associated with liver disease.

## AT A GLANCE: COMPREHENSIVE PROGRAM FOR LIVER SUPPORT

| SELF-CARE PLAN | |
| --- | --- |
| Evaluation | Before starting a self-care plan, with possible liver disease, make sure you first have a baseline Western evaluation and a Chinese medicine evaluation. Lab tests, imaging, and examination can rule out or determine serious liver disease, diabetes, and cardiovascular issues and determine a proper weight loss plan. |
| Self-monitoring | In addition to the general guidelines, your daily journal should make note of your sugar and carbohydrate intake and the glycemic values, energy levels and fluctuations, signs of cognitive problems, increased abdominal or extremity swelling, physical activity, along with body rhythms, including sleep disruption, changes in elimination, and mood changes. If you are diagnosed with liver disease, ask your doctor what he or she would like you to monitor. |
| Diet | In addition to the First-Step Dietary Therapy Program that removes irritants and toxins and soothes the system, add the concepts of glycemic index and weight loss techniques. Adopt a low-glycemic diet. Eliminate all alcohol. Reduce or eliminate sugar intake. Eliminate all high fructose corn syrup from your diet. Keep your sodium levels low. Reduce caffeine intake. To support your liver, your daily protein consumption should be 90 to 100 grams of protein, primarily from vegetable and sustainable fish sources. Use the Chinese medicine diagnosis given to you by your practitioner to modify your dietary choices. |
| Exercise | Exercise should be focused to move Qi and Xue. If you can, start some moderate aerobic movement. Mild weight-bearing exercises will improve your muscle tone. Use Qi Gong warm-up exercises and walking to stimulate balanced flow. For weight loss, you can walk up to 10,000 steps per day, using a pedometer (such as a Fitbit), and walk instead of driving or taking the bus. Do not do excessive exercise. |
| Meditation | Use the Buddha's Breath exercise to ease Stagnation. Regularly practice the Qi meditation. If you can, begin Zen walking. With severe fatigue, you may start with sitting and lying Qi Gong movements. |
| Moxibustion | Moxa supports the liver, strengthens the Spleen and Stomach Qi, and regulates the Liver Qi. |
| Massage | Start with Qi Gong abdominal massage to dispel Dampness and Stagnation. Perform acupressure on Liver 3, Spleen 6, and Stomach 36 to reduce Stagnant Liver Qi and strengthen the Spleen and Stomach. Use ear massage to support digestion and decrease fatigue. |
| Soaks and saunas | Saunas, soaks, and compresses are all effective ways to decrease abdominal discomfort and keep the Qi and Xue flowing harmoniously. |

*(continued)*

| | |
|---|---|
| Nutritional supplements | Follow the nutritional supplement plan with the modifications made in this chapter. Make sure you take a regular dose of *Lactobacillus acidophilus*. Especially focus on vitamin D and omega-3 fatty acid intake. Unless prescribed by your doctor for true deficiencies, do not take iron or vitamin A supplements. |
| **ASSEMBLING THE HEALING TEAM** | |
| Obtaining a Western baseline | If you are overweight, have diabetes, high blood pressure, or signs of metabolic syndrome, make sure you have regular liver tests and other examinations. It's important to rule out serious liver disease, including cirrhosis, liver cancer, and liver failure. If you already have later stage liver disease, see a hepatologist for any other examinations and treatment associated with your stage of disease. |
| Obtaining Chinese medicine diagnosis and treatment | When you go to a Chinese medicine practitioner, it's important to establish communication between the Chinese and Western doctors. Preventive and therapeutic routines may include acupuncture, moxibustion, acupressure, and herbal medicine. |
| Bringing in other modalities | Support your liver and whole mind/body/spirit through regular massage, nutritional and dietary counseling, liver support groups, and exposure to other Eastern and Western healing traditions. |

# CANCER SUPPORT
## A Comprehensive Approach from Diagnosis to Survivorship

When you are diagnosed with cancer, life changes completely. On the day of diagnosis, you begin to walk down a different path with different destinations than the day before diagnosis. Cancer can be a devastating diagnosis for any woman or man, for her or his family, friends, and coworkers, and for anyone else whose life he or she touches. I have also heard people diagnosed with cancer describe it as a turning point in their lives, leading them in new directions.

People who have been diagnosed with cancer need a tremendous amount of support from many different realms—in all aspects of mind/body/spirit.

Many people diagnosed with cancer use all kinds of healing and medicine, from Western diagnosis and treatment to Chinese traditional medicine.

Chinese medicine can offer a full set of tools to help you when you have been diagnosed with cancer and are embarking on one of the most difficult journeys of your life.

## THE NEW CHINESE MEDICINE APPROACH TO CANCER SUPPORT

There are many different types of cancer, with many stages of disease in each type. Some are imminently life-threatening, such as late-stage pancreatic cancer and ovarian cancer, while others are eminently curable with immediate Western treatment, such as certain skin cancers and early stage breast cancer.

According to the American Society of Clinical Oncology, there are more than 120 types of cancer and related hereditary syndromes.[1]

Studies cited by the American Cancer Society show that the lifetime risk of being diagnosed with cancer is slightly more than 40 percent for men and slightly less than 40 percent for women. The lifetime risk of dying from cancer is slightly over 20 percent for men and slightly under 20 percent for women.[2]

In 2011, the Centers for Disease Control and Prevention (CDC) and the National Cancer Institute (NCI) reported that the number of cancer survivors in the United States increased to 11.7 million in 2007. There were 3 million cancer survivors in 1971 and 9.8 million in 2001.

The CDC defines a cancer survivor as anyone who has been diagnosed with cancer, from the time of diagnosis through the balance of his or her life.[3] The National Coalition for Cancer Survivorship led the way with this, creating the phrase "cancer survivorship" to describe the broad experience on the cancer continuum—living with, through, and beyond a cancer diagnosis.

Many cancer survivors now prefer the term "thriver," focusing on living as well as possible. They believe that every person with cancer should be empowered with the resources to thrive.

Approaches to cancer treatment and care vary widely. Although there is standard care for some cancers, cancer treatment varies widely depending upon the type of cancer, where you live, which doctors you are connected to, the type of practitioners to whom you have access, the hospital or center where you are diagnosed and treated, second opinion practitioners you have sought out, and, most important, the philosophy of the care team.

The New Chinese Medicine approach is most in line with the approaches by practitioners and centers in the field of integrative oncology. New Chinese Medicine advocates use complementary and alternative medicine in conjunction with conventional treatment. The U.S. National Institutes of Health Office of Cancer Complementary and Alternative Medicine (OCCAM) defines integrative medicine and complementary and alternative medicine as the following:[4]

- Complementary and alternative medicine (CAM): Any medical system, practice, or product that is not thought of as standard care

- Complementary medicine: A CAM therapy used along with standard medicine

- Alternative medicine: A CAM therapy used in place of standard treatments

- Integrative medicine: An approach that combines treatments from conventional medicine and CAM for which there is some high-quality evidence of safety and effectiveness

Integrative oncology is a subset of integrative medicine. A lot of debate exists as to what, as well as who, exactly defines integrative oncology. Some practitioners see that integrative medicine—as it is usually practiced in the United States—tends to be a medicine that is centered in Western medicine, defined by Western medicine practitioners, and brings in bits and pieces of other types of medicines and cultures. This is rather than incorporating the philosophical base of the medicines from which the practices are drawn.

Therefore, I define my practice, especially within complex areas such as cancer, as Integrated Chinese Medicine. We bring the philosophy of Chinese medicine to the forefront. Chinese medicine defines the milieu, the underpinning of the healing practices. We can interface with Western medicine, with other Eastern practitioners, and with complementary and alternative medicine practitioners while standing our ground in Chinese medicine philosophy.

## THE STAGES OF CANCER SURVIVORSHIP

Cancer survivorship has three distinct phases: living with, through, and beyond cancer. Thanks to the MD Anderson Cancer Center for this compilation.

**Living with cancer** refers to the experience of receiving a cancer diagnosis and any treatment that may follow. During this time:

- Patients will undergo treatment and may be asked to join a clinical trial to study new cancer therapies.

- Patients and their caregivers may be offered services to help cope with emotional, psychological, and financial concerns.

**Living through cancer** is the period following treatment in which the risk of cancer recurring is relatively high. Many patients are relieved that treatment is over, but they feel anxious about no longer seeing their cancer doctors on a regular basis. During this stage:

- Patients typically see their cancer doctor two to four times a year, depending on their circumstances.

**Living beyond cancer** refers to post-treatment and long-term survivorship. While two out of three survivors say their lives return to normal, one-third report continuing physical, psychosocial, or financial consequences. During this stage:

- Most survivors go back to the care of their primary physician.

- Ideally, survivors will have developed a long-term health care plan with their cancer doctor to be implemented by their primary physician.

If you are diagnosed with cancer, you may be supported and treated with Integrated Chinese Medicine at the time of your diagnosis, throughout the course of conventional Western treatments, in conjunction with alternative treatment programs, and after remission or cure.

Treatment at the time of diagnosis will include treatment of symptoms and preparation for conventional therapies, such as surgery, chemotherapy, and radiation. It is optimal to be as highly prepared as possible for all the possible effects of the Western treatment.

Treatment with Integrated Chinese Medicine during conventional Western treatments must be well monitored, taking into account the side effects of drugs and other therapies, drug-herb-supplement interactions, and changes in Western therapies. The Chinese medicine practitioner and Western cancer treatment team need to be in close contact during this time.

Treatment with Integrated Chinese Medicine after all cancer treatment is completed often is focused on supporting the immune system, mitigating side effects that linger such as neuropathy, and dealing with health issues as they come up once Western treatment is completed. In addition to Western monitoring for signs of cancer recurrence, there must be a focus on identifying, preventing, and controlling any long-term and late effects associated with cancer and its treatment.

If necessary, during hospice care, treatment with Integrated Chinese Medicine will focus on support of the Shen, emotional support, pain issues, and allowing the person to be as present as he or she would like at the end of life.

# PART ONE: SELF-CARE PLAN FOR PREVENTION AND THERAPEUTIC TREATMENT

## Step One: Adopt the Comprehensive Program for Strengthening Organ Qi and Protective Qi

A general, supportive health care routine that includes a balanced diet, regular exercise and meditation, self-massage, and other stress-reduction techniques is essential in cancer support and prevention. The Comprehensive Program for Cancer Support integrates the Comprehensive Program for Basic Good Health and a Strong Immune System (see page 223), with specific cancer support needs.

## Step Two: Expand Your Daily Journal

When starting a Comprehensive Program for Cancer Support, the first step is to expand your daily journal. The journal will help alert you to the development or improvement of any disharmonies.

The journal should include additional information on the following:

- Appetite increase or decrease as well as changes in tastes of foods as well as food cravings. Watch for waxing and waning of these symptoms.

- Alcohol and caffeine consumption

- Energy levels and ability to exercise. Note if there is an increase or decrease before or after chemotherapy or radiation treatments.

- Times when fatigue, pain, constipation or diarrhea, depression, or weakness make it difficult to exercise, concentrate, or work

- Physical symptoms you suspect are associated with cancer or your Western treatment, such as fatigue, neuropathy (tingling or numbness in your extremities), blood sugar problems, changes in sleep patterns, swelling in any area, and pain over the liver area

- Cognitive problems, such as "brain fog," excessive forgetfulness, changes in moods, and emotional lability

- During treatment, any immediate changes that are alarming or are a red flag for any practitioner. (Immediately report these to your Western medicine cancer team!)

- If you are not on active cancer treatment, due to no additional treatment, refusal of treatment, or being in remission, note any changes that may require additional support or a visit to the doctor.

Paying close attention to this information over time can reveal very important information about your overall health as well as your response to cancer treatment and supportive therapies. This information indicates how you can control or eliminate some of the troubling symptoms and if there is disease progression or regression. This will help you report to your Chinese medicine practitioner and your Western providers about improvement or worsening of symptoms. This is the best way you can thrive with a cancer diagnosis.

## Step Three: Adding Dietary Guidelines

In addition to the diet guidelines outlines in the Comprehensive Program for Basic Good Health and a Strong Immune System (see page 223), you may tailor your diet to support Spleen and Stomach Qi, remove Toxic Heat, promote a balanced flow of Qi and Xue, support your digestion, and remove foods or herbs that may interact with prescribed medicines. It is best to normalize weight because cancer risk is much higher in overweight and obese people.

- Eat a diet of warm, cooked foods. Reduce cold and raw foods to a minimum. Eat soups and easily digested foods—especially during cancer treatment. Congees are a great supportive food to which you can add herbs that are approved by your treatment team.

- Eliminate or drastically reduce dairy products, to decrease and strengthen the Spleen and Stomach Organ Systems.

- Reduce alcohol intake. Eliminate alcohol completely during cancer treatment. Some drug therapies interact with alcohol, so ask your treatment team for a list. Excessive alcohol consumption increases risk for certain types of cancer.

- Reduce caffeine if it increases symptoms.

- Keep at a healthy weight or lose weight healthfully if you are overweight. Do not go on a crash diet of any sort because that can lead to deterioration of your health. It is best not to start a weight loss program during active cancer treatment. A healthy BMI is between 18.5 and 24.9 (see "Tip" on page 299 for more information).

- Eat a diet moderately high in protein, especially fish and plant-based proteins. You can add protein powders (with no sugar added) such as organic grass-fed whey (contains dairy) protein or hemp protein to your diet by combining with other foods or creating shakes that are not cold and do not have added sugar.

- Adopt a diet focused on balancing high-glycemic foods with lower-glycemic foods and proteins. Visit www.glycemicindex.com and www.nutritiondata.com/topics/glycemic-index for glycemic index information on all foods; use this as a guide for keeping your meals on the low end of the glycemic index. In general, adopt a diet focused on balancing high-glycemic foods with lower-glycemic foods to reduce issues with metabolic syndrome and insulin resistance. Insulin resistance is associated with some types of cancer.

- Try to eliminate any foods that contain high fructose corn syrup.

## AMERICAN CANCER SOCIETY 2012 GUIDELINES

The American Cancer Society's 2012 nutrition guidelines to help reduce cancer risk recommend choosing foods and beverages in amounts that help you get to and stay at a healthy weight.

- Eating a balanced diet that includes 2½ cups (around 250 g) of vegetables and fruits each day and choosing whole grains over refined grains and sugar-sweetened products should be part of this plan.

- Limiting intake of red meats and processed meats, such as bacon, sausage, lunch meats, and hot dogs, is also recommended to help reduce cancer risk. A good way to do this is to choose fish, poultry, or beans for some meals rather than beef, pork, lamb, or processed meats.

- The guidelines note that although eating fish is linked to a lower risk of heart disease, the evidence regarding cancer is limited.

## Step Four: Implementing an Exercise Plan

With a cancer diagnosis, it is important to exercise. Prevention of cancer is also associated with proper exercise and movement. It is especially important to exercise to your capability during cancer treatment, especially to prevent weight gain and improve energy levels. Survival rates in breast cancer are improved with exercise as well as lung cancer in men. Improving insulin sensitivity also improves outcomes of treatment and reduces risk of first diagnosis and recurrence.

However, if you are already suffering from fatigue, it is particularly important that you don't overexercise. To stay as healthy as possible, it is important to oxygenate your system and maintain muscle tone. Exercise should really be according to your level of disease and energy. To regulate and move Qi and Xue so they flow smoothly, do moderate exercise. Use the Qi Gong warm-up exercises (see page 182) and walking to stimulate balanced flow.

If you need to lose weight, you can walk 10,000 steps per day to meet the exercise goal. For example, if you walk a lot at work or to and from work, you may want to wear a pedometer (such as a Fitbit) to monitor your walking. This will help in your weight loss goals.

To support your Spleen and prevent further Deficient Spleen Qi, weight lifting should be done a maximum of three times a week.

You may practice Tai Chi, Qi Gong, or moderate Yoga exercises every day to increase muscle strength, improve balance, and support all your Organ Qi.

## Step Five: Implementing a Meditation Plan

Meditation can alleviate the stress and diminish associated symptoms. First, just start with taking a deep breath. Use Buddha's Breath and Taoist's Breath (see page 179) to infuse your body with Qi. Regular practice of the Qi Meditation (see page 186) can produce constitutional improvements that will do much to restore harmony. Even if you have severe fatigue, Qi Gong breathing and Qi-stimulating movements can be done with minimal effort and still produce great results. (You can even lie down to do them!)

If you are going through chemotherapy treatment, you may also want to use the Lotus Blossom Meditation (see page 189) during your sessions.

As your strength returns, you can increase your routine. Add Zen walking and more aerobic activities for ten minutes a day. Always include the breathing exercises. To decide if you are strong enough to add more vigorous exercise, ask yourself, "Could I walk comfortably at a steady pace for ten minutes? How about for twenty minutes?" If the answer is yes, a daily ten- or twenty-minute Qi Gong workout can provide the Qi nurturing and stimulation you need.

## Step Six: Using Self-Massage and Moxibustion for Preventive Care

Massage and acupressure are extremely helpful after a cancer diagnosis and during Western treatment. For example, you can implement any and all steps of the Ten-Step Qi-Xue Self-Massage (see page 191).

You may also use reflexology on the hands and feet, focusing on the specific parts of your body that are most in need (see pages 210 and 211).

For support of the Stomach and Spleen Qi and to reduce fatigue and digestive problems, perform acupressure on Stomach 36 and Spleen 6 (see page 163). To relieve pain and nausea, you can press on Pericardium 6.

Ear massage is also very helpful for decreasing fatigue, pain, and nausea. Follow these suggestions for a total of ten minutes once a day. For fatigue with digestion problems, use Ear Stomach and Ear Spleen. For fatigue related to negative side effects of medications, use Ear Liver (see the ear chart on page 203).

Shiatsu Partnered Massage (see page 204) can bring you and your loved ones closer together and provide relaxation and relief from symptoms.

### Step Seven: Using Soaks, Saunas, and Compresses for Self-Healing

In general, warming compresses and brief soaks can ease discomfort, calm the Shen, and invigorate you. Don't make the water too cold or too hot.

Use Sleep Ease or Latte Deluxe to Calm the Shen to decrease stress (see pages 212 and 213). Enjoy these soaks for up to half an hour. You can also prepare and use Ginger Bath soaks (see page 213) and Gingerly compresses (see page 217).

### Step Eight: Taking Nutritional Supplements

Much controversy exists among the oncology field over the use of supplements during Western treatment protocols. Some physicians completely oppose supplementation while others cite evidence to support the use of particular supplements during chemotherapy and radiation treatment. For example, some doctors veto the use of coenzyme $Q_{10}$ ($CoQ_{10}$) during chemotherapy and radiation treatment, while others support its use.

Ask your practitioner for specific supplement and dosing recommendations. Your regimen should include taking omega-3 fatty acids and eating healthy sustainable seafood. Visit www.seafoodwatch.org for accurate health and ecological information on seafood. You may take krill oil for omega-3 fatty acids.

Daily *Lactobacillus acidophilus* can also be taken to keep your digestive tract healthy. The Mayo Clinic recommends that "1 x 109 living *L. acidophilus* cells by mouth in divided doses daily is an adequate dose for most people."[5]

## PART TWO: ASSEMBLING THE TEAM

When it comes to cancer support, you need to include both Western-trained and Eastern-trained practitioners to optimize your health care plan. When you use practitioners of both types of medicine in concert, it will give you the opportunity to create an individualized comprehensive treatment plan, share diagnoses, reduce side effects, make better choices for treatments and self-care, and attain the best outcomes.

### Western Medicine

There are a number of screening tests available for cancer (see page 235). If you are diagnosed with cancer, it is likely you are already under the care of a specialized treatment team. It is imperative that you continue that relationship and care no matter what other treatments you get, from Chinese medicine to naturopathic doctors to Western herbalism. If your doctors are not willing to consider support of your Chinese medicine or other treatments of your choice, you may want to change physicians because many are willing to work with a qualified integrative oncology physician or Integrated Chinese Medicine practitioner. It is important to monitor insulin resistance and blood glucose levels along with calculating your BMI. You may need support for weight loss or maintenance before, during, and after Western treatments.

## Eastern Medicine

Chinese medicine is particularly effective for treating the symptoms associated with your cancer treatment and those that linger post-cancer. It can help you maintain metabolic balance. Fatigue, weakness, brain fog, swelling, and other issues are often improved or resolved with Chinese medicine treatment and self-care along with Western therapies. For as much time as you can prior to surgery, chemotherapy, or radiation treatment, you should receive acupuncture, Chinese herbs, massage, dietary support, and other recommendations. Specific Chinese medicine treatment will often change in response to your Western treatment. In our clinic, we have specialized protocols for supporting people who are going through conventional Western treatment. Drug-herb interactions are highlighted as well as specific individualized acupuncture and herb plans to support your Western treatment for the best outcomes.

## Step One: Obtaining a Western Baseline

Maintain your relationship with your Western oncology team. If you are diagnosed with cancer, it is likely you are already under the care of a specialized treatment team. It is imperative that you continue that relationship and care no matter what other treatments you get or practitioners you see, from Chinese medicine to naturopathic doctors to Western herbalism.

If you are overweight, creating a weight loss and weight management program is the best step toward improving health. You may need a medical program, a program such as Weight Watchers or Overeater's Anonymous, therapy groups, individualized therapy, a structured exercise program, or any combination of these to be able to lose weight effectively. Chinese medicine therapies can be used for support in weight loss as well.

Always tell your oncologists and your Western treatment team that you are seeking Chinese medicine therapy or other treatments that may affect your overall treatment plan. By seeing a Chinese medicine doctor, you can benefit from the balancing powers of acupuncture, herbs, and other Chinese medicine therapies. It is best if the members of each team can be introduced to each other and for them to communicate closely.

## Step Two: Obtaining a Chinese Medicine Diagnosis and Treatment

The Chinese medicine practitioner will conduct an interview and use the Four Examinations (see page 76) to determine what disharmonies are present and to find out what symptoms are troubling you. Using this set of traditional diagnostic techniques, the practitioner will design a course that will restore harmony to your Organ Systems and Essential Substances and, as a consequence, alleviate your symptoms, support your immune system, help you lose weight if necessary, and improve your metabolic health. In addition, it is best if your Chinese medicine doctor can also read the lab tests, imaging reports, and biopsy reports from the oncologist or other Western physician for information on your overall health from a Western medicine perspective.

If the practitioner is using Integrated Chinese Medicine, he or she will correlate your Chinese diagnosis with your Western diagnosis and develop a treatment plan that can be shared with you, your oncologist, your Western treatment team, and all your practitioners.

Treatment for severe fatigue, neuropathy, nausea, weakness, weight loss, lowered blood cell counts, and other symptoms associated with cancer and cancer treatment must be tailored to your individual diagnosis. It is likely that ongoing intensive treatment for several months will be recommended. Your practitioner will help you determine the frequency of treatment to maintain strength and vigor and to deal with side effects and support your immune system. Moxibustion will follow the individualized diagnosis that guides acupuncture.

### ACUPUNCTURE

Treatment to strengthen the Spleen and Stomach Qi, tonify Qi and Xue, regulate Qi and Xue, clear Heat Toxins, and remove Dampness will be the main foci of your treatment. Your practitioner must be able to understand all of the complexities to diagnose and treat correctly.

If you have cancer or are in remission, a good idea is for you to ask your practitioner how much experience he or she has in treating people who have been diagnosed with cancer; how much Western knowledge he or she has of lab reports, imaging, and other testing; and if he or she will open a line of communication with your Western practitioners.

## MOXIBUSTION

You can strengthen Spleen and Stomach Qi, tonify Xue, support your immune system, help digestion, and reduce nausea and other symptoms and side effects with moxibustion. You may moxa Stomach 36, Spleen 6, Gallbladder 39, and Ren 6 along with other acupuncture points as directed by your practitioner.

## HERBAL TREATMENTS

Prior to Western cancer treatment and after treatment, a number of herbal formulas can be recommended, guided by your Traditional Chinese Medicine diagnosis. Most herbal formulas are generally designed to treat specific disharmonies that are diagnosed by your Chinese medicine practitioner.

During Western treatment, limitations exist for both the type of formulas and when formulas can be given, based on possible drug-herb interactions and other considerations.

It is imperative that your Chinese medicine practitioner understands how to determine any currently known drug-herb interactions and knows if any herbs are contraindicated.

The Western treatment team and pharmacologist should review the herbal formulas before you take them.

This is a great time to use Integrated Chinese Medicine to its fullest extent.

## Integrated Chinese Medicine During Chemotherapy

In Integrated Chinese Medicine, there are three steps in the chemotherapy cycle during the course of treatment:

1. Circulate

2. Stabilize (detoxify)

3. Tonify

Variations occur in how these steps are used, according to the type of cancer, the type of chemotherapy, and the length of the cycles. However, the conceptual process remains the same.

In addition, we use acupuncture and herbal treatment that address current symptoms.

## EXAMPLE OF CHINESE HERBAL SUPPORT DURING CHEMOTHERAPY

The practioner has investigated drug-herb interactions to the fullest extent that they exist at this time. Use these formulas *only* with the permission of your Western treatment team and oncologist. Please have them contact your Chinese medicine practitioner for more detailed information. Note that this is an example of a possible plan and may not be suitable for everyone.

| DAY | FORMULA | DOSAGE | REASON FOR FORMULA |
|---|---|---|---|
| Circulate 1–7 | Marrow Plus | As prescribed | Vitalize and tonify (Xue) Blood, tonify Qi, strengthen Spleen and Kidney, help offset side effects of medications that suppress white or red blood cells and platelets |
| | Quiet Digestion (if needed) | As prescribed | Regulate digestion, disperse Wind and Damp, resolve Spleen Dampness and regulate the Stomach, resolve Phlegm |
| | Circulate Formula such as *Xue Fu Zhu Yu Tang* | As prescribed | Circulate Qi and Xue (Blood) |
| 8–10 | | Continue Marrow Plus. Your practitioner should closely monitor your blood work and may increase your dose of Marrow Plus if your blood counts begin to drop. You may continue to take Quiet Digestion if you experience nausea or digestive upset. | |
| 8–15 Stabilize | Stabilizing Formula such as *Yin Chai Hu, Yi Ren, Ban Zhi Lian, Gan Cao* | As prescribed | Clear Heat and Clean Toxins |
| 16–21 Tonify | | Continue Marrow Plus and Quiet Digestion as needed, discontinue stabilizing formula and start tonification formula | |
| | Tonification Formula #1 such as Enhance | As prescribed | Tonify Qi, blood, Yin, and Yang; clear Heat, Toxins, and Phlegm; strengthen Spleen, Stomach, and Kidneys |
| | Tonification Formula Cordyceps PS | As prescribed | Tonify Kidney Yang, nourish Lung Yin, strengthen Protective Qi, transform Phlegm |

## Step Three: Bringing in Other Modalities

Your treatment plan can be expanded in several ways. You may want to include other forms of Eastern meditations, biofeedback, hypnosis, or psychotherapy. You might want to use some form of bodywork, such as reflexology, to alleviate symptoms such as neuropathy, alleviate pain, and help improve overall energy.

### AT A GLANCE: COMPREHENSIVE PROGRAM FOR CANCER SUPPORT

| SELF-CARE PLAN | |
|---|---|
| Evaluation | Before starting a self-care plan, make sure your Western treatment team and Chinese medicine practitioner communicate with each other to make sure there is agreement on the type of care that you can do. Both teams should have access to lab tests, imaging, and any other examinations. Also, if you need to lose weight, there should be a proper plan in place that takes into account your cancer diagnosis. |
| Self-monitoring | In addition to the general guidelines, your daily journal should make note of energy levels and fluctuations, signs of cognitive problems, your sugar and carbohydrate intake and the glycemic values, any swellings, changes in tumor size if appropriate. Observe and write down your physical activity, along with body rhythms, including sleep disruption, changes in elimination, and mood changes. Also ask your oncologist or primary care doctor what he or she would like you to monitor. |
| Diet | In addition to the First-Step Dietary Therapy Program that removes irritants and toxins and soothes the system, add the concepts of glycemic index and weight loss techniques if appropriate. Adopt a low-glycemic diet. Eliminate all alcohol. Reduce or eliminate sugar intake. Eliminate all high fructose corn syrup from your diet. Reduce caffeine intake. Your daily protein consumption should come primarily from plant-based and sustainable fish sources. During Western treatment, to get enough nourishment, you can eat congees and soups that are easily digestible and tasty. Use the Chinese medicine diagnosis given to you by your practitioner to modify your dietary choices. |
| Exercise | Exercise should be moderate, focused on strengthening Stomach and Spleen Qi as well as regulating Qi and Xue. If you can, start some moderate aerobic movement. Mild weight-bearing exercises will improve your muscle tone. Use Qi Gong warm-up exercises and walking to stimulate balanced flow. For weight loss, you can walk up to 10,000 steps per day, using a pedometer, and walk instead of driving or taking the bus. Do not do excessive exercise. If you are too tired, you may do sitting Qi Gong. |

*(continued)*

| SELF-CARE PLAN *(continued)* | |
|---|---|
| Meditation | Start with Buddha's Breath and Taoist's Breath to infuse your body with Qi. Regularly practice the Qi Meditation. During chemotherapy, use the Lotus Blossom Meditation. If you have enough energy, begin Zen walking. With severe fatigue, you may start with sitting and lying Qi Gong movements. |
| Moxibustion | Use moxa to strengthen the Spleen and Stomach Qi and tonify Xue through moxa on Stomach 36, Spleen 6, Gallbladder 39, and Ren 6. |
| Massage | Partnered Shiatsu massage can be very soothing and invigorating. For self-massage, use any or all of the portions of the Ten-Step Qi-Xue Self-Massage. Perform acupressure on Spleen 6 and Stomach 36 to strengthen the Spleen and Stomach. Use ear massage to relieve nausea, support digestion, and decrease fatigue. Focus on the areas of need using reflexology. |
| Soaks and saunas | Saunas, soaks, and compresses are all effective ways to decrease abdominal discomfort and keep the Qi and Xue flowing harmoniously. |
| Nutritional supplements | Follow the nutritional supplement plan with the modifications made in this chapter. Make sure you take a regular dose of *Lactobacillus acidophilus*. |
| ASSEMBLING THE HEALING TEAM | |
| Obtaining a Western baseline | It is likely you are already under the care of a specialized treatment team. Continue that relationship; get lab tests and exams as necessary. Report any changes, positive or negative, to your treatment team. If you are overweight, create a practical weight loss and weight management program under the supervision of your practitioners. Introduce your oncologist and Western team members to your Chinese medicine practitioner and support communication among them. |
| Obtaining Chinese medicine diagnosis and treatment | When you go to a Chinese medicine practitioner, it's important to establish communication between the Chinese and Western doctors. Preventive and therapeutic routines may include acupuncture, moxibustion, acupressure, and herbal medicine. Make sure your practitioner is fully aware of drug-herb interactions and how to manage herbs during chemotherapy and radiation treatment. |
| Bringing in other modalities | You may get support before Western treatment, during treatment, and post-treatment through regular massage, nutritional and dietary counseling, cancer support groups, and exposure to other Eastern and Western alternative healing traditions. |

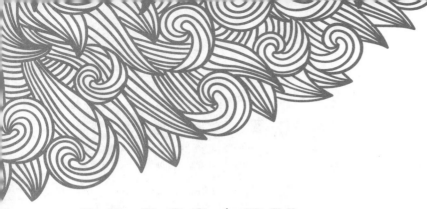

# GLOSSARY

**Acupuncture:** Acupuncture is the art and science of manipulating the flow of Qi and Xue through the body's Channels, the invisible aqueduct system that transports the Essential Substances to the Organ Systems, tissues, and bones. Manipulation of the Qi and Xue is accomplished by the stimulation of specific acupuncture points along the Channels where these Essential Substances flow close to the skin's surface.

**Channels:** Also called vessels and meridians, Channels are the conduits in the vast aqueduct system that transports the Essential Substances to the Organ Systems. They contain the acupuncture points that are stimulated through acupuncture and acupressure.

**Disharmony:** In Chinese medicine, when the Essential Substances, Organ Systems, and/ or Channels are not balanced and functioning optimally, they are said to be in disharmony. Disharmony can be created by the Six Pernicious Influences or the Seven Emotions.

**Eight Fundamental Patterns:** Paired as Interior, Exterior; Heat, Cold; Excess, Deficiency; and Yin, Yang, the Eight Fundamental patterns describe the way in which the Six Pernicious Influences and Seven Emotions create disharmony in the mind/body/spirit.

**Essential Substances:** This refers to the fluids, essences, and energies that nurture the Organ Systems and keep the mind/body/spirit in balance. They are identified as Qi, the life force; Shen, the spirit; Jing, the essence that nurtures growth and development; Xue, which is often translated as "blood," but which contains more qualities than blood and transports Shen; and Jin-Ye, which is all of the fluids that are not included in Xue.

**Five Phases or Five Elements:** This is a traditional theory and systems used by Worsley School acupuncturists and many Japanese and Korean practitioners to describe the physiology of the mind/body/spirit and to guide diagnosis and treatment.

**Jin-Ye:** All fluids other than Xue, including sweat, urine, mucus, saliva, and other secretions such as bile and gastric acid are considered Jin-Ye. Jin-Ye is produced by digestion of food. Organ Qi regulates it. Some forms of refined Jin-Ye help produce Xue.

**Jing:** Often translated as "essence," Jing is the fluid that nurtures growth and development. We are born with Prenatal or Congenital Jing, inherited from our parents. Along with Original Qi, it defines our basic constitution.

**Moxibustion:** The use of burning herbs, placed on or near the body, to stimulate specific acupuncture points and warm the Channels. It is used to stimulate a smooth flow of Qi and Xue.

**Organ Systems:** Unlike the Western concept of organs, Chinese medicine describes Organ Systems. An Organ System includes the central organ plus it's interaction with the Essential Substances and Channels. For example, the Heart System is responsible for the circulation of what Western medicine calls blood, and it also acts as the ruler of Xue and is in charge of storing Shen.

**Qi:** The basic life force that pulses through everything, living and inanimate. Qi warms the body, retains the body's fluids and organs, fuels transformation of food into other substances such as Xue, protects the body from disease, and empowers movement, including physical movement, the circulatory system, thinking, and growth.

**Qi Gong:** The ancient Chinese art of exercise and meditation that stimulates and balances the mind/body/spirit.

**Qi Gong Massage:** An extension of Qi Gong exercise/meditation that also helps balance Qi and harmonize the mind/body/spirit.

**Seven Emotions:** Joy, Anger, Grief, Sadness, Fear, Fright, and Pensiveness/Worry are internal triggers of disharmony in the mind/body/spirit.

**Shen:** Shen, or spirit, includes consciousness, thoughts, emotions, and senses that make us uniquely human. It's transmitted to a fetus from the parents and must be continuously nourished after birth.

**Six Pernicious Influences:** These include Heat, Cold, Wind, Dampness, Dryness, and Summer Heat. They are associated with the development of disharmony and disease in the mind/body/spirit.

**Tao:** The Tao is a philosophical concept and orientation. The word is sometimes translated as the "infinite origin" or the "Unnameable." This philosophy sees the universe and each individual as part of the same process. That process moves all things toward unity and into opposition. In the Tao, there is no beginning and no end, yet whatever has a beginning has an end. Everything changes; nothing is static or absolute.

**Xue:** Although commonly translated as "blood," Xue is not confined to the blood vessels, nor does it contain only plasma and red and white blood cells. The Shen, which courses through the blood vessels, is carried by Xue. Xue also moves along the Channels in the body where Qi flows.

**Yin/Yang:** The dynamic balance between opposing forces is known as Yin/Yang. It is the ongoing process of creation and destruction, the natural order of the universe, and of each person's inner being.

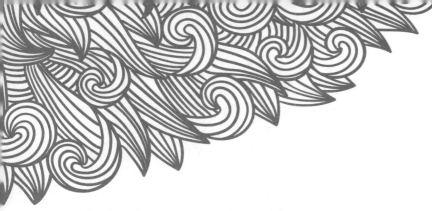

# APPENDIX

## How to Find Practitioners, Supplements and Herbs, and More

### HOW TO FIND A LICENSED QUALIFIED CHINESE MEDICINE PRACTITIONER

**National Commission for the Certification of Acupuncture and Oriental Medicine (NCCAOM)**

http://mx.nccaom.org/FindAPractitioner.aspx

76 South Laura Street, Suite 1290 · Jacksonville, FL 32202

Phone: 904-598-1005 · Fax: 904-598-5001

NCCAOM certifies practitioners in acupuncture, herbs, Oriental medicine, and Asian bodywork. The NCCAOM certification meets national standards for beginning competence in these fields.

The website provides a voluntary practitioner directory for the public to find practitioners as well as a registry for licensing bodies to use for verifying NCCAOM certification. There is also a section on state licensing requirements. NCCAOM practitioners are not necessarily licensed in any state. Each state has its own licensure rules. Check with the licensing or registration body in states that require licensure to find out the status of any individual's license. You may call the practitioner directly to inquire about licensure and additional training.

**Acufinder.com**

www.acufinder.com

Acufinder.com provides the consumer with the ability to find a practitioner within any geographical area in the United States and Canada as well as some other countries. The site shows licensure, state organizations, and organizations to which a practitioner belongs as well as areas of expertise and style of acupuncture.

### American Board of Oriental Reproductive Medicine

www.aborm.org

Email: inquiry@aborm.org

The ABORM is a nonprofit 501(C)6 corporation devoted to teaching, research, and the practice of Oriental medicine in the treatment of reproductive disorders. The ABORM respects the training and lineage of all practitioners who work with reproductive disorders. Practitioners listed on their website have demonstrated competency and advanced knowledge in both Western and Oriental reproductive medicine by passing a rigorous advanced certification examination.

### Misha Ruth Cohen Education Foundation

www.TCMEducation.org

2339 3rd Street, Suite 48, 3R  ·  San Francisco, CA 94107

415-864-7234

Email: TCMEducation@gmail.com

The Misha Ruth Cohen Education Foundation is a 501(c)3 nonprofit organization dedicated to providing resources and education to medical professionals, patients, and the community. The foundation focuses on integrating Western and Eastern medicine, specifically Chinese traditional medicine, in the treatment of complex health issues, including HIV/AIDS, hepatitis B and C, cancer support, gynecological problems, and chronic viral diseases. You may find a list of Hepatitis C Professional Certified Practitioners on the website.

### Misha Ruth Cohen, O.M.D., L.Ac.

Chicken Soup Chinese Medicine

www.docmisha.com

2325 3rd Street, Suite 342  ·  San Francisco, CA 94107

Phone: 415-861-1101  ·  Fax: 415-644-0614

Email: ChickenSoupChineseMedicine@docmisha.com

Chicken Soup Chinese Medicine is the Integrated Chinese Medicine clinical practice of Misha Ruth Cohen, O.M.D., L.Ac., and her clinical team. She and her team provide comprehensive treatment programs to people seeking support for such complex medical challenges as viral hepatitis, fatty liver, liver disease, HIV, cancer support, metabolic issues such as diabetes or high cholesterol, gynecological conditions, and reproductive health. The website has a great deal of information and resources for the general public and practitioners.

### Where to Study Chinese Medicine

**The Accreditation Commission for Acupuncture and Oriental Medicine (ACAOM)**

www.acaom.org

8941 Aztec Drive · Eden Prairie, MN 55347

Phone: 952-212-2434 · Fax: 301-313-0912

Email: coordinator@acaom.org

ACAOM is the national accrediting agency recognized by the U.S. Department of Education for the accreditation of Chinese medicine colleges in the United States. ACAOM establishes policies and standards that govern the accreditation process for acupuncture and Oriental medicine programs.

You may find more information on the accrediting process and status of Chinese medicine colleges at the ACAOM website.

# WHERE TO FIND CHINESE HERBS AND NUTRITIONAL SUPPLEMENTS

*Note:* Chinese herbs should only be used upon the recommendation of a trained Chinese herbalist.

A limited number of herbs (some mentioned in "The Medicine Cabinet" on page 230) may be ordered over the counter without a recommendation from a licensed practitioner. However, because we recommend that a practitioner follow you, this section will include trusted herb companies that we use in our clinic. Many practitioners use these companies and other high-quality companies. You should always ask your practitioner about the qualifications of the herb companies and products they use. (Refer back to chapter 8 for detailed information on Chinese herbal medicine.)

**Crane Herb Company/Crane Herb Pharmacy, Inc.**

www.craneherb.com

745 Falmouth Road · Mashpee, MA 02649

Phone: 508-539-1700 · Fax: 508-539-2369

Email: info@craneherb.com

**Crane-West Herb Pharmacy, Inc.**

www.craneherb.com

515 South Main Street · Sebastopol, CA 95472

Phone: 707-823-5691 · Fax: 707-823-2462

Email: crane-west@craneherb.com

Crane offers products that meet rigorous standards of testing and clinical effectiveness. Crane encourages vendors to make their products with the highest traditions of Chinese herbal medicine. Herb companies represented by Crane include Blue Poppy, Chinese Modular Solutions, Classical Herbs, Dr. Shen's, Golden Flower, Health Concerns, Kan Herb, KPC Herbs, Mycoherb, Pacific Biologics, Spring Wind, and Yin-Care. The Crane Herb companies limit their sale of herbal products to licensed or certified practitioners, to students of Chinese medicine, and to patients with prescriptions from registered practitioners.

**Health Concerns**
www.healthconcerns.com
8001 Capwell Drive  ·  Oakland, CA 94621
Phone: 800-233-9355  ·  Fax: 510-639-9140
Email: service@healthconcerns.com

Health Concerns, founded by herbalist Andrew Gaeddert, is the first company in the United States to manufacture prepared Chinese herbs for practitioners that meet rigorous standards of testing to ensure optimum effectiveness, consistent potency, and maximum bioavailability. I have designed herbal formulas for Health Concerns, including Enhance and other products mentioned in this book.

   Health Concerns' products are almost exclusively sold to licensed health care professionals. In a consumer-oriented section of the website, you will find information about Health Concerns and their products. Health Concerns strongly encourages that their products be used under the direction of a licensed practitioner, so they also provide assistance in locating a practitioner in your area.

**Mayway**
www.mayway.com
Mayway Corporation
1338 Mandela Parkway  ·  Oakland, CA 94607
Phone: 800-2MAYWAY  ·  Fax: 800-909-2828
Email: info@mayway.com

Mayway is a family business that has been importing and distributing traditional Chinese medicines since 1969. Mayway began as a small herb shop in San Francisco's Chinatown, and it has become an internationally known company. Mayway promotes quality standards in their sourcing of herbs and in the manufacturing of herbal products. Mayway's most well-known line is the Plum Flower brand. Mayway sells products to health care practitioners, health-related businesses, and students of Chinese medicine. Proof of licensure or certification is required to open an account.

**Spring Wind Herbs Inc.**
www.springwind.com
2325 Fourth Street, Suite 6 · Berkeley, CA 94710
Phone: 800-588-4883 · Fax: 510-849-4886

Spring Wind specializes in external topical formulas—ointments, crèmes, salves, and liniments—designed by Andrew Ellis, an accomplished master herbalist and teacher. Spring Wind also supplies herbal concentrates and bulk herbs to practitioners. Spring Wind brought the issue of the use of incorrect species of herbs to the forefront and was the first company to introduce a lot-based testing system for a comprehensive list of pesticide residues. Spring Wind also now carries a large and growing selection of USDA NOP Certified Organic herbs.

# WHERE TO STUDY CHINESE HERBAL MEDICINE

**Rocky Mountain Herbal Institute (RMHI)**
www.rmhiherbal.org
Attn: Roger W. Wicke, Ph.D., director
PO Box 579 · Hot Springs, MT 59845
Phone: 406-741-3811

RMHI offers distance learning, interactive game software, clinical reference databases, self-study guides, seminars, and comprehensive international certification programs. HerbalThink-TCM provides an interactive way to learn many aspects of Chinese herbology—explanatory, taking you step-by-step from the theory of Chinese herbology to clinical applications.

**Institute of Chinese Herbology**
www.ich-herbschool.com
1440 Washington Boulevard, #A-2 · Concord, CA 94521
Phone: 800-736-0182
Email: info@ich-herbschool.com

ICH offers distance learning in Chinese herbology for licensed acupuncturists and people who want to study Chinese herbology as a sole practice. Three programs are offered: foundation courses, professional courses, and clinical training in Chinese herbology.

# WHERE TO BUY SUPPLEMENTS

*Note:* Nutritional supplements are best used upon the recommendation of a trained practitioner, doctor, or nutritionist.

Supplements should be recommended by a practitioner after an evaluation. Sometimes there are deficiencies that need to be addressed as well a therapeutic doses than can be used for specific conditions. Because we recommend that a practitioner follow you, this section will include trusted supplement companies. Many practitioners use these companies and other high-quality companies. You should always ask your practitioner about the qualifications of the supplement companies and products they use.

**Karuna Corporation**
www.karunahealth.com
42 Digital Drive  ·  Novato, CA 94949
Phone: 800-826-7225  ·  Fax: 415-382-0142
Email: info@karunahealth.com

Karuna carries a wide variety of supplements and herbs for practitioner distribution only. Karuna herbal and nutritional supplements are free of preservatives, excipients, or other additives problematic for the allergic or sensitive patient. Tablets and capsules contain no sugars, artificial flavorings, or preservatives. We use this local brand in our clinic for all basic supplements. They also provide practitioner information to patients by phone and email.

## The following companies are recommended by Lyn Patrick, N.D.

**Thorne Research, Inc.**
www.thorne.com
P.O. Box 25  ·  Dover, ID 83825
Phone: 800-228-1966  ·  Fax: 800-747-1950
Email: info@thorne.com

Thorne Research is recognized as a manufacturer of hypoallergenic dietary supplements for severely allergic, chemically sensitive, and immune-compromised patients. Thorne Research has been inspected and approved by Australia's Therapeutic Goods Administration (TGA), the Australian pharmaceutical regulatory agency. They use all non-GMO ingredients and have an in-house laboratory for quality control. They carry a wide variety of supplements.

**Pure Encapsulations**
www.pureencapsulations.com
490 Boston Post Road · Sudbury, MA 01776
Phone: 800-753-2277 · Fax: 888-783-2277

Pure Encapsulations produces a complete line of research-based, hypoallergenic nutritional supplements. Products do not contain hidden fillers, coatings, artificial colors, or other excipients. Formulas are free of wheat, gluten, nuts, and hydrogenated oils. Only licensed health care professionals may order from Pure Encapsulations.

**GAIA Herbs**
www.gaiaherbs.com
101 Gaia Herbs Drive · Brevard, NC 28712
Phone: 800-831-7780 · Fax: 800-717-1722
Email: info@gaiaherbs.com

GAIA's mission is to create and nurture healthy connections between plants and people. They do that "through finding and maintaining strong global relationships in addition to championing personal and environmental sustainability here at home, on our own organic farm."

**Integrative Therapeutics**
www.integrativepro.com
825 Challenger Drive · Green Bay, WI 54311
Phone: 800-931-1709 · Fax: 800-380-8189

Integrative Therapeutics sells exclusively to health care professionals. It is a leading manufacturer and distributor of science-based nutritional supplements. They have several different lines of products meeting various nutritional needs to be used in conjunction with lifestyle and diet recommendations.

# FINDING LICENSED PRACTITIONERS OF NATURAL MEDICINE AND THERAPY

## Naturopathic Medicine Doctors

### The Council on Naturopathic Medical Education (CNME)
PO Box 178 · Great Barrington, MA 01230
Phone: 413-528-8877

CNME is the accrediting agency recognized by the U.S. Department of Education for the accreditation of naturopathic medical education programs that voluntarily seek recognition in the United States and Canada. Students and graduates of programs accredited or pre-accredited (candidacy) by CNME are eligible to apply for the naturopathic licensing examinations administered by the North American Board of Naturopathic Examiners (NABNE), and they are generally eligible for state and provincial licensure in the United States and Canada.

**American Association of Naturopathic Physicians (AANP)**

www.naturopathic.org

818 18th Street, NW, Suite 250 · Washington, DC 20006

Phone: 866-538-2267 · Fax: 202-237-8152

Email: member.services@naturopathic.org

AANP's physician members are graduates of naturopathic medical schools accredited by the Council on Naturopathic Medical Education (CNME). CNME is recognized by the U.S. Department of Education as the national accrediting agency for programs leading to the Doctor of Naturopathic Medicine (N.D. or N.M.D.) or Doctor of Naturopathy (N.D.) degree.

## Doctors of Chiropractic

**The Council on Chiropractic Education (CCE)**

www.cce-usa.org

8049 North 85th Way · Scottsdale, AZ 85258

Phone: 888-443-3506 · Fax: 480-483-7333

Email: cce@cce-usa.org

CCE is the national accrediting body for Doctor of Chiropractic programs and chiropractic solitary purpose institutions of higher education recognized by the United States Department of Education.

**American Chiropractic Association (ACA)**

www.acatoday.org

1701 Clarendon Boulevard, Suite 200 · Arlington, VA 22209

Phone: 703-276-8800 · Fax: 703-243-2593

Email: memberinfo@acatoday.org

The American Chiropractic Association is the largest professional association in the United States representing doctors of chiropractic. You can search for a chiropractor in your area on the ACA website.

## Massage and Bodywork

### American Massage Therapy Association (AMTA)
www.amtamassage.org
500 Davis Street, Suite 900 · Evanston, IL 60201
Phone: 877-905-0577
Email: info@amtamassage.org

AMTA professional members are massage therapists who have demonstrated their competency by completing one or more of the following: graduation from a minimum 500 in-class hour, entry-level massage therapy school; proof of current state or provincial licensure (where applicable); or certification by the National Certification Board for Therapeutic Massage and Bodywork.

### Associated Bodywork and Massage Professionals (ABMP)
www.abmp.com
25188 Genesee Trail Road, Suite 200 · Golden, CO 80401
Phone: 800-458-2267 · Fax: 800-667-8260
Email: expectmore@abmp.com

ABMP members at the certified or professional levels must possess a valid massage license from a regulated state, have completed 500 approved educational hours, or be certified through the National Certification Board for Therapeutic Massage and Bodywork. Licensed nurse and physical therapists may qualify for membership at either the certified or professional level with a minimum of 50 hours of additional massage therapy training.

# BOOKS AND PUBLICATIONS

## Book Distributors and Publishers

### Redwing Book Company
www.redwingbooks.com

Redwing provides books, electronic media, and charts for practitioners and the general public. Categories include Chinese medicine, acupuncture, bodywork, nutrition, integrative medicine, complementary and alternative medicine, and other health-related areas.

### Paradigm Publications
www.paradigm-pubs.com

Paradigm Publications provides information about Traditional Chinese Medicine and acupuncture, Japanese acupuncture, and other complementary and alternative healing systems to

English-speaking readers. Publications are for both professionals and the layperson. Their work honors both the East Asian respect for language, tradition, and nature and the West's commitment to science.

**Blue Poppy Enterprises, Inc.**
www.bluepoppy.com
1990 57th Court North, Unit A · Boulder, CO 80301
Phone: 800-487-9296 · Fax: 303-245-8362
Email: info@bluepoppy.com

Blue Poppy provides a wide variety of books and publications aimed at both practitioners and the public.

**Eastland Press**
www.eastlandpress.com
1240 Activity Drive, #D · Vista, CA 92081
Phone: 800-214-3278 · Fax: 800-241-3329

Eastland Press provides books to practitioners in osteopathy, bodywork, and Oriental medicine.

**Eastwind Books**
www.eastwindbooks.com
1435A Stockton Street · San Francisco, CA 94133
Phone: 415-772-5888 · Fax: 415-772-5885
Email: contact@eastwindbooks.com

923 Westwood Boulevard · Los Angeles, CA 90024
Phone: 310-824-4888 · Fax: 310-824-4838
Email: info_la@eastwindbooks.com

Eastwind Books has an extensive selection of resources on Asian and Asian-American issues.

## Recommended Books

Donald I. Abrams and Andrew Weil, *Integrative Oncology*, 2nd Edition (Oxford, UK: Oxford University Press, 2014). This text is part of a series of books for clinicians on several health conditions. *Integrative Oncology* is edited by Andrew Weil, M.D., professor and director of the Arizona Center for Integrative Medicine at the University of Arizona. *Integrative Oncology* uses cases histories, tables, and clinical pearls to discuss integrative interventions complementary to conventional treatments in cancer care.

Lise N. Altshuler, N.D., F.A.B.N.O., and Karolyn Gazella, *The Definitive Guide to Thriving After Cancer: A Five-Step Integrative Plan to Reduce the Risk of Recurrence and Build Lifelong Health*

(Berkeley, CA: Ten Speed Press, 2013). A companion to *The Definitive Guide to Cancer*, this fully revised guide outlines a five-step plan integrating both conventional and alternative therapies for cancer survivors. Dr. Altshuler is widely recognized as an expert in cancer treatment and prevention. She is the founding board member of the Oncology Association of Naturopathic Physicians. Karolyn A. Gazella is the publisher of the *Natural Medicine Journal*, a peer-reviewed medical journal for health care practitioners.

Harriet Beinfield and Efrem Korngold, *Between Heaven and Earth: A Guide to Chinese Medicine* (New York: Ballantine Books, 1991). This book focuses strongly on the philosophy of the Five Phases.

Dan Bensky, Steven Clavey, and Erich Stöger, with Andrew Gamble, illustrations compiled and translated by Lilian Lai Bensky, *Chinese Herbal Medicine: Materia Medica*, 3rd Edition (Vista, CA: Eastland Press, 2004). *Chinese Herbal Medicine: Materia Medica*, 3rd Edition is one of the main books used in the West by Chinese herbal practitioners. It covers more than 530 of the most commonly used herbs in the Chinese pharmacopoeia. This book is essential in the library for anyone studying or practicing Chinese herbal medicine.

Jill Blakeway and Sami S. David, *Making Babies: A Proven 3-Month Program for Maximum Fertility* (New York: Little, Brown and Company, 2009). *Making Babies* is an accessible book that helps you determine your "fertility type" developed by the authors, who combine Chinese medicine and Western medicine to improve the chances of becoming pregnant.

Keith Block, *Life Over Cancer: The Block Center Program for Integrative Cancer Treatment* (New York: Bantam Dell, 2009). Dr. Keith Block, an internationally recognized expert in integrative oncology for more than thirty-five years, presents the Block program for fighting cancer to people who are at different places along the cancer continuum: for those who've been recently diagnosed, to those in treatment, to those who've concluded treatment and need to remain vigilant to prevent recurrence. Dr. Block's program is explained in easy-to-understand language and format. Patients can implement the program themselves or with the assistance of their health care providers.

Boston Women's Health Book Collective, *Our Bodies, Ourselves*, 9th edition (New York: Touchstone, 2001). This is the fortieth anniversary of this women's health bible, one of *Library Journal's* best books of 2011. It offers information about reproductive health, menopause and aging, sexuality, relationships, gender identity, and domestic violence.

John K. Chen, Tina T. Chen, and Laraine Crampton, *Chinese Medical Herbology and Pharmacology* (City of Industry, CA: Art of Medicine Press, 2004). *Chinese Medical Herbology and Pharmacology* is a widely used practitioner herb manual. It covers traditional and modern uses of Chinese herbs, clinical studies and research, safety data and toxicology, and Western pharmacological and herb-drug interactions.

Misha Ruth Cohen, O.M.D., L.Ac., and Robert G. Gish, with Kalia Doner, *The Hepatitis C Help Book: A Groundbreaking Treatment Program Combining Western and Eastern Medicine for Maximum Wellness and Healing*, Revised Edition (New York: St. Martin's Griffin, 2007). Two experts on hepatitis C teamed up to write the first comprehensive guide to orthodox and alternative treatment options. *The Hepatitis C Help Book* includes programs for self-care, nutritional and fitness plans, and a comprehensive Western and Chinese medical treatment program for people affected by HCV.

Misha Ruth Cohen, O.M.D., L.Ac., and Kalia Doner, *The HIV Wellness Sourcebook: An East/West Guide to Living with HIV/AIDS & Related Conditions* (New York: Henry Holt & Company, 1998). *The HIV Wellness Sourcebook* shows how to incorporate herbs, acupuncture, diet, nutritional supplements, stress reduction, and massage into a sensible comprehensive medical plan, which also addresses the spiritual, mental, and emotional needs of people with HIV/AIDS. It features targeted comprehensive programs combining Chinese and Western medicine for treating digestive disorders, respiratory problems, diarrhea, skin problems, fatigue, pain, anemia, depression, and other maladies.

Peter Deadman, Mazin Al-Khafaji, with Kevin Baker, *A Manual of Acupuncture*, 2nd Edition (Hove, UK: Journal of Chinese Medicine Publications, 2007). *A Manual of Acupuncture* is the primary reference in the west for the study of acupuncture points and Channels. There is a companion flash card set, Acupuncture Point Cards. It is also available as an app.

Ted Kaptchuk, *The Web That Has No Weaver: Understanding Chinese Medicine* (New York: McGraw Hill, 1983, 2000). The 1983 edition of this book was the first widely popular book on Chinese medicine theory published in the West. It has been used as a textbook for beginning practitioners.

Rebecca Katz and Mat Edelson, *The Cancer-Fighting Kitchen: Nourishing, Big-Flavor Recipes for Cancer Treatment and Recovery* (Berkeley, CA: Ten Speed Press, 2009). This book includes recipes that stimulate the appetite and address treatment side effects, the "Cancer-Fighting Tool Kit" for what caregivers and friends need to keep loved ones eating during treatment, advice on putting together a culinary support team, a culinary pharmacy that reveals the peer-reviewed science behind every ingredient in the book, plus strategies for food and lifestyle choices that help patients stay energized, along with food shopping, preparation, storage, and serving tips.

Toni Wechsler, *Taking Charge of Your Fertility, 10th Anniversary Edition: The Definitive Guide to Natural Birth Control, Pregnancy Achievement, and Reproductive Health* (New York: William Morrow, 2006). Toni Weschler has developed the Fertility Awareness Method for birth control without chemicals or devices, to maximize a woman's chances of conception, expedite fertility treatment, and gain control of her sexual and gynecological health.

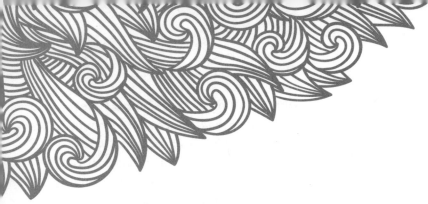

# GENERAL RESOURCES AND REFERENCES

**National Institutes of Health (NIH)**
www.nih.gov
National Institutes of Health
9000 Rockville Pike · Bethesda, MD 20892

NIH's mission is to seek fundamental knowledge about the nature and behavior of living systems and the application of that knowledge to enhance health, lengthen life, and reduce illness and disability. The NIH provides leadership and direction to programs designed to improve the health of the nation by conducting and supporting research:

- in the causes, diagnosis, prevention, and cure of human diseases
- in the processes of human growth and development
- in the biological effects of environmental contaminants
- in the understanding of mental, addictive, and physical disorders
- in directing programs for the collection, dissemination, and exchange of information in medicine and health, including the development and support of medical libraries and the training of medical librarians and other health information specialists

Two institutes within NIH have major research programs in complementary and alternative medicine (CAM) and integrative medicine, the National Center for Complementary and Integrative Health and the Office of Cancer Complementary and Alternative Medicine.

**National Center for Complementary and Integrative Health (NCCIH)**
http://nccam.nih.gov
Phone: 888-644-6226

NCCIH's mission is to define, through rigorous scientific investigation, the usefulness and safety of complementary and integrative health approaches and their roles in improving health and health care.

### Office of Cancer Complementary and Alternative Medicine (OCCAM)

http://cam.cancer.gov/cam

Phone: 240-276-6595 • Fax: 240-276-7888

Email: ncioccam1-r@mail.nih.gov

OCCAM is an office of the National Cancer Institute (NCI) in the Division of Cancer Treatment and Diagnosis. OCCAM is responsible for NCI's research agenda in complementary and alternative medicine (CAM) as it relates to cancer prevention, diagnosis, treatment, and symptom management.

### Centers for Disease Control and Prevention

www.cdc.gov

1600 Clifton Road • Atlanta, GA 30329

Phone: 800-CDC-INFO (800-232-4636)

The CDC's priorities are to improve health security at home and around the world; better prevent the leading causes of illness, injury, disability, and death; and strengthen public health and health care collaboration.

CDC conducts scientific research and provides health information that protects the nation against expensive and dangerous health threats, and it is responsible for responding when these arise. You can find up-to-date information on the CDC's website regarding, cancer, diabetes, hepatitis, HIV/AIDS, obesity, arthritis, heart disease, stroke, and many other public health concerns.

### ClinicalTrials.gov

ClinicalTrials.gov is a service of the U.S. National Institutes of Health. ClinicalTrials.gov is a registry and results database of publicly and privately supported clinical studies of human participants conducted around the world. It is run by the United States National Library of Medicine at the National Institutes of Health, and it is the largest clinical trials database, currently holding registrations from more than 130,000 trials from more than 170 countries in the world. You may find information about clinical studies and search for current and past clinical trials and their results in any disease. The database and searches includes acupuncture trials, herb trials, supplement trials, and other integrative medicine studies as well as conventional Western medicine trials.

### Consumer Lab

www.ConsumerLab.com

Consumer Lab is a subscription-based website that provides up-to-date product quality ratings and comparisons of hundreds of vitamins, supplements, herbs, and other health products. Independent testing is conducted by ConsumerLab.com. In addition to the products that it selects to be tested, ConsumerLab.com allows manufacturers/distributors to request the testing of their own products for a fee through a voluntary testing program. All such products are purchased on the market by ConsumerLab.com and are not supplied by the manufacturer/distributor. These products undergo the same testing and evaluation as other products. Most products reviewed are consumer brands, not practitioner-based brands.

**Natural Medicine Comprehensive Database: Consumer Version**
http://naturaldatabaseconsumer.therapeuticresearch.com/home.aspx?cs=&s=NDC
3120 West March Lane · Stockton, CA 95219
Phone: 209-472-2244 · Fax: 209-472-2249

The Natural Medicine Comprehensive Database: Consumer Version is a subscription-based website with the goal of providing reliable information on herbal remedies, dietary supplements, vitamins, minerals, and other natural products. Many products contain several ingredients. When considering the possible health benefits, safety, and possible side effects of any product, be sure to consider each separate ingredient. The database provides the consumer with information and tools to help evaluate natural products. Through collaboration with Consumer Reports, this information is available to consumers who use ConsumerReportsMedicalGuide.org.

**Natural Medicine Comprehensive Database: Professional Version**
http://naturaldatabase.therapeuticresearch.com/home.aspx?cs=NEWORDER&s=ND
3120 West March Lane · Stockton, CA 95219
Phone: 209-472-2244 · Fax: 209-472-2249

The Natural Medicines Comprehensive Database is a subscription-based website for health professionals that is composed of multiple databases. The core database contains the detailed, evidence-based monographs on individual natural ingredients (such as glucosamine, echinacea, etc.). There are currently almost 1,100 monographs on these individual natural ingredients. The database contains information on effectiveness, drug/herb/supplement interactions, nutrient depletion issues, diseases, colleague interactions, and continuing education for professionals.

**Society for Integrative Oncology (SIO)**
www.integrativeonc.org
Phone: 347-676-1746

The mission of the Society for Integrative Oncology is to advance evidence-based, comprehensive, integrative health care to improve the lives of people affected by cancer. SIO publishes practice guidelines for integrative oncology and provides information for practitioners and patients. SIO sponsors a yearly international integrative oncology conference that includes all disciplines.

On the website, you can search for integrative oncologists, Chinese medicine practitioners and acupuncturists, naturopathic doctors, researchers, lifestyle coaches, nutritionists, bodyworkers, patient advocates, and more.

**Caring Ambassadors Program, Inc.**
www.caringambassadors.org
PO Box 1748 · Oregon City, OR 97045
Phone: 503-632-9032 · Fax: 503-632- 9038

Caring Ambassadors Program is a nonprofit organization with a singular mission: to help improve the lives of people affected by challenging health conditions through advocacy, information, and support.

They have two main programs: Lung Cancer and Hepatitis C. Also, My Journey, My Choices is the Caring Ambassador's site for people to create, track, and research their own journey to wellness.

**Progressive Medical Education (PME)**
www.progressivemedicaleducation.com
14795 Jeffrey Road, Suite 101 · Irvine, CA 92618

Progressive Medical Education is a service created by integrative health care providers, led by Lyn Patrick, N.D., for any provider interested in integrative and alternative medicine. In addition to working as clinicians for many years, the founders have worked in the field of continuing medical education, coordinating international conferences and lecturing to providers from the fields of integrative medicine, naturopathic medicine, and Traditional Chinese Medicine (TCM). The PME site provides access to online education for medical providers. The areas of specialty are environmental illness and toxins, hepatology, hepatitis C, the microbiome, herbal medicine, and more.

# NOTES

## CHAPTER TWO

[1]   "Understanding the Mind/Body/Spirit" in *A Complete Translation of the Yellow Emperor's Classic and the Difficult Classic.* Translated by Henry C. Lu, Ph.D.

[2]   Ibid.

[3]   Jing, the basic life essence, is often said to come into existence "before" Yin and Yang. But its character is said to be Yin. This dialectical view accepts the fact that Jing can exist before Yin and Yang and have Yin qualities, and that Yin itself possesses Yin and Yang aspects.

[4]   "Difficulty 38 of the Nan Jing" in *A Complete Translation of the Yellow Emperor's Classic of Internal Medicine and the Difficult Classic.* Translated by Henry C. Lu, Ph.D.

[5]   Five Phases diagnoses are not part of what has come to be called Traditional Chinese Medicine (TCM). TCM is based on the Eight Fundamental Patterns and the Essential Substances, Organ Systems, and Channels. These elements form the basis for herbal therapy and the type of acupuncture provided by TCM practitioners. Therefore, Five Phases practitioners do not generally use herbal therapy unless they are also trained in TCM.

## CHAPTER FIVE

[1]   *When You Visit a Chinese Medicine Practitioner*, derived from the work of Miriam Lee, used by permission of the author.

[2]   www.acaom.org. From the ACAOM website: The Accreditation Commission for Acupuncture and Oriental Medicine (ACAOM) is the national accrediting agency recognized by the U.S. Department of Education for the accreditation and pre-accreditation ("Candidacy") throughout the United States of first-professional master's degree and professional master's-level certificate and diploma programs in acupuncture and Oriental medicine, and professional post-graduate doctoral programs in acupuncture and in Oriental medicine (DAOM), as well as freestanding institutions and colleges of acupuncture and Oriental medicine that offer such programs. The Commission fosters excellence in acupuncture and Oriental medicine education by establishing policies and standards that govern the accreditation process for acupuncture and Oriental medicine programs. Currently, ACAOM has over 60 schools and colleges with accreditation or Candidacy status.

[3]   Find an NCCAOM practitioner at www.nccaom.org.

## CHAPTER SIX

[1]   You Are What You Eat: www.glycemic.com/GlycemicIndex-LoadDefined.htm.

[2]   www.wholegrainscouncil.org/whole-grains-101/gluten-free-whole-grains.

[3]   Oats are inherently gluten-free, but they are frequently contaminated with wheat during growing or processing. Several companies (Bob's Red Mill, Cream Hill Estates, GF Harvest, Avena Foods [Only Oats], Legacy Valley [Montana Monster Munchies], and Gifts of Nature) currently offer pure, uncontaminated oats. Ask your physician if these oats are acceptable for you.

      Visit www.befreeforme.com/blog/?p=2119 for a discussion on oats in the gluten-free diet or visit Health Canada's website for an extensive technical review at www.hc-sc.gc.ca/fn-an/securit/allerg/cel-coe/oats_cd-avoine-eng.php on the safety of oats in the gluten-free diet.

[4]   Ibid.

[5]   Translation taken from *All the Tea in China*, by Kit Chow and Ione Kramer (San Francisco: China Books and Periodicals, Inc., 1990).

[6]   M. Mukhtar and N. Ahmad, "Tea Polyphenols: Prevention of Cancer and Optimizing Health," *American Journal of Clinical Nutrition* 71, no. 6 (2000): 1698–1702.

## CHAPTER SEVEN

[1]   M. Rose, et al., "Arsenic in Seaweed—Forms, Concentration, and Dietary Exposure," *Food and Chemical Toxicology* 45, no. 7 (2007): 1263-7.

[2]   R. Chowdhury, et al., "Association of Dietary, Circulating, and Supplement Fatty Acids with Coronary Risk: A Systematic Review and Meta-Analysis," *Annals of Internal Medicine* 160 (2014): 398–406.

[3]   Derived from Mary Austin, *The Textbook of Acupuncture Therapy* (New York: ASI Publishers 1972).

[4]   www.mayoclinic.org/drugs-supplements/acidophilus/background/hrb-20058615.

[5]   www.dhaomega3.org/Overview/Differentiation-of-ALA-plant-sources-from-DHA-+-EPA-marine-sources-as-Dietary-Omega-3-Fatty-Acids-for-Human-Health.

[6]   www.consumerreports.org/cro/2012/05/are-krill-oil-pills-as-good-as-fish-oil/index.htm.

## CHAPTER EIGHT

[1] An example of a manufacturing process for granulated herbs is KPC Herbs at www.kpc.com/index. php/manufacturing-process.

[2] Adapted from *Oriental Materia Medica: A Concise Guide* (Long Beach, CA: Oriental Healing Arts Institute, 1986).

[3] D. Bensky, et al., *Chinese Herbal Medicine: Materia Medica*, 3rd Edition (Seattle, WA: Eastland Press, 2004).

[4] V. Scheid, et al., *Chinese Herbal Medicine: Formulas and Strategies*, 2nd Edition (Seattle, WA: Eastland Press, 2009).

[5] J.K. Chen, T. T. Chen, and L. Crampton, *Chinese Medical Herbology and Pharmacology*, Vol. 369. (City of Industry, CA: Art of Medicine Press, 2004).

[6] NCCAOM State Licensure Requirements, http://mx.nccaom.org/StateLicensing.aspx.

[7] NCCAOM Find a Practitioner, http://mx.nccaom.org/FindAPractitioner.aspx.

[8] Cancer Institute of the Chinese Academy of Medical Sciences, "Astragalus Update," *Professional Health Concerns* 102 (1988): 2.

[9] M. Zhou, et al. "Therapeutic Effect of Astragalus in Treating Chronic Active Hepatitis and the Changes in Immune Functions," *Medical Journal of Chinese People's Liberation Army* 7, no. 4 (1982):242–44.

[10] *Oriental Materia Medica: A Concise Guide*, 523.

[11] R.K. Zee-Cheng, "Shi-quan-da-bu-tang (ten significant tonic decoction), SQT. A potent Chinese biological response modifier in cancer immunotherapy, potentiation and detoxification of anticancer drugs," *Methods and Findings in Experimental and Clinical Pharmacology*, 9 (1992): 725–36.

[12] H. Yeung, *Handbook of Chinese Herbs and Formulas*, (London: Institute of Chinese Medicine, 1985), 89.

[13] Ibid., 126.

[14] H.F. Chiu, et al., "Pharmacological and Pathological Studies on Hepatic Protective Crude Drugs from Taiwan," *American Journal of Chinese Medicine* 20, 3–4 (1992): 257–64.

[15] B.E. Shan, et al., "Stimulating Activity of Chinese Medicinal Herbs on Human Lymphocytes in Vitro," *International Journal of Immunopharmacology* 21, 3 (1999): 149–159.

[16] Clear Heat Clean Toxin herbs are herbs that work against the Epidemic Factor Toxic Heat. Toxic Heat is often associated in modern times with viral and bacterial infections and inflammation associated with cancers and other diseases.

[17] L. Chenghai, "Effect of Fuzheng Huayu Formula and Its Actions against Liver Fibrosis," *Chinese Medicine* 4, 12: (2009).

[18] N.F. Ji, et al., "Polysaccharide of Cordyceps sinensis enhances cisplatin cytotoxicity in non-small cell lung cancer H157 cell line," *Integrative Cancer Therapies* 10 4 (2011): 359–36.

[19] J.W. Jeong, et al., "Induction of Apoptosis by Cordycepin via Reactive Oxygen Species Generation in Human Leukemia Cells," *Toxicology in Vitro* 25 (2011): 817–24.

[20] R.M. Thorat, et al., "Phytochemical and Pharmacological Potential of Eclipta Alba: A Review," *International Research Journal of Pharmacy* 1, 1 (2010): 77–80.

[21] B. Singh, et al., "In Vivo Hepatoprotective Activity of Active Fraction from Ethanolic Extract of Eclipta Alba Leaves," *Indian Journal of Physiology Pharmacology* 45, no. 4 (2001): 435–41.

[22] C. Chih-Jung, et al., "Ganoderma Lucidum Stimulates NK Cell Cytotoxicity by Inducing NKG2D/NCR Activation and Secretion of Perforin and Granulysin," *Innate Immunity* 20 (2014): 301–11.

[23] D. Silva, "Ganoderma Lucidum (Reishi) in Cancer Treatment," *Integrative Cancer Therapies* 2, no. 4 (2003): 358–64.

[24] T. Willard, *Reishi Mushroom: Herb of Spiritual Potency and Medical Wonder*, (Sylvan Press, 1990) 12.

[25] Z.B. Lin, et al., "Anti-Tumor and Immunoregulatory Activities of *Ganoderma lucidum* and Its Possible Mechanisms," *Acta Pharmacologica Sinica* 25, no. 11 (2004):1387–95.

[26] F. Scaglione, et al., "Immunomodulatory Effects of Two Extracts of Panax ginseng C.A. Meyer," *Drugs Under Experimental and Clinical Research* 16, no. 10 (1990): 537–42.

[27] S.H. Park, "*An 8-Week, Randomized, Double-Blind, Placebo-Controlled Clinical Trial for the Antidiabetic Effects of Hydrolyzed Ginseng Extract*," *Journal of Ginseng Research* 38, no. 4 (2014): 239–43.

[28] H.X. Li, et al., "The Saponin of Red Ginseng Protects the Cardiac Myocytes Against Ischemic Injury *in Vitro* and *in Vivo*," *Phytomedicine* 19, no. 6 (2012): 477–483.

[29] B.C. Enger and E.R. Long, eds., *AIDS, Immunity, and Chinese Medicine*, (Long Beach, CA: Oriental Healing Arts Institute, 1989).

[30] T. Hatano, et al., "Two New Flavonoids and Other Constituents in Licorice Root : Their Relative Astringency and Radical Scavenging Effects," *Chemical and Pharmaceutical Bulletin* 36 no. 6 (1988): 2090–7

[31] M. Shinada, et al., "Host-parasite interaction/immunology/microbiology/virology," *Proceedings of the Society for Experimental Biology and Medicine* 181, no. 2 (1986): 205–10.

[32] J. Eisenburg, "Treatment of chronic hepatitis B. Part 2: Effect of glycyrrhizic acid on the course of illness," *Fortschritte der Medizin* 110, no. 21 (1992): 395–8.

[33] V. Chen, et al., "Identification and Analysis of the Active Phytochemicals from the Anti-Cancer Botanical Extract Bezielle," *PLOS One* 7, no. 1 (2012).

[34] J.S. Seak, "Chemoprevention of *Scutellaria barbata* on Human Cancer Cells and Tumorigenesis in Skin Cancer," *Phytotherapy Research* 21, no. 2 (2007): 135–41.

[35] Bensky, *Chinese Herbal Medicine: Materia Medica*, 269.

## CHAPTER NINE

[1]   C. Chace, "A Response to the Dao," *Journal of the National Academy of Acupuncture and Oriental Medicine* 2, no. 2 (1995): 17–24 (in response to Sean Marshall's Essay "Classic Chinese Medicine: The Science of Biological Forces and Their Therapeutic Application").

[2]   "NIH Complementary and Integrative Health Agency Gets New Name," NIH, December 17, 2014, https://nccih.nih.gov/news/press/12172014.

[3]   www.acupunctureresearch.org.

[4]   J. David and L. Yin, "Acupuncture Past and Present," *The FDA Consumer*, May 1973.

[5]   D. Lytle, "An Overview of Acupuncture," Center for Devices and Radiological Health, the U.S. Department of Health and Human Services, Public Health Service, Food and Drug Administration, May 1993.

[6]   C.A. Moss, "Acupuncture Stimulation of the Endogenous Opioids and Effects on the Immune System," *The AAMA Review 2*, no. 1 (1990).

[7]   W. Huang, et al., "Characterizing Acupuncture Stimuli Using Brain Imaging with fMRI: A Systematic Review and Meta-Analysis of the Literature," *PLOS ONE* 7, no. 4 (2012).

[8]   A.J. Vickers, et al., "Acupuncture for Chronic Pain: Individual Patient Data Meta-Analysis," *Archives of Internal Medicine 172*, no. 19 (2012).

[9]   www.mayoclinic.org/tests-procedures/acupuncture/basics/risks/prc-20020778, updated September 2014.

[10]  *Acupuncture: Review and Analysis of Reports on Controlled Clinical Trials*, download PDF at http://apps.who.int/iris/bitstream/10665/42414/1/9241545437.pdf?ua=1.

[11]  Lorraine Wilcox, *Moxibustion: A Modern Clinical Handbook* (Boulder, CO: Blue Poppy Press, 2009).

## CHAPTER TEN

[1]   Watch Sifu Larry Wong teach Parting Clouds on YouTube: www.youtube.com/watch?v=xMoucUXR054.

## CHAPTER ELEVEN

[1]   Massage routine adapted from traditional texts, the wise counsel of Larry Wong, my teacher Dr. Koichi Nakamura, and longtime personal experience as a massage practitioner.

[2]   www.nationaleczema.org/eczema/treatment/alternative-therapies/bleach-baths.

## CHAPTER THIRTEEN

[1]   M.R. Cohen, R. Gish, and K. Doner, *The Hepatitis C Help Book: A Groundbreaking Treatment Program Combining Western and Eastern Medicine for Maximum Wellness and Healing*, Revised Edition (New York: St. Martin's Griffin, 2007).

[2]   M.R. Cohen with K. Doner, *The HIV Wellness Sourcebook: An East/West Guide to Living with HIV/AIDS and Related Conditions* (New York: Holt Paperbacks, 1998).

## CHAPTER FOURTEEN

[1]   A. Sinclair, et al., "Omega-3 Fatty Acids and the Brain: Review of Studies in Depression," *Asia Pacific Journal of Clinical Nutrition* 16, S1 (2007): S391–7.

[2]   www.bidmc.org/YourHealth/TherapeuticCenters/Depression.aspx?ChunkID=40045, updated April 2014.

[3]   www.globalhealingcenter.com/natural-health/folic-acid-foods, updated June 2014.

[4]   A. Ströhle, "Physical Activity, Exercise, Depression, and Anxiety Disorders," *Journal of Neural Transmission* 116, no. 6 (2009): 777–84.

[5]   G.I. Papakostas and J.E. Alpert, "S-adenosyl-methionine in Depression: A Comprehensive Review of the Literature," *Current Psychiatry Reports* 5, no. 6 (2003): 460–6.

[6]   G.A. Ebey and K.L. Ebey, "Rapid Recovery from Major Depression Using Magnesium Treatment," *Medical Hypotheses* 67, no 2. (2006): 362–70.

[7]   M. Berk, et al., "Vitamin D Deficiency May Play a Role in Depression," *Medical Hypotheses* 69, no. 6 (2007): 1316–9.

## CHAPTER FIFTEEN

[1]   W.C. Chumlea, et al., "Age at Menarche and Racial Comparisons in US Girls," *Pediatrics* 111, no. 1 (2003): 110–3.

[2]   NIH National Institute on Aging, www.nia.nih.gov/health/publication/menopause, updated May 2014.

[3]   Ibid.

[4]   www.cdc.gov/physicalactivity/everyone/guidelines/adults.html, updated March 3, 2014.

[5]   American Cancer Society recommendations, www.cancer.org/cancer/breastcancer/moreinformation/breastcancerearlydetection/breast-cancer-early-detection-acs-recs, revised January 2014.

[6]   Adapted from Susun Weed, "The Art of Herbal Breast Massage," *Supplement to New Age Journal*, July/August 1995.

[7] www.mayoclinic.org/drugs-supplements/acidophilus/dosing/hrb-20058615.

[8] American Cancer Society recommendations, www.cancer.org/cancer/cervicalcancer/detailedguide/cervical-cancer-prevention, updated August 2014.

[9] www.nlm.nih.gov/medlineplus/druginfo/natural/934.html, updated July 21, 2011.

[10] P.O. Chocano-Bedoya, et al., "Intake of Selected Minerals and Risk of Premenstrual Syndrome," *American Journal of Epidemiology* 177, no. 10 (2103): 1118–27.

[11] Ibid.

[12] A.F. Walker, et al., "Magnesium Supplementation Alleviates Premenstrual Symptoms of Fluid Retention," *Journal of Women's Health* 7, no. 9 (1998): 1157–65.

[13] www.cancer.org/cancer/news/expertvoices/post/2012/08/02/the-bottom-line-on-soy-and-breast-cancer-risk.aspx, updated August 2, 2012.

[14] www.iofbonehealth.org/calcium-rich-foods.

[15] www.mayoclinic.org/diseases-conditions/menopause/in-depth/hormone-therapy/art-20046372.

[16] H.Y. Chiu, et al., "Effects of Acupuncture on Menopause-Related Symptoms and Quality of Life in Women on Natural Menopause: A Meta-Analysis of Randomized Controlled Trials," *Menopause* 22, no. 2 (2015): 234–44.

[17] www.cdc.gov/reproductivehealth/Infertility/index.htm#a.

[18] Ibid.

[19] Licensed acupuncturist Caylie See, a Chinese medicine fertility expert, contributed to this section on tracking fertility for women.

[20] W.E. Paulus, et al., "Influence of acupuncture on the pregnancy rate in patients who undergo assisted reproduction therapy," *Fertility and Sterility* 77, no. 4 (2002): 721–4.

[21] A. El Refaeey, A. Selem,, A. Badawy, "Combined coenzyme Q10 and clomiphene citrate for ovulation induction in clomiphene-citrate-resistant polycystic ovary syndrome," *Reproductive BioMedicine Online* 29, no. 1 (2014): 119–24.

[22] www.ncbi.nlm.nih.gov/pubmed/15149558.

[23] www.ncbi.nlm.nih.gov/pubmed/19447425.

## CHAPTER SEVENTEEN

[1] D. Preiss and N. Sattar, "Non-Alcoholic Fatty Liver Disease: An Overview of Prevalence, Diagnosis, Pathogenesis and Treatment Considerations," *Clinical Science* 115, no. 5 (2008): 141–50.

[2] www.niddk.nih.gov/health-information/health-topics/liver-disease/nonalcoholic-steatohepatitis/Pages/facts.aspx, updated November 2014.

[3] M.F. Abdelmalek, et al., "Increased Fructose Consumption Is Associated with Fibrosis Severity in Patients with Nonalcoholic Fatty Liver Disease," *Hepatology* 51, no. 6 (2010): 1961–71.

[4] M. Kong, et al., "Vitamin D Deficiency Promotes Nonalcoholic Steatohepatitis through Impaired Enterohepatic Circulation in Animal Model," *American Journal of Physiology: Gastrointestinal and Liver Physiology* 307, no. 9 (2014): G883–93.

[5] N. Chalasani, et al., "The Diagnosis and Management of Non-Alcoholic Fatty Liver Disease: Practice Guideline by the American Association for the Study of Liver Diseases, American College of Gastroenterology, and the American Gastroenterological Association," *Hepatology* 55, no. 6 (2012): 2005–23.

[6] J.S. Bajaj, et al., "Randomised Clinical Trial: Lactobacillus GG Modulates Gut Microbiome, Metabolome and Endotoxemia in Patients with Cirrhosis," *Alimentary Pharmacology Therapeutics* 39, no. 10 (2014): 1113–25.

[7] www.mayoclinic.org/drugs-supplements/acidophilus/dosing/hrb-20058615.

[8] M. Cohen, R. Gish, and K. Doner, *The Hepatitis C Help Book: A Groundbreaking Treatment Program Combining Western and Eastern Medicine for Maximum Wellness and Healing*, Revised Edition (New York: St. Martin's Griffin, 2007).

## CHAPTER EIGHTEEN

[1] From the American Society of Clinical Oncology, www.cancer.net/cancer-types.

[2] From the American Cancer Society, www.cancer.org/cancer/cancerbasics/lifetime-probability-of-developing-or-dying-from-cancer, updated September 2014.

[3] MMWR report from CDC 2011, www.cdc.gov/media/releases/2011/p0310_cancersurvivors.html.

[4] http://cam.cancer.gov/health_definitions.html, updated November 2012.

[5] www.mayoclinic.org/drugs-supplements/acidophilus/dosing/hrb-20058615, updated November 2013.

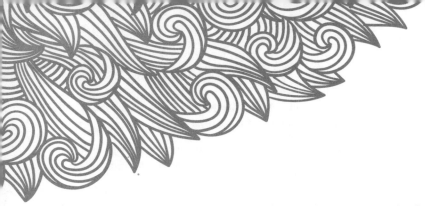

# ABOUT THE AUTHOR

Misha Ruth Cohen, a doctor of Oriental medicine and licensed acupuncturist, is the clinical director of Chicken Soup Chinese Medicine, executive director of the Misha Ruth Cohen Education Foundation, and research specialist of Integrative Medicine at the University of California Institute for Health and Aging, all in San Francisco. She is a member of the board of directors of the Society for Integrative Oncology. Dr. Cohen has been practicing traditional Asian medicine for the past forty years.

After attending Oberlin College, Misha Cohen was trained in acupuncture at Lincoln Hospital's Detox Program in the South Bronx under the auspices of the Quebec School of Acupuncture. After moving to California, she continued her studies in Chinese traditional medicine, acupuncture, and Chinese herbal medicine at the San Francisco College of Acupuncture and Oriental Medicine. She received her doctorate in gynecology from SFCAOM in 1987.

She is nationally certified in acupuncture and herbal medicine. She has developed treatment protocols for people with HIV/AIDS, hepatitis C, liver disease, and cancer support. She was a member of the Ad Hoc Subpanel on Alternative and Complementary Therapy Research of the NIH Office of AIDS Research and in 1996 was selected by *POZ* magazine as one of fifty top AIDS researchers.

Dr. Cohen has written and been the subject of numerous professional and public-oriented articles, been an author for several peer-reviewed journal publications, appeared on national radio and TV, and published several books. She is the author of *The Chinese Way to Healing: Many Paths to Wholeness* (New York: Putnam Perigee, 1996; iUniverse, 2006), *The HIV Wellness Sourcebook: An East/West Guide to Living Well with HIV/AIDS and Related Conditions* (New York: Henry Holt, 1998), and *The Hepatitis C Help Book* (New York: St. Martin's Press, 2000, 2001, and 2007). She was the Complementary and Alternative Medicine Editor for *NUMEDX* magazine (numedx.com) and was featured as a columnist in *Hepatitis Magazine/Liver Health Today* for several years.

Dr. Cohen is recognized internationally as a senior teacher and leading expert in Chinese traditional medicine. She was invited several times by the Chinese government to present her programs, and her articles on HIV/AIDS were officially translated for use in China.

Dr. Cohen designed the HIV Professional Certification Program for Licensed Acupuncturists and the Hepatitis C Professional Training Program for Licensed Acupuncturists. She regularly trains Chinese medicine practitioners, including medical doctors, in Europe and the U.S. in cancer support, gynecology, HIV, hepatitis, and other subjects. She frequently attends and presents at international AIDS, hepatitis, and cancer symposiums, as well as many Chinese medicine and lay conferences.

She has presented her research projects at many scientific conferences, most notably the International AIDS Conference, the Society for Integrative Oncology, and the Society for Acupuncture Research.

Dr. Cohen has created Chinese medicine treatment protocols for PMS, infertility, hepatitis, HIV, endometriosis, HPV-related diseases, and menopausal syndromes that are used by many practitioners of Asian medicine. She has also developed herbal formulas for HIV, hepatitis C, chronic viral illness, cancer support, fibromyalgia, and the common cold.

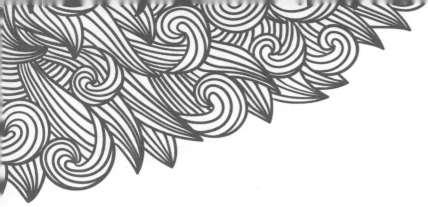

# ACKNOWLEDGMENTS

This book is dedicated to all of my loving friends, family, clients, teachers, mentors, students, mentees, colleagues, guides, and adversaries—living and passed on. Each one of you has helped me to understand the intricate balance of Yin and Yang and to perceive wholeness and wellness as a continuous and unending journey.

Particular mention goes to Craig Mitchell, once a student, now an old friend and famous Chinese medicine author, educator, and leader, who, when asked to write this book, told my publisher that the book they wanted should be written by me. And there began this journey.

Thanks to Jill Alexander, my editor, who saw the full potential for this book and kept me on track through the whole process, bringing me back to center when I strayed.

I want to thank my early teachers Koichi Nakamura; the teachers at Lincoln Detox: Mutulu Shakur, Walter Bosque, Richard Delaney, Wafiya, and Mario Wexu; the teachers at the San Francisco College of Acupuncture and Oriental Medicine: Andrew Tseng, Stuart Kutchins, Efrem Korngold, Bui Tam; and the many more who taught me as the years went by.

Special mention goes to the students of acupuncture at Lincoln Detox, especially Mark Seem, who translated materials from French that we used as part of our training, and the rest who understood that acupuncture can be used any place, for anyone, and at any time to alleviate suffering.

Thanks to all of the patients at Lincoln Detox, who were never shy about exactly how, why, and where they wanted to be needled. And to all the patients in the Tenderloin of San Francisco, where I was able to practice Shiatsu and acupuncture for marginally housed people and others who would have had no other place to get treated. This influenced me deeply to take the path that I did.

I want to acknowledge all of the practitioners at Chicken Soup Chinese Medicine and Quan Yin Healing Arts Center who walked this path with me, landing in many different places and treating tens of thousands of people. I especially want to recognize the practitioners and apprentices who spent countless hours developing treatment plans, communicating with Western medicine teams, and helping me carry out the comprehensive programs that are detailed in this book: Elisa Angelone, K.C. Chamberlain, Sebastian Fey, Cindi Ignatovsky, Nancy Legato, Corrina Rice, Jerome White, and more. A special thank you to Linda Robinson-Hidas for graciously setting up the raw herb pharmacy twenty-five years ago that still serves many clients in my clinic.

Deep appreciation goes to the Western doctors, practitioners, and researchers with whom I have directly worked, some of whom have mentored me, who believed in the process enough to refer and accept referrals and work with my team to truly integrate treatment and support research: Donald Abrams, Fritz Weiser, Jane Melnick, Jeff Burack, Joel Palefsky, Karen Smith-McCune, Laura Esserman, Lee May Chen, Lisa Catalli, Lyn Patrick, Marina Kasavin, Marion Peters, Maurizio Bonacini, Michael Berry, Nancy Harris, Naomi Jay, Natalie Bzowej, Norah Terrault, Rainer Weber, Rob Taylor, Robert Gish, Ruedi Luthy, Silvio Schaller, Stefanie Ueda, Stewart Cooper, Sue Dibble, and Todd Frederick, along with other physicians, oncologists, and hepatologists; plus the many enthusiastic laypeople who have helped further the understanding between medicines of East and West.

Gratitude to all of my Asian medicine colleagues, natural medicine colleagues, and herbalists who have supported research, been co-investigators, taught me, studied with me, supported publications, funded projects, and made the practice of integration possible: Andrew Ellis, Andrew Gaeddert, Anne Biris, Anne Fonfa, Beth Burch, Carla Wilson, Caylie See, Cindy Langhorne, Howard Moffett, Jack Miller, Jill Blakeway, John Chen, Larry Wong, Lorne Brown, Lorren Sandt, Lyn Patrick, Mike Smith, Subhuti Dharmananda, Thomas Garran, Todd Luger, Tom Sinclair, and the hundreds of practitioners who were certified through the Quan Yin and MRCEF Hepatitis C and HIV Professional Certification Programs, and many more who cannot be mentioned here. A special mention goes to Health Concerns, Spring Wind Herb Company, Fungi Perfecti, and Mayway for research support and donations.

A unique salute to all the research, education, and treatment organizations that have trusted me as a leader, teacher, and researcher and who have supported integration through research and education: National Cancer Institute, Gateway for Cancer Research, University of California San Francisco, Society for Integrative Oncology, Society for Acupuncture Research, Caring Ambassadors Program, Oregon College of Oriental Medicine, Pacific College of Oriental Medicine, American College of Traditional Chinese Medicine, Five Branches University, Humanitarian Acupuncture Project, and Quan Yin Healing Arts Center.

A deep bow to the thousands of clients at Quan Yin Acupuncture and Herb Center, Quan Yin Healing Arts Center, and Chicken Soup Chinese Medicine, who have been through all of our ups and downs—the Loma Prieta earthquake, the writing of many books and journal articles, moves, and more—from whom I learn this medicine every day.

A million thanks to friends and manuscript readers Katharine Woodruff, Alice Osiecki, and Tracy Sola for helping me make fewer mistakes and reach more people. Warmness to Kalia Doner, who helped me write my first four books and to whom I largely owe my improved writing skills.

A special appreciation to the staff of Chicken Soup Chinese Medicine and the Misha Ruth Cohen Education Foundation: Mark Ryan, Simmone Guerrero, and Hannah Cohen, along with all of the clinic assistants and interns for taking up the slack and bearing with me during the months of intensive writing. Thanks to former staff Gary Smith, Mercedes Abraham, and Meghan Francisco, who held steady during both good and difficult times.

This book is especially dedicated to my family of birth, especially my mother, Jackie, who fought cancer and illness for many years with great stoicism and finally died in peace; my grandfather Harold, who, after his death, awakened me to the concept of death simply as another transition; my grandmother Ethel, who valiantly struggled with cancer before she died; my grandmother Lucille, who taught yoga for many years and was rarely ill; my aunt Zelda, who lived for years in a wheelchair with a spinal tumor, swam every day, and lived well; my aunt Jane, who lived a full life with a zest that was a joy to behold; my sister Susan, who is the bedrock of the family and supports me in myriad ways; my nephews Eric and Aaron, who have grown into wonderful young men; and my father, Bart, who supported my early interest in science and all of my endeavors and continues to be a source of encouragement.

A big woof to Frida and Yoshi, who remind me of the fragility of life and make each day a pleasure.

Special gratitude and love goes to my life partner, Carla Wilson, for all the support through the writing and publishing process, and without whose sustenance this book would never have come to fruition.

Finally, this book is dedicated to people diagnosed with HIV/AIDS, hepatitis C, cancer, and other life-threatening or serious illnesses who have accompanied me on this journey. You have given me courage, encouragement, support, and knowledge. Every day, I am wondrous at how you have helped me open my heart and mind, perceive new possibilities, and live life knowing that it is a gift.

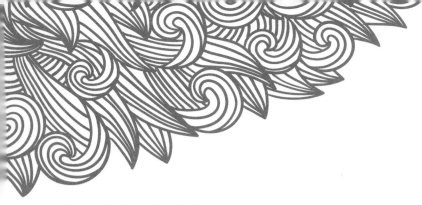

# INDEX

## A

Accreditation Commission for Acupuncture and Oriental Medicine (ACAOM), 86
Acquired Jing, 22
acupressure
  for anxiety, depression, 243
  for cancer support, 322
  for digestive disorders, 291
  for fatty liver disease, 307
  for gynecological health, 267
  for preventive care, 228
  use of, 89
acupressure massage, 197–203
acupuncture
  for anxiety, depression, 244
  for cancer support, 325
  Channels and, 31
  common questions, 169–171
  conditions treated with, 168, 170–171
  described, 89, 154
  for digestive disorders, 295
  for fatty liver disease, 310–311
  functions of, 157–158
  for gynecological health, 260, 269, 281–282
  mind/body/spirit in, 160
  practitioner credentials, 86–87
  for preventive care, 236
  risks and side effects, 170
  science of, 160–162
  treatment considerations, 159–160
  types of, 155–157
acupuncture points
  channels, 163–167
  ear, 203
  head, 201
  for moxibustion, 174
  for Shiatsu massage, 206
adzuki beans, 105
age considerations
  in acupuncture, 159–160
  in dietary principles, 107–109
  in infertility, 271
AIDS, 16, 88, 147–148
Air Qi, 21
Akabane test, 156
alcohol abuse, alcoholism, 132, 155, 298
alertness, acupoints for, 197–198
allergies, 130, 229
alternative medicine, 316
American Cancer Society, 321
American ginseng (*Xi Yang Shen*), 150
anatomy. *See* physiology and anatomy
Ancestral (Extraordinary) Organs, 30–31, 69
Ancestral Qi, 21
anemia, 128, 133, 147
*Angelica sinensis* (Dang Gui), 148
anger, 44, 52
anxiety and depression
  case studies, 12, 245
  comprehensive program, 240–248
  dietary therapy for, 133
  herbs for, 149
appendicitis, 69
appetite loss, 147
arrhythmia, 66
assisted reproduction technologies, 276–277
asthma, 64, 127, 149
astragalus (*Huang Qi*), 145–146
atractylodes (*Bai Zhu*), 146

## B

back pain, 198–199, 200
back self-massage, 202
bacterial infections, 150
*Bai Zhu* (atractylodes), 146
*Ban Zhi Lian* (scutellaria), 152
*Bao Gong* (uterus), 30–31, 69
barley, 103
beans, 105–106
Belt (Dai Mai) Channel, 41, 73
bile, 31
black beans, 105
Bladder Channel of Foot–Taiyang, 35, 71, 74, 166
bleach soak, 215
bleeding, herb for, 151
blood sugar, 149
Blood Vessels, 31
body language evaluation, 81
body mass index (BMI), 299
bones, 30
Brain, 30, 69
breast health, 132, 257–258, 259
breathing exercises, 179, 185, 243
brown rice cereal, 114
bruising, 134
Buddha's Breath, 179
buplerum (*Chai Hu*), 146–147, 148

## C

caffeine, 109, 110
calcium, 137. *See also* nutritional supplements
cancer support
  comprehensive program, 318–329
  herbs for, 145, 152
  New Chinese Medicine approach, 315–318

cancer survivors, 316, 317
Chace, Charles, 155
*Chai Hu* (buplerum), 146–147
Channel Qi, 21
Channels (meridians)
    defined, 19, 31
    disharmonies in, 70–74
    Eight Extraordinary, 38–41
    Fifteen Collaterals, 42
    functions of, 32
    Twelve Primary, 32–38
charisma, 28
chemotherapy, 326–327
chicken broth recipe, 119–120
chicken soup recipes, 120–121
chickpeas, 105
Chinese medicine. *See* New
    Chinese Medicine; Traditional
    Chinese Medicine (TCM)
Chinese medicine practitioners
    examination by, 78–85
    selection of, 85–88
    training and credentials of, 86–87
    treatment modalities, 88–90
    Western practitioners and,
        220–221, 233–234
Chinese mugwort (moxa), 89
cholesterol, 149
Chong Mai (Penetrating) Channel,
    41, 73
chronic fatigue, 127
Circulation Sex, 45
cirrhosis, 134
cleansing diet, 113–114, 225
climate, in acupuncture, 159
codonopsis (*Dang Shen*), 147
Cold
    compresses for, 216–218
    described, 48–49
    disharmony pattern, 56
    in Liver System, 63
    soak recipes for, 213
    stages of, 50–51
colds and flu, 230
colitis, 128, 130, 294
Collapsed (Sinking) Qi, 57, 60
collateral channels, 42, 73–74
complementary medicine, 316
comprehensive program overviews.
    *See also specific health issues*
    anxiety and depression, 248
    cancer support, 328–329

digestive disorders, 296–297
fatty liver disease, 313–314
gynecological health, 283–287
preventive care, 238–239
compresses
    for anxiety, depression, 244
    for cancer support, 323
    for digestive disorders, 291
    for fatty liver disease, 307
    for gynecological health, 258, 279
    for preventive care, 228
    recipes for, 216–218
conception, 31. *See also* infertility
Conception Channel. *See* Ren Mai
    (Conception) Channel
congee recipes, 117–119
Congenital Jing, 22
congestive heart failure, 66
connective tissue theory, 161
constipation, 132, 133, 198
Constitutional (Korean)
    acupuncture, 157
cordyceps (*Dong Chong Xia Cao*),
    147–148
coughs, 130, 147, 150, 217
couscous, 104
Crohn's disease, 129, 130

**D**
Dai Mai (Belt) Channel, 41, 73
Damp Cold, 61, 129
Damp Heat
    Large Intestine System, 69
    Liver System, 63
    Spleen System, 62, 130
    Triple Burner System, 68
    Urinary Bladder System, 69
Damp-Heat Dysentery, 69
Dampness
    compresses for, 216–218
    described, 49
    dietary therapy for, 129
    in Lung system, 64
Dang Gui (*Angelica sinensis*), 121,
    148
*Dang Shen* (codonopsis), 147
*Da Qing Ye* (isatis), 150
decoctions, 139–140
Deep Touch Head Massage,
    200–201

Deficiency patterns
    described, 56
    dietary therapy for, 127–130
    in Heart System, 65
    Jing, 59
    Jin-Ye, 59
    in Kidney System, 59–60
    in Liver System, 62–63
    in Lung system, 64–65
    in Marrow, 69
    Qi, 57, 131
    in Spleen System, 60–61, 65
    in Stomach System, 67
    Xue, 58, 133, 228
depression. *See* anxiety and
    depression
diabetes, 100, 133, 299, 302
diagnostic evaluations
    acupuncture, 157–158
    body language, 81
    facial color, 81–83
    pulse, 84–85
    questions, 77
    smell, 84
    tongue, 78–81
    touch sensitivity, 85
    voice, 83–84
diarrhea, 128, 129, 147, 198
dietary principles
    age adjustments, 107–109
    balance and moderation, 97–102
    disharmony and, 53, 67
    eating habits, 92–93
    food as medicine, 107
    food diary, 102
    food flavors and energetics,
        93–96, 225
    glycemic index, 100–102
    grains and legumes, 102–106
    importance of, 91
    meal plan guidelines, 99–100
    seasonal foods, 97
    tea, 109–111
dietary therapy. *See also* nutritional
    supplements
    for anxiety, depression, 241
    for cancer support, 320–321
    common questions, 124–126
    for dampness, 129–130
    for deficiencies, 127–131, 133
    described, 89
    for digestive disorders, 289–290

for dryness, 132, 133
for excess heat, 132
for fatty liver disease, 304–305
First-Step program phases, 113–115
general guidelines, 113
for gynecological health, 255, 262–263, 266, 278
for Phlegm, 130
for preventive care, 225–226
for Stagnant Liver, 131, 132–133
warning, 124
digestion, digestive disorders
acupoints for, 197
comprehensive program, 288–297
dietary therapy for, 122–123, 132
herbs for, 147, 151
medicines for, 230–231
in travelers, 232
diseases
diagnoses and disharmonies, 54–55
Epidemic Factors in, 51–52
Yin/Yang symptoms, 18
disharmony
in Channels, 70–74
in Chinese Medicine theory, 13
Eight Fundamental Patterns, 55–56
Epidemic Factors, 51–52
in Essential Substances, 57–59
excessive physical activity, 53
excessive sex, 53
in Organ Systems, 59–69
poor nutrition, 53
Six Pernicious Influences, 48–51
Western disease associations, 54–55
Yin/Yang, 18–19
Disturbed Shen, 58, 241
Dong Chong Xia Cao (cordyceps), 147–148
Dryness
described, 49
dietary therapy for, 132, 133
herbal oils for, 216
Du Channel, 40
Du Mai (Governing) Channel, 41, 72, 74
dysentery, 129

E

ear massage. See also Qi Gong massage
for anxiety, depression, 243
for cancer support, 322
for digestive disorders, 291
for fatty liver disease, 307
for gynecological health, 267
instructions for, 202
for preventive care, 228
Earth Phase, 46, 134
eclipta (Mo Han Lian), 148–149
edema, 129
Eight Extraordinary Channels, 38–41, 72–73
Eight Fundamental Patterns, 55–56
emotions, 43, 52–53
endometriosis, 15, 134
endorphins theory, 161
enemas, 141
enteritis, 128
Epidemic Factors (Li Qi), 51–52
Essential Fatty Acids, 136. See also nutritional supplements
Essential Substances, 19, 20–25, 57–59
examinations. See Four Examinations
Excess patterns
described, 56
in Heart System, 66
Jin-Ye, 59
in Lung System, 63–64, 65
Qi, 57
in Spleen System, 61–62
Xue, 58
exercise. See also Qi Gong
for cancer support, 321–322
for digestive disorders, 290
excessive, 53
for fatty liver disease, 305
for gynecological health, 256, 267, 278–279
for preventive care, 226–227
Exterior patterns of disharmony, 55
External Pernicious Influences, 21
Extraordinary (Ancestral) Organs, 30–31, 69
eyes, 28, 130

F

facial color evaluation, 81–83
fallopian tube patency, 270
fatigue, 131, 147, 149, 151
fatty liver disease
comprehensive program, 302–314
defined, 298–299
risk and diagnosis, 299–300
fear, 53
fever, 218
fibrocystic breasts, 132
fibroid tumors, 260
fibrosis, 134
Fifteen Collaterals, 42, 73–74
Fire Phase, 44, 134
Five Element Worsley Acupuncture, 157
Five Phases or Element (Wu Xing), 42–47, 134
folic acid, 241
food dairy, 102
Food Energetics, 92, 97, 225. See also dietary principles; dietary therapy
food flavors, 93–96
food poisoning, 128
foot bath, 216
foot reflexology, 211
forgetfulness, 149
Four Examinations
inquiring, 77
listening/smelling, 83–84
looking, 77–83
touching, 84–85
frozen foods, 92
Fu (Yang) Organs, 18, 26, 29–30. See also specific organ systems

G

Gallbladder Channel of Foot-Shaoyang, 37, 72, 74, 167
Gallbladder System
described, 29, 31
disharmonies in, 68
Wood Phase and, 44
Gan Cao (licorice root), 150–151
ganoderma (Ling Zhi), 149
garbanzo beans, 105
gastritis, 128
gastroenteritis, 129

gate theory, 161
geographic location, in
    acupuncture, 159
geographic tongue, 81
GI (glycemic index), 100–102, 306
ginger compresses, 217, 291
ginger soak, 213
ginseng (Ren Shen), 149
ginseng, American (Xi Yang Shen),
    150
gluten, gluten intolerance, 103
glycemic index (GI), 100–102, 306
goiter, 132
Governing Channel. See Du Mai
    (Governing) Channel
Grain (Gu) Qi, 21, 91, 102
grains, 102–104, 126
grief, 52
groin swelling or lumps, 132
Gua sha, 89
Gu (grain) Qi, 21, 91, 102
gynecological health. See
    also infertility; menopause;
    menstruation, menstrual problems;
    PMS
    acupressure for, 200
    Chinese vs. Western approach,
        249–252
    comprehensive program,
        253–263
    screening recommendations, 259

H
hand reflexology, 210
hara massage, 291
headaches, 132, 133, 198
head massage, 200–201, 243. See
    also Qi Gong massage
health maintenance. See preventive
    care
health practitioners. See also
    Chinese medicine practitioners
    for cancer support, 323–328
    for digestive disorders, 293–296
    for fatty liver disease, 308–311
    for gynecological health,
        259–261, 267–268, 280–281
    for preventive health care,
        233–234
hearing, 27

Heart Channel of Hand-Shaoyin, 34,
    71, 74, 165
heart disease, 125
Heart System
    described, 28–29
    disharmonies in, 65–66
    emotions and, 52
    facial color and, 82
    Fire Phase and, 44
    Xue and, 24
Heat
    described, 49
    dietary therapy for, 132
    disharmony pattern, 56
    in Lung system, 64
    soak recipes for, 214
    stages of, 51
hepatitis
    case study, 220–221
    Damp Heat of Liver System and,
        63
    dietary therapy for, 128, 129, 130,
        132
    herbs for, 146, 148, 151
    NASH, 299
    practitioner selection and, 88
    term defined, 299
herbal medicine
    for anxiety, depression, 245–246
    for cancer support, 326–327
    characteristics of, 138–139
    common herbal formulas, 153
    decoction preparation, 142
    described, 90
    for digestive disorders, 294–295
    for fatty liver disease, 311–312
    forms of, 139–141
    for gynecological health, 261,
        263–264, 268, 281
    herb combinations, 143
    herb/drug interactions, 234
    herb profiles, 145–152
    practitioner credentials, 87, 144
    for preventive care, 236–237
    reference books, 142
    side effects, 145
    use caution, 138
high blood pressure, 155
high fructose corn syrup (HFCS),
    125, 303
hijiki, 124
HIV/AIDS, 16, 88, 147–148

homeopathic medicines, 230–231
Huang Qi (astragalus), 145–146

I
immersion therapies, 212–218
immune system
    acupoints for, 197, 198
    herbs for, 145–146, 149
    preventive program, 223–239
    weakened, 238
impotence, 147
infertility
    assisted reproduction
        technologies, 276–277
    case studies, 60, 270
    causes, 69, 269–271
    Chinese vs. Western approach,
        272–275
    comprehensive program, 277–283
influenza, 65
inquiring examination, 77
insomnia, 149, 213
integrative medicine, 7, 316–317
Interior patterns of disharmony, 55
Intestinal Abscess, 69
irritability, 150
irritable bowel syndrome, 65
isatis (Da Qing Ye), 150

J
Japanese acupuncture, 156
jet lag, 232
Jing
    described, 19, 22–23
    dietary therapy for, 91
    disharmonies, 59
Jing Luo Zhi Qi, 21
Jin-Ye, 19, 25, 59
Ji Xue Teng (spatholobus), 152
journaling
    for cancer support, 319
    for digestive disorders, 288–289
    for fatty liver disease, 302–304
    food diary, 102
    for gynecological health, 254,
        265, 277
    for preventive care, 223–224
joy, 28, 52
Jueyin stage, 51

## K

kicharee, 116
kidney beans, 105
Kidney Channel of Foot-Shaoyin, 36, 72, 74, 166
kidney disease, 128, 147
Kidney System
    described, 27
    disharmonies in, 59–60
    emotions and, 53
    facial color and, 83
    Water Phase and, 45
Kong Qi, 21
Korean (Constitutional) acupuncture, 157
krill oil, 136

## L

Lack of Shen, 58, 241
*Lactobacillus acidophilus*, 135, 229
Large Intestine Channel of Hand-Yangming, 33, 70, 73
Large Intestine System, 29, 45, 69
lentil broth, 114
lentils, 106
lethargy, 131
licorice root (*Gan Cao*), 150–151
lima beans, 106
*Ling Shu* (Upper Burner), 30, 68
*Ling Zhi* (ganoderma), 149
lips, 27
*Li Qi* (Epidemis Factors), 51–52
listening/smelling examination, 83–84
Liver Channel of Foot–Jueyin, 37, 72, 74, 167
liver disease, 148. *See also* fatty liver disease; hepatitis
Liver System
    described, 27–28
    dietary therapy for, 131, 132
    disharmonies in, 62–63
    emotions and, 52
    facial color and, 82
    Gallbladder System and, 29
    Wood Phase and, 44
    Xue and, 24
longevity, 126, 178
looking examination, 77–83
loose stools, 128, 151

lotus blossom meditation, 189
Lower Burner, 30, 68
Lung Channel of Hand-Taiyin, 33, 70, 73, 163
Lung System
    described, 28
    disharmonies in, 63–65
    emotions and, 52
    facial color and, 83
    Metal Phase and, 45

## M

magnesium, 137. *See also* nutritional supplements
malaria, 146
manic behavior, 132
Marrow, 30, 69
Marrow Washing Qi Gong, 178
massage
    acupressure, 197–203
    for anxiety, depression, 243–244
    for cancer support, 322
    for digestive disorders, 291
    for fatty liver disease, 307
    for gynecological health, 256–257, 267, 279
    during pregnancy, 191, 198
    Qi Gong, 190–197
    Shiatsu partnered, 204–209
    use of, 89
    warnings, 191
    Western reflexology, 210–211
massage oils, 231
meal plan guidelines, 99–100
meat, 124–125
medical history, 56
medicine cabinet, 230–231
meditation
    for anxiety, depression, 242
    for cancer support, 322
    for digestive disorders, 290
    for fatty liver disease, 306
    for gynecological health, 256
    for preventive care, 226–227
    recommendations, 186–189
men, Jing and life stages, 23
menopause, 253, 265–269
menstruation, menstrual problems
    Chinese vs. Western approach, 249–252

dietary therapy for, 132, 133, 134
herbs for, 148, 152
infertility and, 270
menarche, 253
Organ System balance and, 31
tongue characteristics and, 80–81
Uterus disharmony and, 69
mental illness, 240
meridians. *See* Channels (meridians)
metabolic syndrome, 101, 301
Metal Phase, 45, 134
Middle Burner
    Damp Heat in, 68
    described, 30
    diet and, 107, 108
millet, 104
mind/body/spirit, 11–13, 159–160
miraculous meridians. *See* Eight Extraordinary Channels
miscarriages, 275
miso broth, 113
miso soup recipes, 122–123
*Mo Han Lian* (eclipta), 148–149
moxa (Chinese mugwort), 89
moxibustion
    for cancer support, 322, 326
    described, 89, 171
    for digestive disorders, 291, 295
    for fatty liver disease, 311
    for gynecological health, 261, 267, 269, 280, 281–282
    instructions for, 172–174
    for preventive care, 228, 236

## N

National Center for Complementary and Integrative Health (NCCIH), 160
National Certification Commission for Acupuncture and Oriental Medicine (NCCAOM), 86–87, 144
Nei Dan exercises, 181
nervousness, 133
New Chinese Medicine
    benefits of, 15
    described, 7–9, 13–14
    preventive focus, 17
    as pursuit of wholeness, 15–16
night sweats, 150

Normal Qi, 21
nutrition. *See* dietary principles; dietary therapy
nutritional supplements
    for anxiety, depression, 244
    for cancer support, 323
    for digestive disorders, 292–293
    for fatty liver disease, 307–308
    for gynecological health, 258, 263, 282–283
    for preventive care, 229
    recommended types, 135–137
Nutritive Qi, 21

### O

obesity and overweight
    cancer and, 320, 324
    fatty liver and, 299, 302, 309–310
observation, in diagnosis, 77–83
Omega-3 fatty acids, 136, 241. *See also* nutritional supplements
organic foods, 93
Organ Qi, 21, 223–239
organ removal, 28
Organ Systems. *See also specific organ systems*
    defined, 19
    disharmonies in, 59–69
    Fu (Yang), 18, 26, 29–30
    Xue and, 24
    Zang (Yin), 18, 26–29
Original Qi, 21
O-ring test, 156
overeating, 92

### P

pain relief, 134, 151, 152, 199
palpitations, 149
panic attacks, 245
parasites, 129
Pectoral Qi, 21
pelvic inflammatory disease, 134
Penetrating (Chong Mai) Channel, 41, 73
peppermint soak, 214
Pericardium Channel of Hand-Jueyin, 36, 72, 74, 164
Pericardium System, 29, 67
perimenopause, 253

Pernicious Influences, 21, 48–51, 215–216
Phlegm
    described, 49
    dietary therapy for, 130
    in Heart System, 66, 67
    in infants, 108
physiology and anatomy
    Channels (meridians), 31–42
    Essential Substances, 20–25
    Organ Systems, 26–31
    overview, 19
pinto beans, 106
PMS
    comprehensive program, 262–264
    dietary therapy for, 132
    Western approach, 252
pneumonia, 150
pregnancy
    case study, 63
    contraindicated treatments, 151, 152, 174
    diet during, 125
    Excess patterns during, 58
    massage warnings, 191, 198
Prenatal Jing, 22
preventive care
    as acupuncture function, 158
    for cancer support, 318
    as Chinese Medicine focus, 17
    comprehensive program, 223–239
    for fatty liver disease, 302
    for gynecological health, 253–258
processed foods, 93
progesterone cream, 264
Protective Qi, 21, 223–239
protein powder, 115
psychoneuroimmunology, 252
pu-erh tea, 109
pulse evaluation, 84–85

### Q

Qi
    described, 19, 20
    dietary therapy for, 91, 119–121, 127, 130, 131
    disharmonies, 57

flow in Twelve Primary Channels, 38
    forms of, 20–21
    Jing and, 22
    soak recipe for, 213
    Xue and, 24
Qi Gong
    for anxiety, depression, 242
    basic techniques, 178–179
    breathing in, 179, 185
    described, 90, 176–177
    effects of, 177–178
    exercises, 179–185
    historic uses, 176
    vs. Western exercise, 175
Qi Gong massage, 190–197
Qi meditation, 186–188
Qi stage, 51
questions, in diagnosis, 77
quinoa, 104

### R

raw foods, 92
Rebellious Qi, 57
recipes
    bath soaks, 212–216
    beans, 105–106
    compresses, 217–218
    grains, 103–104
    tea, 111
    therapeutic foods, 116–123
recurrent pregnancy loss, 275
Refined Jin-Ye, 25
reflexology
    for anxiety, depression, 243
    for digestive disorders, 291
    for gynecological health, 257, 279
    instructions for, 210–211
Ren Channel, 40
Ren Mai (Conception) Channel, 41, 73, 74
*Ren Shen* (ginseng), 149
repetitive use syndrome, 71
reproductive health. *See* gynecological health; infertility; menopause; menstruation, menstrual problems; PMS

## S

sadness, 52
salt soak, 215
*San Jiao. See* Triple Burner System
San Qi, 121, 151–152
SAR (Society for Acupuncture Research), 161
saunas
    about, 218
    for cancer support, 323
    for fatty liver disease, 307
    for gynecological health, 258
    for preventive care, 228
sciatica, 158
scutellaria (*Ban Zhi Lian*), 152
Sea of Marrow, 30
Sea of Qi and Xue, 41
seasons
    in acupuncture, 159
    in dietary principles, 97
sea vegetables, 124
self-care practices
    for anxiety, depression, 240–244
    for cancer support, 318–323
    for digestive disorders, 288–293
    for fatty liver disease, 302–308
    for gynecological health, 253–258
    importance of, 14
    preventive care, 223–232
self-massage. *See* massage
Seven Emotions, 43, 52–53
Severe Dampness, 49
sex, excessive, 53
Shao Yang, 146
Shao Yang stage, 50
Shaoyin stage, 51
Shen
    calming program, 241–247
    described, 19, 22
    dietary therapy for, 91
    disharmonies, 58, 240–241
Shen Cycle, 43
Shiatsu partnered massage, 204–209, 322
shingles, 168
shoulder, acupoints for, 199
signs (term), 127
Sinking (Collapsed) Qi, 57, 60
sinus congestion, 130, 214, 230

Six Pernicious Influences, 48–51, 215–216
skin, organ systems and, 28, 29
skin disorders
    dietary therapy for, 130, 132, 133
    medicine for, 231
    soaks for, 212
Small Intestine Channel of Hand-Taiyang, 35, 71, 74, 165
Small Intestine System
    described, 29
    disharmonies in, 68
    Fire Phase and, 44
smell evaluation, 84
soaks
    for anxiety, depression, 244
    for cancer support, 323
    for digestive disorders, 291
    for fatty liver disease, 307
    for gynecological health, 258, 267, 279
    for preventive care, 228
    recipes for, 212–216
Society for Acupuncture Research (SAR), 161
soybeans, 106
spatholobus (*Ji Xue Teng*), 152
Spleen, Great Collateral of, 74
Spleen Channel of Foot-Taiyin, 34, 71, 74, 163
Spleen System
    described, 27
    dietary therapy for, 107, 127–130
    disharmonies in, 60–62, 65
    Earth Phase and, 46
    emotions and, 52
    facial color and, 82–83
    Stomach System and, 29
    Xue and, 24
split peas, 106
Stagnation patterns
    compresses for, 216–218
    in Heart System, 66
    in Liver System, 62, 131, 132
    Qi, 57
    Xue, 58, 134–135
steatosis. *See* fatty liver disease
Stomach Channel of Foot-Yangming, 33, 70, 74, 163
Stomach Heat, 67
Stomach System
    described, 29

dietary therapy for, 107, 128
    disharmonies in, 67
    Earth Phase and, 46
strength, regaining, 117–119
stress, 231, 240–248
sugar, 125
Summer Heat, 50
sweating, spontaneous, 147
swelling, 128
symptoms (term), 127

## T

Taiyang stage, 50
Taiyin stage, 50
Tao, 17–19
Taoist's Breath, 179
tea, 109–111
thyme soak, 214
tinctures, 141
tongue evaluation, 78–81
touching examination, 84–85
touch sensitivity, 85
Traditional Chinese Medicine (TCM)
    acupuncture, 156
    fertility in, 272–273
    Five Phases and, 42
    New Chinese Medicine and, 13–14
    physiology and anatomy of, 19
    power of, 13
    women's health in, 249–250
trauma, 231
travel, healthy, 232
Triple Burner Channel of Hand-Shaoyang, 37, 72, 74, 164
Triple Burner System
    Circulation Sex and, 45
    described, 28, 29–30
    disharmonies in, 67–68
tuberculosis, 147
Twelve Primary Channels, 32–38, 70–72
type A personality, 132

## U

ulcers, 128, 129
Upper Burner (*Ling Shu*), 30, 68
Urinary Bladder System, 29, 69
urinary incontinence, 127
uterine contour, 271

uterine fibroids, 134
Uterus (*Bao Gong*), 30–31, 69

**V**

vegetable broth, 113
vegetables, steamed, 123
viral meningitis, 150
Vitamin D, 136. *See also* nutritional
  supplements
voice evaluation, 83–84

**W**

Water Phase, 45, 134
weakness, 147, 149
Wei Dan exercises, 180
Wei Qi, 21
Wei stage, 51
Western medicine
  for anxiety, depression, 246–247
  baseline examinations, 233–236,
    259, 293, 309–310, 324–325
  Chinese medicine and, 220–221,
    233–234
  diseases and disharmonies,
    54–55
  fertility in, 273–275
  women's health in, 251–252
Western reflexology, 210–211
Wind, 44, 50
women, Jing and life stages, 22
women's health. *See* gynecological
  health
Wong, Larry, 176–185
Wood Phase, 44, 134
worry, 52
Worsley, J. R., 157
*Wu Xing* (Five Phases), 42–47

**X**

*Xi Yang Shen* (ginseng, American),
  150
Xue
  described, 19, 23–24
  dietary therapy for, 91, 116, 119–121,
    133, 134–135
  disharmonies, 58
Xue stage, 51
Xue Stasis, 58

**Y**

Yangming stage, 50
Yangqiao (Yang Heel) Channel, 39,
  41, 73
Yangwei (Yang Linking) Channel, 39,
  41, 73
Ying Qi, 21
Ying stage, 51
Yinqiao (Yin Heel) Channel, 39, 41,
  73
Yinwei (Yin Linking) Channel, 39,
  40, 41, 73
Yin/Yang
  described, 18–19
  disease symptoms, 18
  disharmonies, 56
  Organ Systems, 18, 26–30
Yuan Qi, 21

**Z**

Zang-Fu Zhi Qi, 21
Zang (Yin) Organs, 18, 26–29. *See
  also specific organ systems*
Zheng Qi, 21
Zong Qi, 21